Fixed Restorative Techniques

Dental Laboratory Technology Manuals

Fixed Restorative Techniques

Dental Laboratory Technology Manuals

Henry V. Murray, B.S., D.D.S.

Troy B. Sluder, D.D.S., M.S.

Roger E. Barton, D.D.S., EDITOR

REVISED EDITION

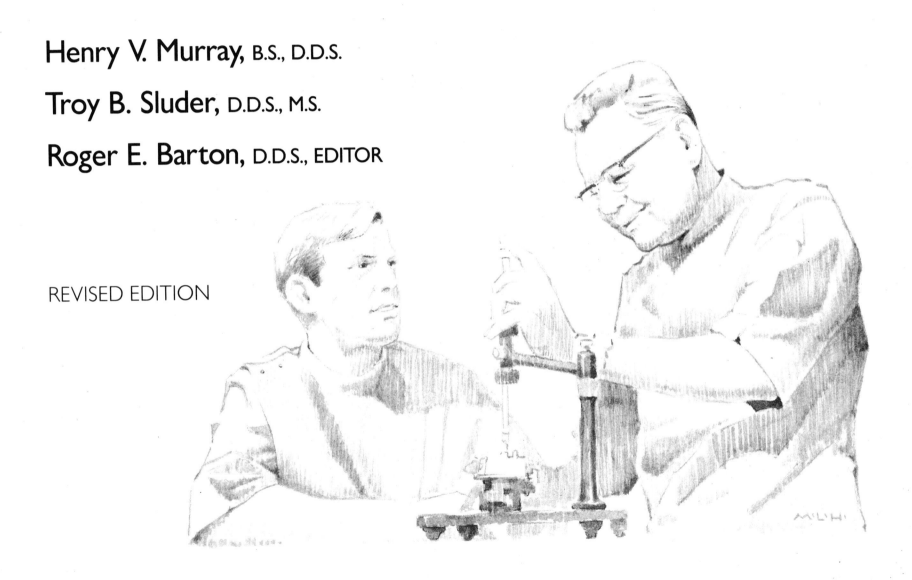

The paper in this book meets the guidelines for permanence and durability of the Committee on Production Guidelines for Book Longevity of the Council on Library Resources.

10 09 08 07 06   9 8 7 6 5

Printed in the United States of America

Library of Congress Cataloging-in-Publication Data

Murray, Henry V.
   Fixed restorative techniques / Henry V. Murray, Troy B. Sluder; Roger E. Barton, editor. — Rev. ed.
      p.   cm. — (Dental laboratory technology manuals)
   Includes index.
   ISBN-13: 978-0-8078-4250-8 (pbk.: alk. paper)
   ISBN-10: 0-8078-4250-8 (pbk.: alk. paper)
   1. Dental casting—Laboratory manuals. 2. Gold alloys—Laboratory manuals. I. Sluder, Troy B. II. Barton, Roger E., 1922–   . III. Title. IV. Series.
   [DNLM: 1. Dental Restoration, Permanent—methods—laboratory manuals. WU 500 M982f]
   RK658.M87   1989
   617.6′9—dc 19
   DNLM/DLC
   for Library of Congress   88-39479
                                                                      CIP

Dental Laboratory Technology Manuals:

Dental Anatomy

Gerald M. Cathey, B.S., D.D.S., M.S.

Fixed Restorative Techniques
Revised Edition

Henry V. Murray, B.S., D.D.S.
Troy B. Sluder, D.D.S., M.S.

Laboratory and Clinical Dental Materials

Karl F. Leinfelder, D.D.S., M.S.
Duane F. Taylor, B.S.E., M.S.E., Ph.D.

Removable Prosthodontic Techniques
Revised Edition

John B. Sowter, D.D.S., M.Sc.

CONTENTS

PREFACE

This manual is one of a series intended to help train individuals in basic dental laboratory techniques. It is designed to acquaint the student dental technician with the procedures involved in making cast restorations with gold alloys.

Gold has been an important and preferred dental material for more than a century. Its physical properties have not been duplicated in other alloys. However, the cost of gold has prompted the development of numerous low-precious and nonprecious alloys. These metals are not described in this manual, but the techniques used to make gold alloy castings are basically applicable to nonprecious alloys.

Many of the castings now used in dentistry have porcelain bonded to their surfaces to make them esthetic. Because of the complexity and scope of materials and techniques associated with porcelain-fused-to-metal restorations, they are not included in this particular manual.

All sections of the manual have been extensively revised, and some—Occlusion, Post/Core Foundations, and Interconnectors and Telescopic Construction in Fixed Bridges—have been completely rewritten. There are also many new photographs and technical drawings. A new feature of this edition is the inclusion of a few review questions at the end of each section. These questions cover the primary objectives of the section and are intended to encourage review.

The technical procedure photographs reused from the first edition were done by Mr. William G. Blanton, C.D.T.; the original art work was rendered by Mr. James C. Handy. The new photographs and art work were produced by Mr. Tom Edwards and Mr. Warren McCollum of the Learning Resources Center of the School of Dentistry of the University of North Carolina at Chapel Hill under the direction of Mr. David L. Raney.

Dr. Henry V. Murray, Jr., is a professor in the Fixed Prosthodontics Department at the University of North Carolina School of Dentistry. He received his degrees from the University of North Carolina. As a teacher and practitioner he is respected by both colleagues and students for his abilities and devotion to the dental profession.

Dr. Troy B. Sluder, Jr., is a professor in the Operative Department at the University of North Carolina School of Dentistry. He received his dental degree from the University of North Carolina and his Master of Science degree in dental materials from the University of Michigan. He has contributed to the second edition of the textbook *The Art and Science of Operative Dentistry* and is recognized as a very thorough and competent teacher and practitioner.

Roger E. Barton
Editor

Fixed Restorative Techniques

Dental Laboratory Technology Manuals

SECTION I

Introduction to Fixed Restorative Techniques

Fixed restorative techniques are the procedures required for constructing cast metal restorations that are rigidly attached (cemented) to the teeth. This manual includes the techniques that involve cast gold restorations in combination with manufactured porcelain facings or custom-made resin facings. The areas of dentistry commonly associated with fixed restorative techniques are operative dentistry and fixed prosthodontics.

DEFINITIONS ASSOCIATED WITH FIXED RESTORATIVE TECHNIQUES

Operative dentistry is the branch of oral health service concerned with replacing lost tooth structure with suitable materials.

Fixed prosthodontics, also known as crown and bridge prosthodontics, is "the science and art of providing suitable substitutes for the coronal portions of teeth or for one or more lost or missing natural teeth and their associated parts in order that impaired function, appearance, comfort, and health of the patient may be restored." (Current Clinical Dental Terminology)

Prosthodontics is "the branch of dental arts and science pertaining to the restoration and maintenance of oral function by the replacement of missing teeth and structures by artificial devices." (CCDT) The term *prosthodontics* is a combination of the words *prosthesis* and *dentistry* and is used synonymously with *prosthetic dentistry*. A *prosthesis* is defined as "the replacement of an absent part of the human body by an artificial part." (CCDT)

By definition, any type of dental restoration placed in or on a tooth is a prosthesis, because it replaces a "missing part of the body." In common usage, a "dental prosthesis" is a device or restoration that replaces one or more lost teeth, the entire crown of a tooth, or a portion thereof. A removable dental prosthesis may be inserted and removed by the patient; a cast gold restoration or fixed partial denture (fixed bridge) is firmly held in place and cannot be removed by the patient.

TYPES OF FIXED RESTORATIONS

This manual is concerned with three types of fixed dental restorations: inlays and onlays, crowns, and bridges.

An inlay (Figure 1) is a dental restoration that fits *into* a prepared cavity in a tooth and is secured therein by cement. Inlays (and other "fillings") are placed within a cavity preparation cut into a part of the clinical crown of a tooth and are therefore referred to as *intracoronal* restorations. Retention of an inlay within the tooth is accomplished by (1) cutting the cavity preparation with near parallel walls; (2) making a casting that fits very accurately between these walls; and (3) cementing the restoration into place. Thus *retention* (resistance to displacement) is developed between the casting and the *internal* walls of the prepared cavity in the tooth.

An inlay is used to restore *individual* tooth contours and function. On rare occasions inlays are used to support an adjacent artificial tooth (fixed bridge).

There are two commonly used modifications of the inlay, the *onlay*

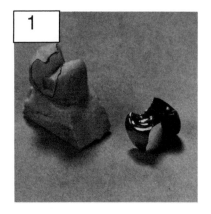

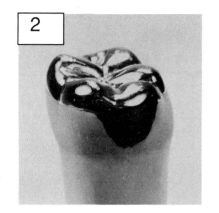

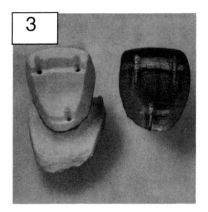

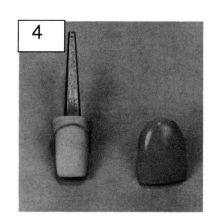

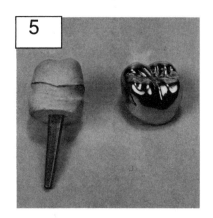

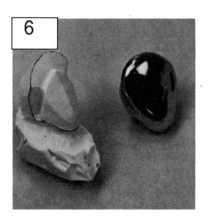

and the *pinlay* or *pinledge*. An onlay (**Figure 2**) is a dental restoration that covers the entire occlusal surface of the tooth as well as fitting into a prepared cavity in the tooth. It gains retention from intracoronal cavity form. By virtue of covering the entire occlusal surface, it protects the tooth from fracture due to biting forces. Onlays normally involve the mesial, distal, and occlusal surfaces of a posterior tooth and are used when the occlusal surface requires alteration and/or the tooth requires protection against fracture. Because of the incidence and danger of tooth fracture with inlays, onlays have become the dominant form of intracoronal cast restorations. Accordingly most subsequent categoric references in this manual use the term *onlay*. An onlay may also be used as a retainer for a fixed partial denture, particularly if the patient is relatively immune to caries.

A pinlay (or pinledge) (**Figure 3**) is a thin cast restoration that covers the lingual surface and one or both proximal surfaces of an anterior tooth. It has two or three parallel pins, approximately 1.5 to 2.0 millimeters long, that penetrate the lingual dentin for retention. Frequently, a proximal groove is used in lieu of one of the pins. The thinness of the casting and the small diameter of the pins require that a pinlay be constructed of a hard alloy. A properly constructed pinlay is an esthetic restoration and may be used as a conservative type of retainer for anterior fixed partial dentures.

A crown (**Figures 4 and 5**) is "a restoration which restores all or part of the clinical crown of a tooth, its retention normally being derived primarily from the preparation of the surface of the tooth." (CCDT) Crowns are termed *extracoronal* restorations since they cover all or most of the coronal portion of the tooth and gain their support and retention primarily from this outer surface of the tooth. Retention or resistance to displacement is developed between the inner surface of the casting and the *external* surfaces of the prepared tooth. However, a portion of the tooth surface is uninvolved in some crown preparations (**Figure 6**). To compensate for this reduction in coverage, retentive grooves or boxes are usually cut into the tooth. Such crowns are in part intracoronal restorations.

Conversely, many onlays are extended to cover most of the surfaces of a tooth and are, in part, extracoronal restorations. Consequently, the distinction between the crown and onlay or extracoronal and intracoronal restorations is often more academic than practical.

The crown, being more extensive than other restorations, is used primarily to restore badly "broken-down" teeth, i.e., teeth with extensive decay and/or restorations involving most surfaces. Often a crown is a "last resort" for teeth that have been extensively "filled" and patched over a period of years. Hence crown preparations (teeth pre-

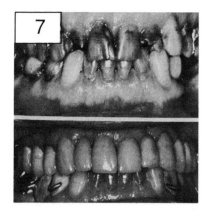
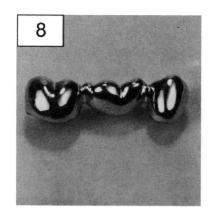
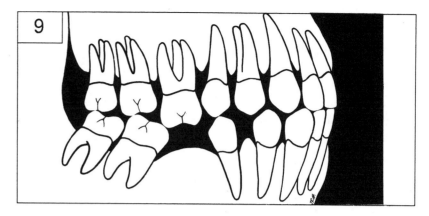

pared to receive crowns) are not often as smooth and well shaped as might be desired, and seldom are they as ideal as those pictured in most texts. The capable dentist not only can save these broken-down teeth, but can restore them as healthy, effective members of the dental arch (**Figure 7**).

Crowns are also important components of most fixed bridges. The various types of crowns and their particular usage as individual restorations or components of fixed bridges are discussed in subsequent sections.

The fixed bridge or fixed partial denture (**Figure 8**) is being used with increasing frequency. The components of the fixed bridge are discussed later; the purpose of the fixed bridge should be explained now. When a tooth is lost, the patient loses the chewing function of the lost tooth and also all or part of the function of the tooth opposing it. In other words, the loss of one tooth means that two teeth are "lost" insofar as chewing or mastication is concerned, because a tooth must have an opponent or "antagonist" to work against. Thus, one of the purposes of a fixed bridge is to *restore chewing function.*

Chewing is not the only function lost when a tooth is removed. Teeth offer mutual support to one another. Each tooth is supported in its position by the teeth on either side of it. When a tooth is lost, some of the support for adjacent teeth is lost, and they tend to tip or drift into the newly opened space.

A tooth is also "supported" by its opponent or antagonist in the opposite arch. If a tooth is lost, its antagonist will probably erupt into the space because there is no opponent to govern or control its position. Thus a second purpose of a bridge is to *support adjacent and opposing teeth.* Failure to maintain or restore this function may result in altered

position of many teeth, and subsequent decay and/or periodontal disease. Thus the loss of one tooth not only affects the adjacent and opposing teeth but very possibly may also affect the health of every other tooth in the mouth unless it is properly replaced. Maintenance of arch integrity is the most important reason to replace a missing posterior tooth. (**Figure 9**)

One obvious result of the loss of a tooth is change in personal appearance, especially if an anterior tooth is lost. Thus a third important purpose of a bridge is *esthetics* or *appearance.* Other factors such as *the effect on speech* (phonetics) and *on tongue habits,* are of varying importance, depending on which tooth or teeth may be missing.

Although the terms *fixed* and *removable* imply a kind of oppositeness, the purposes of fixed and removable dentures are actually the same: restored function, maintenance of oral health, and improved esthetics through the adequate replacement of missing teeth. In fact, in many instances either prosthesis could be used.

The removable partial denture is supported in part by the remaining natural teeth and in part by the edentulous ridge. The fixed partial denture is supported solely by remaining natural teeth. It will become obvious from subsequent discussions that the number and/or position of the remaining natural teeth may contraindicate the use of a fixed partial denture. There are also other conditions that make the removable partial denture preferable. However, where it can be properly employed, the fixed bridge is the prosthesis of choice because it is more stable, requires less bulk, and when properly executed affords better support and protection for the teeth that suspend it.

Fixed partial dentures (or bridges) are indicated whenever a tooth needs to be replaced and a sufficient number of healthy teeth remain to provide adequate support. This situation exists in many mouths and is created daily in many more as a result of the loss of teeth from accidents and disease. As a result of better education and financial resources, more patients with missing teeth are demanding fixed prosthodontic service. Technical advances in dentistry (notably high-speed cutting instruments and improved impression materials and techniques) have facilitated the dentist's ability to provide such services. Thus there is an increasing demand for trained technicians who understand this art and are capable of developing such restorations.

GOLD RESTORATIONS

There are actually two general methods of restoring teeth with gold. One method consists of serially packing small pieces of pure gold directly into the prepared tooth. Such restorations are done directly by the dentist and thus do not involve the services of dental laboratory technicians. In the second method a wax pattern in the exact form of the prepared cavity is made and then surrounded with a heat-resistant material called *investment*, to form a mold. The wax is eliminated by heat, leaving a cavity. Molten alloy is then cast into this cavity. The result is a casting that has the same size and shape as the wax pattern. The dentist attaches the gold casting permanently to the tooth with cement. By such a procedure, disease (caries) is eliminated, the prepared tooth is sealed and protected against the ingress of oral fluids (thus preventing further decay), and the original contours of the tooth are restored. Cast gold restorations are usually developed by technicians and are the focus of this manual.

The gold casting may be an onlay or a crown depending upon the form of the tooth preparation. The dentist authorizes the type of gold alloy to be used, depending on the size and purpose of the restoration. The laboratory technician is responsible for fabrication of the gold casting.

The length of service of onlays and crowns, as well as the life of the teeth they restore, is dependent upon close attention to minute details of construction by both the dentist and the laboratory technician. Each restoration must be carefully designed to restore the patient's damaged masticatory apparatus to a state of optimum health, function, appearance, and comfort.

In order to perform these exacting techniques the dental laboratory technician must have a basic knowledge of dental anatomy and dental materials and must possess the artistic skills and manual dexterity required to reproduce tooth forms. The technician must also have the patience to apply this knowledge diligently.

TERMINOLOGY

Some of the significant terms associated with fixed restorative techniques can be best understood by giving a brief description of the procedures required to make a cast gold alloy restoration. A dentist first "prepares" the tooth or teeth that will be restored. Such teeth are then referred to as *preparations*.

An *impression* (a negative reproduction of a given area of the oral cavity) is made by using a suitable impression material. The impression is then filled with an artificial stone similar to plaster that will harden to form a *cast*, which is a positive reproduction of an area of the oral cavity. Impressions and casts may reproduce hard tissues, soft tissues, or both.

A *die* is a positive reproduction of a tooth that has been prepared to receive a crown or an onlay. It is made of a hard material that will withstand the carving of a wax pattern. A die may be made from an impression of all or part of an arch, or from a small impression of an individual tooth.

A *wax pattern* is carved to the exact form desired for the cast gold restoration. It is used to form a mold into which the gold can be cast. A wax pattern carved outside the mouth on a die is called an *indirect pattern*. A pattern made by a dentist working directly on a tooth in the mouth is called a *direct pattern*. Wax patterns carved partially in the mouth by a dentist and completed by a technician using a die are called *direct-indirect patterns*.

The completed wax pattern is invested in a refractory (heat-resistant) material called *investment*. The pattern and investment are heated, thus volatilizing the wax and leaving a hollow mold cavity in the investment. Molten gold alloy is then *cast* into the hot mold to produce a *casting* the same size and shape as the wax pattern. After the investment is cleaned away, the casting is placed in acid to remove the surface oxides—a process called *pickling*.

If the pattern was made by the indirect method, the casting is carefully test-fitted on the die. After the test fitting on the die, the casting is burnished, finished, polished, thoroughly cleaned, and returned to the dentist, who completes the final marginal adaptation of the casting on the natural tooth.

If the casting was made by the direct method, it is test-fitted directly on the tooth and is then finished, polished, and thoroughly cleaned.

The final step in a fixed restorative technique is *cementation*. There are a variety of cements; the dentist chooses the one that best suits each particular restoration. The cement mix is applied to the tooth and the casting, and the restoration is pressed firmly to place. After the excess cement is removed, the restoration is complete.

DIAGNOSIS AND TREATMENT PLANNING

The construction of onlays, crowns, and bridges requires the coordinated efforts of the dentist and the dental laboratory technician to ensure a successful result. The dentist is responsible for diagnosis and treatment of the patient's dental problems. The technician is responsible for skillful and proficient performance of the laboratory phases.

The first step in providing care is to determine the conditions present in a given patient. A medical and dental history of the patient is necessary. A thorough clinical examination, using available diagnostic aids, is essential. Radiographic (x-ray) evaluation is normally a necessary part of the examination. This examination and patient history frequently enable the dentist to arrive at a complete diagnosis in simple cases. More complicated cases usually require the development of mounted *study casts* and often a trial wax model of the proposed restoration to determine form and occlusal relationships. This latter process is usually referred to as a *diagnostic wax-up*.

The next step is to determine what treatment is to be accomplished. A written *treatment plan* is a blueprint for proposed dental treatment.

The third step in dental care is to accomplish the treatment procedures. The dentist and auxiliary personnel work carefully together to obtain the desired result. When treatment includes the development of a prosthesis or appliances, the laboratory technician is an indispensable member of the dental team.

SEQUENCE OF TREATMENT

Clinical procedures are those accomplished by the dentist in the dental office. *Laboratory procedures,* which may be done in the laboratory by the dental laboratory technician, must be coordinated with clinical procedures in terms of design, material, and time.

Usually the tooth-preparation phase of onlays, crowns, and bridges is preceded by several preliminary appointments. These may include two appointments for the diagnosis and treatment plan. In addition, any needed surgical procedures are accomplished and the oral soft tissues are returned to optimal health before the restorative treatment begins.

A typical sequence of treatment might proceed as described below. Note that laboratory procedures hinge on progress made in clinical procedures.

APPOINTMENT ONE

Clinical Procedures: The history, clinical examination, and radiographic evaluation are completed, and preliminary impressions for diagnostic casts are made.

Laboratory Procedures: The preliminary impressions are poured in plaster or dental stone to produce the study casts.

APPOINTMENT TWO

Clinical Procedures: The treatment plan is presented to the patient, at times using the casts as a visual aid. Often more than one plan of treatment is possible, and these choices may be presented to the patient. A decision is made on the basis of the dentist's preference, the patient's preference, and financial considerations.

Laboratory Procedures: Custom trays may be constructed on the study casts in preparation for future impressions.

APPOINTMENT THREE

Clinical Procedures: Each defective tooth is prepared according to established principles. An impression is made of the prepared teeth and adjacent structures. An impression of the opposing arch may be made to provide an opposing cast. A registration of the jaw relationship is usually obtained as well. Temporary restorations are placed to protect the prepared teeth.

Laboratory Procedures: The dies for each prepared tooth and the master working cast are made as soon as possible from the impression. The method selected to make dies depends upon the impression material, the type of restoration, and the individual preferences of the dentist and the technician. The impression of the opposing arch is poured with a suitable cast material. The master working cast with the dies of the prepared teeth and the opposing cast are mounted on an articulator, using the jaw relationship record. Wax patterns are designed and formed following the dentist's work authorization. The patterns are invested and cast and the castings adjusted and finished. The completed restorations are sent to the dentist on the working cast.

APPOINTMENT FOUR

Clinical Procedures: The temporary restorations are removed from the prepared teeth. The castings are placed on the prepared teeth and are checked carefully for marginal adaptation and relationship to adjacent and opposing teeth and the soft tissues. The castings are adjusted if necessary. If the treatment involves individual onlays or crowns, these restorations may be cemented into place and thus completed during this appointment.

If the castings are retainers for a fixed bridge or need to be soldered together, another impression or registration is taken with the castings in place. The temporary restorations are replaced on the prepared teeth.

Laboratory Procedures: The retainers or castings and their dies are seated in the registration or impression. If additional castings are needed, such as a pontic to be used with already established retainers to develop a bridge, a new working cast is developed from the impression. If the castings that were trial-inserted need only to be united by soldering, the impression or index is used to develop a soldering invest-ment model to facilitate this procedure. The finished work is returned to the dentist.

APPOINTMENT FIVE

Clinical Procedures: The temporary restorations are removed from the prepared teeth. The castings are checked for fit, adjusted, and cemented.

SUMMARY

The essential clinical and laboratory procedures have been outlined to illustrate the basic steps in an actual treatment procedure. Depending upon the complexity of the treatment procedure, the dentist may alter this sequence and may require several more appointments. Laboratory procedures become more complicated as treatment becomes more complex.

It must be recognized that such an arrangement constitutes a team effort. Accordingly, the dentist must provide accurate impressions, registrations, and the information necessary to permit the laboratory technician to develop precise castings. In addition, adequate knowledge must exist to permit mutual understanding of procedures and respect for the challenges involved. The result is optimum treatment for the patient.

REVIEW QUESTIONS

1. Define operative dentistry.
2. Define fixed prosthodontics.
3. What are the types of fixed dental restorations?
4. What is an impression, and what is its purpose?
5. What is the dentist's responsibility, and what is the technician's responsibility, in producing a successful result for the dental patient?

SECTION 2

Types of Fixed Restorations

Since teeth do not have reparative capability as do soft tissues and bone, decayed or broken teeth must be restored if they are to be preserved to ensure continued function and esthetics and to avoid infection and pain. Most missing teeth need to be replaced to prevent shifting of adjacent and opposing teeth as well as to restore function and esthetics. Some teeth are restored or replaced solely for esthetics.

Several different materials are used for such restorations including silver alloy amalgam, resin, porcelain, and gold, or some combination of these materials. Most directly placed restorations are completed by the dentist during a single patient visit. However, as described in Section 1, cast restorations must be made in the laboratory.

Etruscan excavations in central Italy have revealed that these ancient people were able to mold gold into dental appliances. Evidence of advanced dental appliances has also been uncovered in excavations relating to ancient Central American Indians, the Mayans and Aztecs. The first modern crowns were made by adapting gold plate to the prepared tooth and then flowing solder over the plate to close seams and provide contour. In the late 1800s some dentists made inlays by burnishing platinum foil into a cavity preparation and then filling the platinum with gold solder. This was the best method known to make inlays until William F. Taggert perfected the disappearing-wax-pattern ("lost wax") casting technique in the early 1900s. His work opened the door for the development of modern dental casting procedures.

MATERIALS FOR CAST RESTORATIONS

Gold alloys used in dentistry have been standardized by the American Dental Association and the National Bureau of Standards. Onlays and crowns are usually made of one of these alloys, the choice of which is dependent upon the size, complexity, and function of the restoration. For esthetic reasons porcelain may be used to make crowns and inlays for anterior teeth. An onlay that must be extended onto the facial surface may be made more esthetic by developing a "window" in the onlay, which is then filled with a resin material. Crowns are made more esthetic by veneering them with resin or porcelain.

Because of the high cost of gold, nonprecious metal alloys have been developed for use in dental castings. These alloys must be ductile, tarnish-resistant, wear-resistant, and simple to use. Some alterations in technical procedures are necessary if nonprecious alloys are used. However, because of the great number and variety of currently available alloys, coverage of all specific techniques for their use is beyond the scope of this manual.

INLAYS/ONLAYS

Inlays are named according to the specific tooth surfaces that are involved. For example, an occlusal inlay restores the occlusal surface; an MO (mesioocclusal) inlay restores the mesial and occlusal surfaces; an MOD (mesioocclusodistal) inlay restores the mesial, occlusal, and distal surfaces. Inlays are also referred to on the basis of the number of surfaces they involve—a one-, two-, three-, four-, or five-surface inlay.

In addition, inlays/onlays (like other dental restorations) are grouped into six classes according to the character of the involved tooth surfaces and the form of the resulting restorations.

Class I inlays (**Figure 1**) occur on the occlusal surface of the premolars and molars and on the facial and lingual surfaces of other teeth. Decay which originates in pits and fissures of the tooth is repaired by Class I restorations.

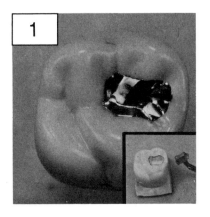

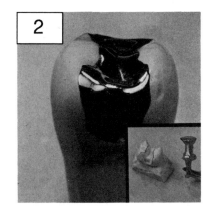

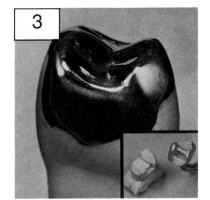

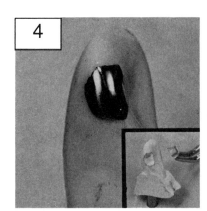

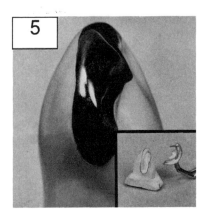

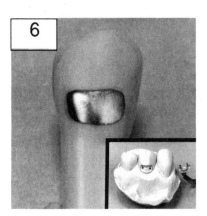

Class II inlays (**Figure 2**) restore the occlusal surfaces *and* the mesial and/or distal surfaces. Examples are MO, DO, and MOD inlays. Class II inlays, and also Class III, IV, V, VI inlays, restore decayed areas that originate on a smooth surface of the tooth in contradistinction to pit and fissure caries.

There are many modifications of Class II inlays. The most common modification is an MOD inlay that *caps* (covers) one or more cusps (**Figure 3**). This is done to protect the tooth from potential fracture due to occlusal forces, or to restore worn surfaces. The restoration is called an *onlay* when some or all of the cusps are capped. As stated in Section 1, onlays have become the commonly used design for intracoronal castings, because they prevent the fracture of teeth that frequently occurs with inlays.

A recent modification known as *skirting* is an extension of the onlay from the proximal surface onto the facial and/or lingual surfaces. Skirting extends the preparation around line angles so that the completed onlay binds the tooth together and is used in conjunction with cusp capping to provide additional protection for the tooth, as shown in **Figure 3**.

Skirting and cusp capping may be used to protect a tooth that has had a root canal filling placed. These procedures prevent fracture of the teeth, which are usually weakened by the caries or prior restorative involvement that made the endodontic treatment necessary and the access entry into the tooth that must be made to accomplish the root canal procedure.

Some Class II onlays gain added retention through the use of pins. The pins are an integral portion of the casting and fit into small holes prepared in the tooth.

A *Class III* inlay (**Figure 4**) restores the mesial or distal surface of an anterior tooth without involving the incisal angle and/or incisal edge. A Class III inlay may utilize a "dovetail" on the lingual surface to give the restoration better retention. Class III inlays are most commonly used on the distal surface of canine teeth.

Class IV inlays (**Figure 5**) involve the mesial or distal surface of an anterior tooth and include the incisal angle and/or incisal edge. Pins may be used to gain added retention. An MID (mesioincisodistal) inlay is an example of a Class IV restoration.

Class V inlays (**Figure 6**) occur on the facial or lingual surface of a tooth near the gingiva. Pins are usually placed to aid retention.

Class VI inlays occur on the worn incisal or occlusal surfaces of teeth. Pin retention is used routinely in this type of restoration.

A *pinlay* (**Figure 7**) combines the principles of Class III, IV, and VI inlays and covers the lingual surface of an anterior tooth and may cover one or both of the proximal surfaces and the incisal edge. Very little

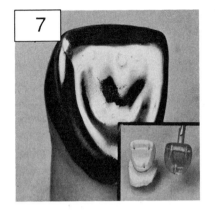
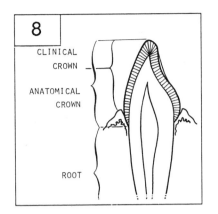
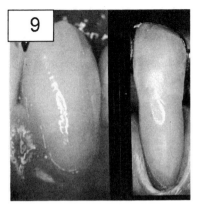
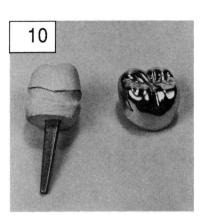

tooth structure is removed when making a preparation for a pinlay. Retention is gained from three or more pins that are placed on the lingual surface, usually including one at the mesiofacial angle, one at the distofacial angle, and one in the cingulum area near the gingiva.

CROWNS

Crowns are extracoronal restorations—dental restorations that cover all or part of the coronal surface of a tooth. *Coronal* means "crown," and the crown of a tooth is the portion that is covered with enamel (**Figure 8**). The restoration termed a *full crown* replaces most or all of the enamel of a tooth—hence the name.

A more significant term involving the word *crown* is *clinical crown*. The clinical crown of a tooth is the part that is not covered by gingival tissue (**Figure 9**). The clinical crown may be somewhat shorter than the anatomic crown, because the gingiva usually covers some of the enamel. However, the clinical crown may be longer than the anatomic crown when the gingiva recedes and some of the root surface is exposed. In any case, the full crown restoration normally covers all of the clinical crown and may extend beneath the edge of the gingiva. Crowns that cover only a part of the clinical crown of a tooth are termed *partial crowns*.

Full Cast Crowns

The most commonly employed type of crown is the full cast crown (**Figure 10**). As the name implies, this restoration covers all of the exposed surface of the tooth. It is made entirely of metal.

A variety of techniques have been used in the past to develop crown restorations because of limitations of the casting process. Today virtually all crowns are developed on a die as a very accurate wax pattern, which is then invested and cast with a suitable alloy.

Veneered Crowns

For esthetic reasons some full crowns are developed with a tooth-colored front or "face." These are termed *faced* or *veneered crowns* and are of two types—resin-faced or porcelain-faced. Resin and porcelain are the two suitable tooth-colored materials available to dentistry today.

Resin-faced Crown (Figure 11) The wax pattern for a resin-faced crown is developed just as for the full cast crown. A "window" is then carved into the wax on the facial surface. Special undercuts, or "locks," are made in the wax pattern to mechanically secure the resin. Resin of the desired shade is placed in the window after the casting is completed. Several types of resin may be used for such facings. Methyl methacrylate was the first resin used, but other resins are becoming more popular.

This type of crown presents certain inherent problems. No resin materials available today are hard enough to withstand the wear imposed by occlusal function. This problem is circumvented by forming the occlusal surface in metal and only the face or front surface of the crown in resin. On anterior teeth the resin can usually be extended to the biting edge far enough to hide the metal without subjecting it to excessive occlusal contact.

A second disadvantage of resins is their permeability, which permits the absorption of oral fluids (including food fluids). Stagnation and

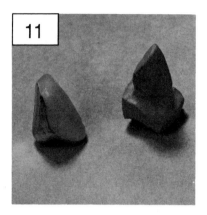
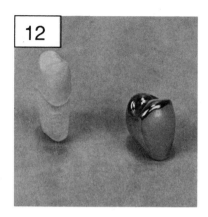

decomposition of these fluids may produce a foul odor and discoloration of the facing.

The same problems occur due to percolation (seepage of fluids between the resin and metal) as a result of lack of adhesion or bonding between the two materials. A major cause of this percolation is the marked difference in thermal expansion between resins and metals. Restorations are subjected to changes in temperature by the intake of hot and cold foods. The metal and resin expand and contract at different rates and hence tend to separate. The mechanical locks that are used to hold resin facings in position cannot entirely resist the thermal forces that lead to percolation.

Resin-faced crowns also have some advantages. The most significant is that resins are comparatively easy to handle and little special equipment is required to apply the resins. Another distinct advantage is the ease with which the dentist can repair the resin facing in the mouth in the event of breakage or other failure. Yet another advantage is their toughness or resistance to breakage: because they are "plastic," they do not often break or crack. However, many dentists have found that failures of resin facings due to wear, percolation, absorption, and insufficient mechanical retention equal or exceed "breakage" of porcelain veneers. The most significant advantage of resin as compared to porcelain is that it is less abrasive and thus does not cause wear of opposing teeth.

Porcelain-faced Crown (Figure 12)   The porcelain-faced crown is a cast crown with a porcelain window or veneer fashioned from a stock tooth or facing. The porcelain facing is shaped and positioned next to the die. A wax pattern is then made to encompass the die and receive the facing. The facing is removed and the pattern cast. Once the casting is finished, the facing is cemented into the crown.

Most of the problems inherent with the resin-faced crown are overcome by the porcelain-faced crown, but other problems come into play. In marked contrast to resins, glazed porcelain does not wear excessively nor does it absorb fluids and discolor, but it can break unless properly handled. In the porcelain-faced crown the facing *must* be protected from occlusal forces by the casting, lest the cement bond fail and the facing be broken or lost. The display of metal along the occlusal or incisal edge is an esthetic disadvantage, although under ideal conditions it can be kept minimal by rounding the facioincisal or facioocclusal angle so that light is not reflected directly off the metal. Breakage of a porcelain facing can only be repaired with self-curing resin.

Another disadvantage, which the porcelain-faced crown shares with the resin-faced crown, is a lack of bond between the two applied materials. The intermediate cement offers some seal, but adequate retention requires mechanical friction and accuracy of fit between the casting and facing, as with an inlay. Although gold and porcelain expand and contract at different rates, the differential is not as great as that between gold and resin and does not often result in failure of the cement bond.

The porcelain-faced crown is difficult to fabricate. Proper occlusion is much less easily achieved than with resin, especially if the display of incisal or occlusal metal is limited. The development of porcelain-fused-to-metal crowns and bridges has made porcelain-faced construction virtually obsolete. Dentistry is now primarily divided between the use of *resin-faced* and *porcelain-fused-to-metal* construction. As stated in the Preface and Section 1, porcelain-fused-to-metal restorations are not covered in this manual.

Partial Crowns

A partial crown covers only part of the crown of a tooth. It is difficult to differentiate between onlays and partial crowns in some instances. As mentioned earlier, the inlay is an intracoronal restoration; the full crown an extracoronal restoration. If the major retention comes from box forms cut into the tooth and is thus provided by the internal surfaces of a preparation, the restoration is intracoronal. If the preparation of the tooth is essentially enamel removal and retention is provided by external surfaces of the preparation, the restoration should be considered extracoronal. It is somewhere between these categories that extensive

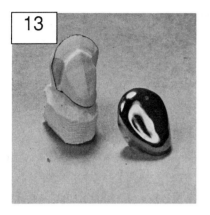
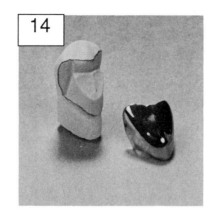
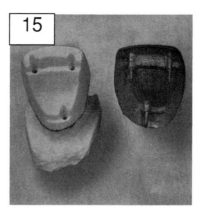
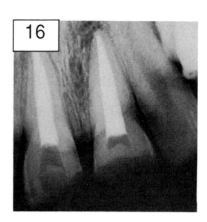

onlays and partial crowns fall, since they involve both intra- and extra-coronal retention.

The most common form of partial crown is the three-quarter crown. This term is actually a misnomer, as the clinical crown of a tooth has five surfaces. Because the standard "three-quarter" crown (**Figure 13**) covers all surfaces except the facial, it is really a "four-fifth" crown. Explanation of this discrepancy is simple enough. In the past the incisal edge of an anterior tooth was not thought of as a surface; in this sense there were only four surfaces, three of which were covered by the crown. The name is still accepted usage.

The three-quarter crown was originally conceived as a more esthetic and conservative retainer than the full metal crown for anterior bridges. The original design displayed a definite border of gold on both proximal surfaces and the incisal edge of the preparation. This form was progressively modified until today the ideal anterior three-quarter crown displays only a fraction of a millimeter of metal along the incisal edge of the tooth. Even so, the standard three-quarter crown with its metal incisal coverage is fast becoming unacceptable to the esthetically conscious public. Many dentists find it necessary to use full crowns with resin veneers or porcelain-fused-to-metal construction to avoid any possible display of gold. Often a modified three-quarter crown can be used that varies from the standard style by the absence of incisal or facial cusp coverage, which results in no display of metal on the facial surface (**Figure 14**).

Pinlays, especially three-pin hoods (**Figure 15**), are also used as retainers for short-span bridges when the abutment teeth are sound and metal display is unacceptable to the patient.

When the design of partial crowns is studied, it becomes readily apparent that as extension of the tooth preparation becomes more conservative, retention is derived less from the surface and more from the deeper, internal areas of the tooth. In these circumstances accuracy and "snugness" of fit become increasingly important. This demand must be faced and met by both dentist and technician in each and every phase of developing such restorations if they are to be successful. When a dentist has made good preparations and impressions, the responsibility for the success or failure lies in the hands of the technician.

Post Crowns

When the pulp of a tooth has been irreparably damaged by caries, trauma, or dental procedures, two choices are available: either remove the tooth, or remove the damaged pulp and fill the pulp canal (or canals) with a suitable material. Endodontics is the field of dentistry that deals with the latter treatment. Thus an endodontically treated tooth is one that has had the root canal filled (**Figure 16**). These teeth have a tendency to be brittle. A crown that adequately restores an endodontically treated tooth must support this brittle tooth structure (both crown and root) and must gain its retention from the remaining tooth structure, which is frequently only the root. Both of these requirements are met by incorporating a metal post that extends into the root canal space (**Figure 17**). Crowns incorporating such posts are termed *post* or *dowel crowns*.

Under heavy occlusal or traumatic loads a post may cause the root to split longitudinally (**Figure 18**). For this reason the dentist prepares the tooth so that it can receive a collar of metal to surround the outer surface of the remaining tooth structure. This collar serves to bind the

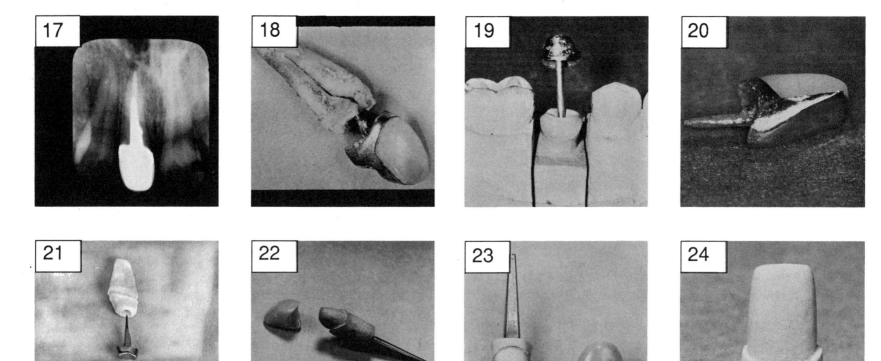

tooth together, rather like a barrel hoop (**Figure 19**).

There are two basic designs for post crowns: a one-piece crown and post (**Figure 20**), or a crown with a separate post, a two-piece design (**Figure 21**). In either case the crown may be all-metal or veneered.

In the two-piece design the post and crown are cast as separate units. Often the post includes a "core" (**Figure 21**) or "thimble" to replace a portion of the prepared tooth form that is missing due to caries, previous restorations, or fracture of the tooth. The result of this post and core is an ideal stump form over which the crown can be cemented.

One of the earliest dowel or post crowns was the Richmond crown, a porcelain-faced post crown of one-piece construction. The two-piece counterpart of the Richmond crown, known as the Davis crown, consisted of a post over which was cemented an all-porcelain crown. Many dentists still refer to post or dowel crowns as Richmond or Davis crowns, regardless of how they are constructed. The technician must be

able to interpret the dentist's terminology even if it is outdated.

Jacket Crowns

The origin of the term *jacket crown* is difficult to explain. Originally, "porcelain jacket crown" referred to the complete veneer, all-porcelain crown that was introduced by Charles H. Land in 1886. After acrylic was introduced to dentistry, complete veneer acrylic crowns were made, and these too were referred to as jacket crowns, or more specifically acrylic jacket crowns. Regardless of its origin, *jacket* is commonly used to refer to both the all-porcelain crown (**Figure 22**) and the all-resin crown (**Figure 23**).

Neither conventional porcelain nor resin can routinely be made into a crown with the marginal accuracy of metal castings. Neither of these materials is strong in thin cross section; thus shouldered or heavily

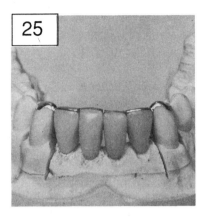
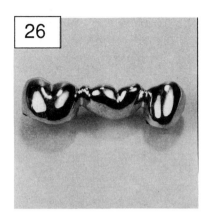
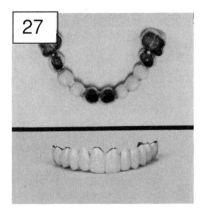
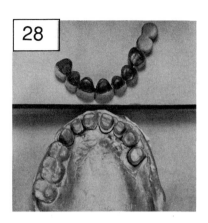

chamfered preparations (**Figure 24**) are made to provide adequate bulk at their margins.

Although jacket crowns are second to the veneered metal crown in marginal adaptation, they are unsurpassed in esthetics. This advantage stems from working solely with tooth-colored materials—tooth, cement, and porcelain or acrylic, with no metal to "mask."

Porcelain is the superior material for jacket crown construction. Acrylic jackets are generally considered to be little more than temporary crowns. This is because acrylic jackets percolate at their margins due to thermal expansion and contraction, are not resistant to abrasion and wear, and absorb mouth fluids with resultant discoloration and odor. Porcelain on the other hand wears well, is impervious to mouth fluids, and is thermostable. One disadvantage of porcelain is its brittleness and its susceptibility to fracture. However, when properly designed and applied, the porcelain jacket is adequate to withstand normal usage for very reasonable periods of time.

The fracture of natural teeth in accidents is a basic reason jacket restorations are necessary. The other reason is extensive decay or repeated failure of filling materials. Present-day use of jacket crowns is limited almost exclusively to the anterior teeth.

Very recent advances in ceramic technology have resulted in both injection-molded and cast ceramic restorations that have exceptional marginal accuracy and good strength. Development of these technologies will unquestionably make the conventional porcelain jacket crown obsolete in the very near future.

THE FIXED BRIDGE (FIXED PARTIAL DENTURE) AND ITS COMPONENTS

A fixed bridge (**Figure 25**) is a restoration replacing one or more missing teeth that gains its support from the remaining natural teeth to which it is cemented. Some missing teeth may be replaced by either a fixed bridge or a removable partial denture. Where there is a choice the fixed bridge is preferred.

Abutments

An *abutment* is a remaining natural tooth or root(s) that gives support to a dental prosthetic appliance. The teeth that are clasped by a removable partial denture and thus give it support are termed abutments. Teeth that support a fixed partial denture are likewise termed abutments or, more generally, "bridge" abutments.

There can be any number of abutments for a fixed bridge, depending on its length or span. The most common bridge replaces one missing tooth and is supported by an abutment on either side of the space. This is termed a *three-unit bridge* (**Figure 26**) because three teeth are involved—two abutments and one replacement. A similar bridge could replace two or three missing teeth and still have only two abutments, one at either end of the bridge. Even more extensive bridges are commonly required and may involve an entire arch (**Figure 27**). A bridge of this magnitude has a minimum of four abutments and conceivably could have thirteen abutments.

On occasion many teeth are joined together within one framework with no replacement tooth. Such an appliance is not a bridge but rather

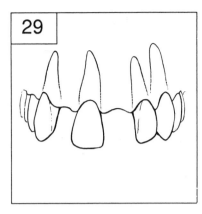

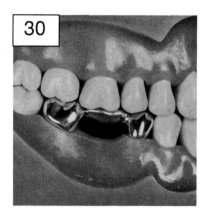

a *fixed splint*. Its purpose is to tie together, or "splint," adjacent teeth to make them stronger when there has been significant loss of supporting bone or when the occlusal forces imposed on the teeth are greater than can be resisted individually. Fixed splints are made in the same fashion as a fixed bridge, the only difference being the absence of replacement teeth. Many appliances are in fact a combination splint and bridge, and it becomes difficult to determine which term should apply (**Figure 28**). If a missing tooth is replaced, the prosthesis is termed a *bridge*. If, in addition, the prosthesis provides significant splinting, it may be called a *splint bridge*.

The opposite extreme is the *one-abutment bridge*. Seldom indicated, this type of bridge involves a restoration on a single abutment tooth with a replacement tooth attached to one side. This prosthesis is also termed a *cantilever* or *wing bridge*. Its most common use is in the replacement of a maxillary or mandibular lateral incisor cantilevered from the adjacent canine. A more sound utilization of the cantilever principle involves two or more abutments with a replacement extended at one end of the appliance (**Figure 28**). Obviously, too great a "lever arm" should not be created.

Though used infrequently, the proper term for an intermediate abutment is *pier*. A pier is an abutment which is located between two other abutments and has a replacement on either side. The smallest bridge incorporating a pier would thus involve five units.

An example may best serve to clarify abutment terminology. Let us imagine a six-unit maxillary anterior bridge extending from right canine to right central to left lateral and canine (**Figure 29**). The right lateral and left central are to be replaced. The right canine is a *terminal abutment*. The right central is an intermediate abutment or *pier*. The left lateral and canine serve essentially as one "two-rooted" tooth, and as such are considered together as the terminal abutment for that end of the bridge. The splinting together of two adjacent teeth to serve as support for a fixed or removable partial denture is termed *double abutting*, and the splinted teeth are termed a *double abutment*.

A few minutes spent studying the model of a dental arch can reveal the almost infinite number of abutment and replacement combinations that could be utilized in the development of fixed partial dentures to replace varying numbers of missing teeth.

Retainers

A *retainer* is that part of a dental bridge which restores the abutment tooth and unites it with the suspended portion of the bridge. In other words, a retainer is the restoration cemented on or in the abutment tooth to which the replacement tooth is attached.

Retainers may be any type of cast restoration—onlay, pinlay, partial crown, or full crown. The retention of a retainer is of vital importance. Retentive requirements are in direct proportion to the extent of the prosthesis and the occlusal forces to which it is subjected. Obtaining adequate retention requires accurate tooth preparations and impressions and precise fabrication. The most important requirement of a retainer is that it adequately restore the abutment tooth. No amount of retention can long prevail against the ingress of decay. Likewise the ultimate in retention and marginal seal cannot save the tooth from the ravages of periodontal disease invoked by poor contour and occlusal disharmony of a restoration.

Pontics

A *pontic* is the portion of a dental bridge that serves as the replacement for the missing tooth or teeth (**Figure 30**). The requirements of a pontic are: (1) maintenance of arch integrity, (2) restoration of occlusal function, and (3) in certain areas of the mouth restoration of tooth form and appearance. The pontic must be designed and fabricated to be biologically acceptable to oral tissues and to facilitate oral hygiene.

Maintenance of intra-arch integrity is accomplished by restoring proximal contact. Teeth within a given dental arch normally offer mutual support to one another through their proximal contact (**Figure 9, Section 1**). When a tooth is lost, the adjacent teeth tend to tip into the resulting space. By rigidly bridging such a void, the pontic serves to maintain space and prevents the drifting and tipping movement of the neighboring teeth. A pontic may also prevent the extrusion of an opposing tooth, which could cause collapse of tooth position within the opposing arch.

The restoration of tooth form and appearance is the least important function of a pontic from the dental standpoint. For the patient, however, this is often its most important function.

Many concepts are involved in considering the biological acceptance of the pontic. For the sake of simplicity these are generally classified in two groups: (1) materials used in construction, and (2) size and form.

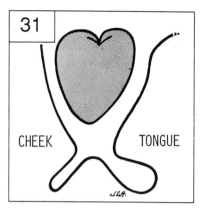
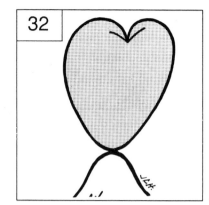

TYPES OF PONTICS: MATERIALS

The materials used in the construction of pontics are the same as those used for the various full crowns, thus the same two major groupings can be identified: (1) all-metal pontics, and (2) faced pontics. The material used to make the pontic takes on added significance when the pontic tip must come into contact with tissue.

Highly glazed porcelain is the best material that can be used in contact with oral tissues. This statement implies a smooth, nonporous, preferably convex surface fired to a natural glaze without the addition of a heavily fluxed overglaze which might be soluble in oral fluids. Second in order of compatibility with oral tissue is a noble metal alloy. The metal tip surface must be smooth, nonporous, and highly polished. Third in the list of available materials are the resins. A dense, well-cured, nonporous surface is essential. Resins tend to absorb mouth fluids after a period of time and become foul.

A junction line or margin between two different materials (such as metal and porcelain or metal and resin) is never desirable in the area of tissue contact. Such margins or junctions always present microscopic voids and irregularities that harbor bacterial plaque.

All-metal Pontics

As with crowns, some pontics are made entirely of metal, usually gold. Metal pontics are normally esthetically unacceptable in the anterior region of the mouth but are usually acceptable in the posterior regions.

The simplest all-metal pontic is the *hygienic pontic*, so termed be-

cause it permits free-cleansing by the patient (see **Figure 30**). The hygienic pontic is essentially a bar of metal that spans the space between abutments. Its gingival surface is contoured to provide maximum self-cleansing efficiency and is *not* extended to contact the soft tissue covering the edentulous ridge. Its occlusal surface is contoured to provide occlusal anatomy and to establish centric and functional occlusion. It is usually restricted in faciolingual width to reduce occlusal loading and to be compatible with the contour of the underlying edentulous ridge.

There should be adequate space between the gingival surface of the hygienic pontic and the crest of the edentulous ridge to provide room for free-cleansing by the patient. The pontic must have at least the minimum cross-sectional diameter that can provide adequate rigidity (**Figure 31**). Thus a significant space is required between the crest of the ridge and the occlusal plane (usually about 5 millimeters). If sufficient space is not available, the pontic should be carried toward the gingiva to contact the soft tissue. Tissue contact may be established in one of two ways: (1) through a heart-shaped contour just contacting the crest of the ridge (**Figure 32**), or (2) through a convex contour contacting the facial aspect of the ridge (**Figure 33**). The heart-shaped contour is preferred. The convex tip contacting the facial aspect of the ridge is indicated only when the vertical clearance is extremely limited (less than 3 millimeters) or when there is a depression in the facial contour of the ridge so that the ridge is displaced lingual to the center of the occlusal surface.

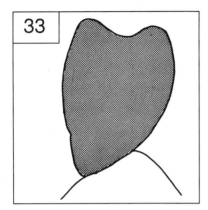 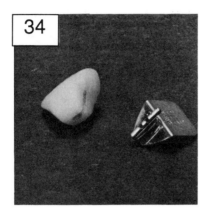 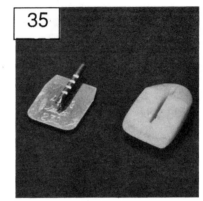 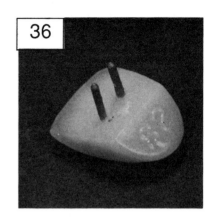

Veneered Pontics

This group includes the porcelain-faced pontic and the resin-faced pontic and also the porcelain-fused-to-metal pontic, though that technique is not covered in this manual. The design of the gingival surfaces or "tips" of faced pontics requires special consideration. Glazed porcelain is the most acceptable material available. Highly polished noble alloys, acrylic, and unglazed porcelain complete the list, in order of decreasing acceptability. Acrylic and unglazed porcelain tips should be avoided if possible. Let us consider then the relationship between materials and design of pontics.

Porcelain-faced Pontics   A porcelain-faced pontic can be made like a porcelain-faced crown: a stock facing can be prepared to form a window in the facial surface, with the gingival surface or tip being formed by gold. Another design has the gingival tip formed of unglazed porcelain. This technique involves the use of a manufactured pontic facing with a porcelain tip, such as the Steele's Trupontic (**Figure 34**). The prefabricated tip form must be ground to contour, thus destroying the manufactured glazed surface. These surfaces can be polished, but they are not as smooth and nonporous as a glazed surface, and they are not as acceptable to the tissue.

Another popular porcelain pontic facing for anterior bridges is the "flatback" or *slot facing* (**Figure 35**). These facings are designed to be interchangeable, so that if one is broken it can be replaced without removing the bridge. Slot facings have a flat lingual surface with a slot or groove extending from the gingival end almost to the incisal. A prefabricated backing containing a post to fit the facing slot can be soldered to the framework; or the post and backing can be waxed and

cast. The interchangeability is very desirable and accounts for the wide use of these facings. However, from the standpoint of biological compatibility these are the worst facings available. The junction between facing and backing occurs in the center of the gingival tip. Especially if a prefabricated backing is used, a marked discrepancy usually occurs at this junction, leaving a groove that traps debris and bacteria. This problem can be overcome by covering the entire tip of the facing with gold, but that solution makes the replacement of the facing more difficult.

The best pontic incorporating a stock facing was the baked-tip pontic using a long-pin facing (**Figure 36**). The stock long-pin facing was ground to contour as necessary, and the gingival end was reduced to leave approximately 1 millimeter clearance between facing and ridge. Porcelain that fuses at a temperature below that of the manufactured facing was then added, slightly in excess of the desired tip contour. After baking, this porcelain tip was ground carefully to final contour and then fired to a glaze. No subsequent changes were made by grinding on this tip surface; thus tissue contact was established in glazed porcelain. Such a pontic tip provides the maximum in tissue acceptance. Unfortunately long-pin facings are no longer marketed.

The porcelain-fused-to-metal pontic affords the same glazed porcelain tip, differing only in that the entire porcelain portion of the pontic is fabricated by the technician rather than being constructed with a manufactured facing. It was the advent of the porcelain-fused-to-metal technique that eliminated the use of pin facings.

Resin-faced Pontics   Resin-faced pontics can likewise be made with either the resin or gold forming the pontic tip. Since highly polished gold is the more stable material, the tip of such pontics should prefer-ably be made of gold rather than resin. This design also permits easier repair or replacement of the pontic facing in the mouth, which may be necessary when acrylic is used (**Figure 37**).

TYPES OF PONTICS: FORMS

The second consideration in biological acceptance of the pontic is size and form. Some factors governing size have been mentioned in the discussion of types of pontic construction. The mesiodistal width of the pontic is determined by the space and is thus unalterable. Faciolingual width is reduced in proportion to the length of span, occlusal relation-ship, and the residual ridge contour.

Narrowing of the occlusal surface is often a requisite for units of posterior bridges in order to reduce occlusal loading and the resultant stresses that are transmitted to the abutment teeth. In any bridge situa-tion the abutment teeth must resist their normal occlusal load plus that of the replacement tooth or teeth. For example, in a three-unit bridge from the mandibular second premolar to second molar, the abutments support their normal load *and* the additional load delivered through the first molar pontic. To keep this load within tolerable limits, the size of the occlusal surfaces of all three units may need to be reduced. Narrow-ing the occlusal table obviously will not effect a decrease in load when biting on hard, unyielding objects. However, restriction of the occlusal table dimension can reduce the total load from chewing normal, plas-tic food masses, by reducing the square millimeters of surface to be loaded. Ideally, then, in this three-unit example, the occlusal surface of each unit should be reduced one-third, thus resulting in the same total loadable surface area that the two abutments had originally.

Maintaining such a proportionate decrease becomes impractical and impossible in bridges of longer span if adequate occlusal surface for stable centric and functional occlusion is to be maintained. Neverthe-less every effort should be made to approximate this proportionate decrease in loading, either by actual reduction of surface area or the development of exaggerated grooves and spillways to promote rapid unloading of the functional surfaces. The goal is to achieve penetration of foodstuff with a biting pressure low enough to prevent overloading the abutment teeth and their supporting tissues.

Reduction in the occlusal surface area of posterior bridges is made by

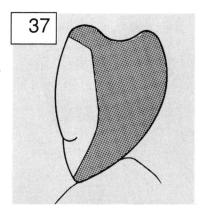

narrowing the surface faciolingually, as mesiodistal distance cannot be altered. On mandibular posterior bridges the reduction in width is done at the expense of the lingual cusp. The facial cusps must maintain their centric and eccentric occlusal contacts. On maxillary teeth some nar-rowing may be done at the expense of the facial cusp, but sufficient horizontal overlap must be maintained to prevent cheek biting. There-fore narrowing of maxillary posterior bridges is done at the expense of both facial and lingual contours. Nevertheless the position of the lin-gual cusp tip must permit maintenance of stable centric contact.

The occlusogingival length of a pontic is determined by the corre-sponding space, the type of pontic tip design, and esthetics.

Most of the factors relating to form or contour are likewise at hand. The occlusal surface is contoured to provide maximum centric and functional occlusion with as much consideration for ideal anatomy as is consistent with good occlusion. Proper horizontal and vertical overlaps must be developed as a product of proper occlusal and facial contour. The one factor relative to contour that is unique to a pontic is tip form.

CONTOUR OF PONTIC TIPS

A pontic tip is the portion of the pontic that approximates or directly contacts the subjacent soft tissues; hence it is the contour that will most directly affect tissue response. Four concepts or forms are recognized for the contour of pontic tips.

The Hygienic Pontic The hygienic pontic has already been de-

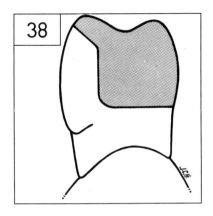

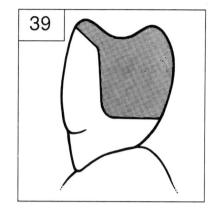

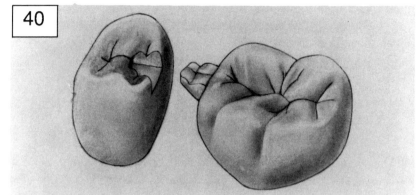

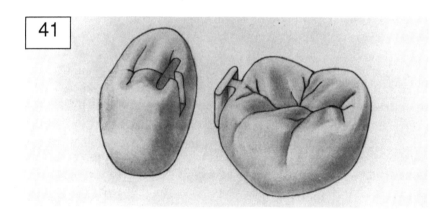

scribed as a pontic that does not approximate the soft tissues, or one that is heart-shaped and possibly just touches the tissue of the crest of the ridge in the center of the edentulous space. This pontic design is the most acceptable to the tissue as it has the least tissue contact. (See **Figures 30–32**).

The Convex Tip   The three remaining types of pontics are normally intended to contact soft tissue. Of these, the convex tip, properly done, is most desirable (**Figure 37**). The convex tip involves *slight* compression of the soft tissue overlying the edentulous ridge. The amount of this compression depends on the character of the tissue and should be determined and indicated by the dentist on the basis of careful evaluation of these tissues in the mouth. The cast may be "relieved" to indicate the desired amount of compression. This relief takes the form of a *slight* concavity carved into the cast, against which the convex tip is adapted. The relief is greatest on the facial aspect of the ridge (usually less than 0.3 millimeter), tapering to none toward the crest of the ridge. Such compression provides firm contact of the pontic tip against the soft tissue and prevents the intrusion of most debris.

The important aspect of this design is that a pontic tip that is convex in all directions can be cleaned, even though the bridge cannot be removed. Convexity permits total surface contact and cleaning with dental floss or tape. The size of the pontic tip and degree of convexity must be compatible with size and contour of the residual ridge and the amount of compression established.

The convex form also minimizes the total area of tissue contact and facilitates access into the gingival embrasures.

The Saddle Pontic Tip   The saddle pontic tip (**Figure 38**) gets its

name from its similarity to the horse saddle. It is the exact opposite of the convex tip, being distinctly concave in at least one dimension. It is the most unacceptable tip design biologically, yet probably the most widely used. Faciolingually this tip forms a concave surface or saddle over the ridge. Mesiodistally it is usually flat to slightly convex. Cleaning of the tissue surface is essentially impossible due to its contour. The saddle form results in the maximum total area of tissue contact and usually limits access into the gingival embrasures.

The Ridge-lap Pontic Tip   The ridge-lap pontic tip (**Figure 39**) is essentially a compromise between the convex and saddle designs. It creates a limited concavity in a faciolingual direction and definite convexity in the mesiodistal dimension. It is relatively amenable to cleaning. This philosophy embodies consideration of hygiene and biological acceptance. The slight to moderate faciolingual concavity presented by the ridge-lap design permits esthetic adaptation without heavy tissue contact—which accounts for many dentists' preference for this design.

Astute clinicians are well aware that the success of many fixed bridges is related to the degree of convexity of their pontic tips.

CONNECTORS

A *connector* is the part of a fixed bridge that unites the pontic to the retainer. It may be rigid or nonrigid. A *rigid connector* is a solid metal union between pontic and retainer, either soldered or cast. A *nonrigid connector* joins the pontic and retainer via mechanical locking of the metal parts without creating a solid union. Semiprecision types are made by carving and machining a female rest in the retainer, then waxing and casting a male lug or key on the pontic to fit closely. Precision types are manufactured to close tolerances and are usually of the "T" or mortise design (**Figure 41**). These are available as prefabricated metal connectors for incorporation in castings, or as plastic patterns that can be incorporated in the wax pattern and cast.

Nonrigid connectors are employed in fixed bridges (1) when the position of the abutments will not permit "draw" or seating of the bridge as a single unit; (2) when it is desirable to segment large bridges to facilitate fabrication and cementation, yet maintain the "splinting" affect of mechanical continuity; and (3) when one retainer is markedly more retentive than the other. In the latter instances the reason for using the nonrigid connector is to relieve some of the stress on the weaker retainer. Such connectors are often termed *stress breakers* and the bridge termed a *broken-stress bridge*. How much stress is "broken" or relieved depends on the type of nonrigid connector used. The dentist should decide whether or not to use a nonrigid connector. In certain instances, however, the technician may recommend their use to facilitate fabrication.

The most commonly used nonrigid semiprecision connector is the *simple lug-rest* (**Figure 40**): a rest in the retainer, and a lug that extends from the pontic to fit into the rest. This is similar to an occlusal rest and lug used in removable partial dentures. Such connectors provide resistance to vertical forces applied to the pontic, but little resistance to lateral and torsional forces.

The *T-shaped keyway* (**Figure 41**) is the most commonly used form of

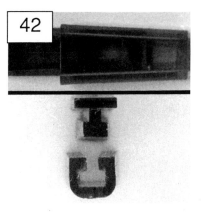 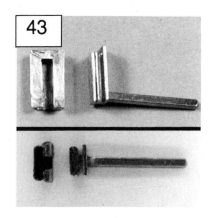

precision connector. It resists vertical forces and to a large extent lateral and torsional stresses. These nonrigid precision connectors may be tapered or parallel-sided. The tapered design is normally used to couple components of fixed bridges and is thus commonly referred to as an *interconnector*. These are available as plastic patterns that can be incorporated in a wax pattern and cast (**Figure 42**).

Parallel-sided connectors are normally precision-manufactured metal components and are generally referred to as *precision attachments*. Although they may be used as interconnectors for fixed bridge components, they are more commonly employed as attachments for removable partial dentures (**Figure 43**).

REVIEW QUESTIONS

1. Name the classes of inlays/onlays. Define each class.
2. Identify the types of crowns. Define each type.
3. Name the components of a fixed bridge. Describe or define each component.
4. Name and describe the types of pontics on the basis of the material used in construction.
5. Identify and describe the types of pontics on the basis of the gingival contour of the pontic tip.

SECTION 3

Basic Concepts of Prepared Tooth Forms

Sections 1 and 2 briefly described the distinctions between intracoronal and extracoronal restorations. The type of restoration that is used depends on the tooth preparation. Conversely, and possibly more logically, the type of tooth preparation depends on the type of restoration desired. Preparations for directly formed restorations (amalgams and resins) are created to provide "locking" of the filling material in the tooth. But preparations for indirectly formed restorations (castings) must be created with smooth, tapered walls that allow placement of the casting into or onto the tooth, as well as its removal from the tooth.

Dental laboratory technicians are concerned only with those restorations that are developed indirectly, that is, outside the mouth. These are cast metal restorations with the exception of the all-porcelain or acrylic jacket and the porcelain inlay or onlay. The major differences in tooth preparation form, as far as the technician is concerned, depend on the extent of the restoration (how much of the tooth is involved) and how it is retained in the tooth.

The dentist bases his decisions about the extent of the preparation and restoration on many factors: (1) the extent of decay and/or previous filling material; (2) the size, shape, and position of the tooth; (3) the type and character of the occlusion; (4) the caries experience of the patient; (5) esthetics; (6) the purpose of the restoration, such as individual tooth restoration, removable partial denture abutment restoration, terminal or intermediate retainer for a fixed partial denture, or segment of a splint; (7) dentally indicated or personally preferred materials; (8) the dentist's preference of preparation form; and (9) specific, unusual tooth conditions, such as a fractured tooth, endodontically treated tooth, or enamel hypoplasia.

Whatever the criteria, preparation form is established before the technician becomes involved. Nevertheless there are several features with which the technician must be thoroughly familiar if adequate restorations are to be made.

Convenience Form: "Draft" or "Draw"

In dentistry the term *convenience form* has several implications. The convenience form referred to here is the taper or convergence of the prepared tooth form, which permits seating and withdrawal of a casting. The term *draw* (contracted from the word *withdraw*) is used to designate this form. The term *draft* refers to the angle of the taper given to the prepared tooth so that the casting can be removed easily; that is, no undercuts are present that prevent the removal of a casting.

The prepared tooth that is to receive any type of cast restoration must "draw." Absolute parallelism is impossible to attain in dental preparations and is not consistent with the accuracy of techniques involved in constructing a restoration. Thus some taper or convergence of the walls of the preparation is indicated (**Figure 1**). Ideally this taper should be in the range of 2° to 5° per surface, or 5° to 10° overall.

The term *undercut* arises at this point as an antonym of *draw*. If the walls of a tooth prepared for a crown diverge occlusally, or a significant portion of one wall is divergent occlusally in relation to the other walls of the preparation, it is said to be undercut, or not to draw (**Figure 2**). Isolated defects, such as voids created in a surface by removal of decay or old restorative material, may be eliminated by filling them with suitable cements before the impression of the preparation is made. Such undercuts may also be "blocked out" on the die with "undercut wax" or other suitable materials.

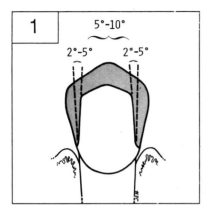

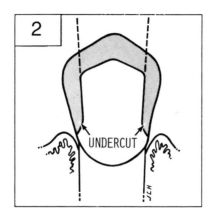

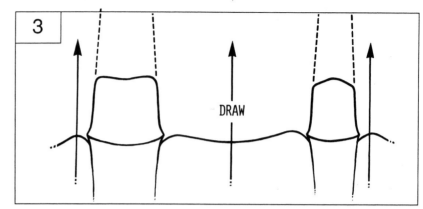

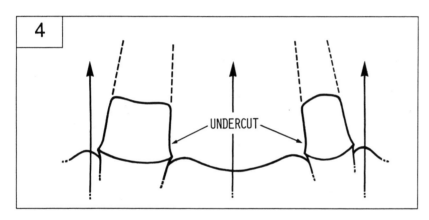

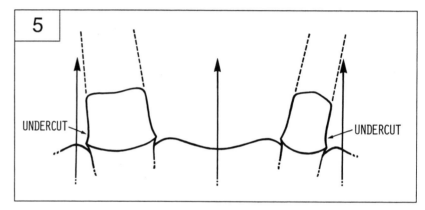

Although draw is absolutely critical in the individual preparation, it takes on added significance in the bridge situation. Here two or more abutment preparations must not only draw individually, but must also draw with each other (**Figures 3, 4, and 5**).

Though draw is a "must," it is best to remember at this point that retention is enhanced by parallelism. The more parallel a preparation can be and still have draw, the better. In other words, ideal draw is 5° to 10° convergence—no more, no less.

MARGINS

Dentally speaking, a margin is any surface junction between tooth and restorative material. The term applies to the finish line developed in the preparation of the tooth (cavosurface angle), as well as to the termination of the restoration that fits this finish line.

Margins are the most critical portion of any restoration for two reasons. First, they seal the breach in the tooth surface created by the preparation. It is the accuracy of fit of the margin that prevents leakage between the tooth and the restoration. The various cements that are available for securing such restorations in or on a tooth are slowly soluble in oral fluids. Thus if a casting is truly to "restore" a tooth, the entire marginal adaptation must be extremely accurate.

Secondly, the margin is critical because it is often placed at or beneath the crest of the gingival tissue surrounding the tooth. Any error in the marginal fit of the casting will leave a discrepancy in normal contour and cause surface roughness. This promotes collection of debris and bacteria, resulting in irritation of the adjacent tissue. The eventual result of such irritation is resorption of supporting bone. Poor-

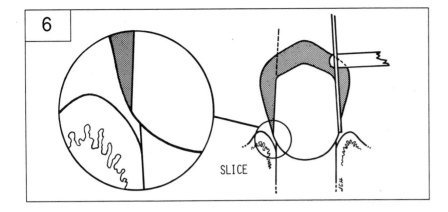

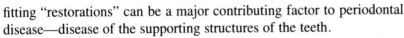

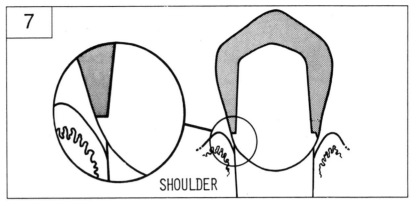

fitting "restorations" can be a major contributing factor to periodontal disease—disease of the supporting structures of the teeth.

The dentist deals with margins of amalgam, resins, and cast alloys. The laboratory technician deals primarily with margins made of cast alloys. The ability to develop accurate margins is the most important skill that the fixed restorative technician can have. A restoration with ideal contour, occlusion, and esthetics will have short-lived usefulness if marginal adaptation is poor.

TYPES OF MARGINS

There are four basic types of margins, defined in terms of their form or shape, and some modifications of these basic forms.

Slice or Feathered Margin

The name is descriptive as this type of margin is created by slicing off the side of a tooth to produce a flat surface (**Figure 6**). This produces a poor margin, because a distinct termination (cavosurface angle) depends on the contour of the tooth surface beyond the preparation. Often the resulting finish line is indefinite on certain areas of a preparation and is difficult to identify in impressions and subsequent dies. This may seriously jeopardize the creation of an accurate margin on the restoration. Also, because the amount of tooth structure removed at the marginal termination is minimal, the gold that replaces this tooth structure must be extremely thin. Owing to the improved quality of cast gold

alloys, cross-sectional thickness of gold in the margin of such castings is not as critical today. Even so, a thin gold margin may bend under mechanical or hydraulic stress during seating and/or cementation of the casting. This danger should be considered when such a pattern is being developed. A dentist often obtains this type of margin, desirable or not, especially when markedly curving or bell-shaped surfaces are prepared—such as posterior interproximal surfaces.

The advantages of the slice margin are ease of preparation and conservation of tooth structure. However "conserving" tooth structure to the extent of jeopardizing the restoration is false economy.

Shoulder Margin

This name is likewise descriptive, as this margin is a ledge or shoulder at the gingival portion of the preparation (**Figure 7**). From the standpoint of sealing the breached tooth, the shoulder, or "butt joint" as it is also termed, is the poorest margin used. This was particularly significant in the early days of dental castings, when compensating techniques were inadequate. Castings generally were too "small," as the early investments did not properly compensate for the shrinkage of the cast alloy. As a result crowns did not seat fully unless the castings were relieved on their internal surfaces. The net result was an open margin or gap between the shoulder on the prepared tooth and that of the casting (**Figure 8**). Erosion of the exposed cement opened direct access to deeper portions of the tooth (dentin), and decay soon invaded. Today casting techniques are essentially adequate, but if for any reason a shouldered crown is not fully seated the result is the same.

The shouldered margins are not as conservative as others. This is a

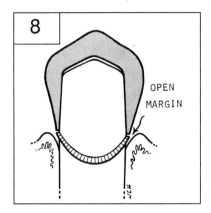

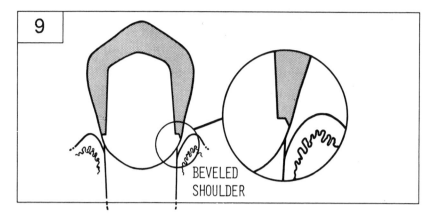

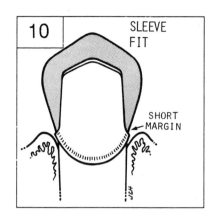

disadvantage insofar as conservation of tooth structure is concerned, but it is usually an advantage when fabrication is considered. This is particularly true if a faced crown or porcelain-fused-to-metal crown is to be made, because the greater thickness of these restorations is needed for strength and esthetics. Some dentists use a shoulder margin for all types of crowns. Though not recommended for cast crowns, it is the margin of choice for porcelain and acrylic jacket crowns. These materials are very weak in thin cross-section and require greater thickness at their margin to provide sufficient edge strength for resistance to fracture.

Beveled Shoulder Margin

This is a shoulder margin that is beveled along the cavosurface angle (**Figure 9**). This modification of the shoulder margin is preferred when forming a metal margin. To overcome the "open gap" discrepancy that occurs with the incompletely seated shoulder crown, the concept of "sleeve fit" or "stovepipe fit" was promoted. The premise here is that the crown, even if inadequately compensated in casting and too small to seat completely, will seal against the tooth at the marginal contact (**Figure 10**). This tapered-sleeve concept embodies the same principle as the stovepipe or metal flue joint—hence the names.

Chamfer Margin

The word *chamfer* means "bevel." As used in dentistry, it implies specifically a curved bevel (**Figure 11**). Varying degrees of chamfer may be produced, ranging from a near-slice margin to an almost-

shouldered margin. In general we speak of light, medium, and heavy chamfer. Thus the chamfered margin falls somewhere in the middle between the slice and shoulder margins. Properly executed, it overcomes the ultraconservative disadvantages of the slice margin without being as gross and difficult to prepare as the shoulder margin.

In actual practice the chamfer preparation may vary from the one extreme to the other—light to heavy—within a single preparation. Because of the varying contour of a tooth, certain chamfered areas or surfaces tend to become a slice whereas other areas on the same tooth tend to become shouldered. The skilled dentist overcomes these tendencies and, in fact, takes advantage of them to reduce some surfaces conservatively while reducing other surfaces more heavily, usually to allow space for greater dimension of restorative materials such as veneers. This versatility, together with the "tapered-sleeve fit" (which is best obtained with the chamfer) and the relative ease of preparation, makes the chamfered margin preferable for routine use by many dentists. In addition, a moderate to heavy chamfer produces better distribution of stress than other marginal configurations.

Summary

Various types of marginal preparations are used, for various reasons. The dentist's preference is based on conservation of tooth structure, the type of restoration, and ability to prepare various types of margins during clinical procedures. The dentist must also accurately record these margins by means of the impression. Regardless of type or character, the technician must recognize the margin and fabricate the restoration to fit that margin accurately.

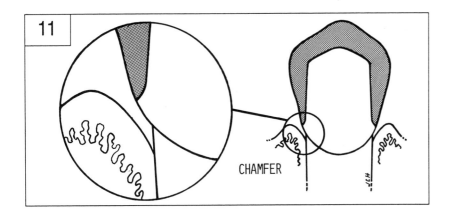

11

CHAMFER

REVIEW QUESTIONS

1. Define margin.
2. What are the two reasons why the margins are the most critical portion of any restoration?
3. What are the four basic types of margins?
4. Describe the four basic types of margins.
5. To what does the term *convenience form* refer?

SECTION 4

Impressions, Casts, and Dies

An *impression* is "an imprint or negative form of the teeth and/or other tissues of the oral cavity made in a plastic material that becomes relatively hard or set while in contact with these tissues. An impression is made in order to produce a positive form or cast of the recorded tissues. Impressions are classified according to the materials of which they are made (e.g., reversible and irreversible hydrocolloid impressions, modeling compound impressions, plaster impressions, wax impressions) and according to the structures included or recorded in the impression material (e.g., edentulous impression, dentulous impression) and according to its purpose (e.g., complete denture impression, partial denture impression, and inlay impression)." (Current Clinical Dental Terminology)

An *impression tray* is "a receptacle or device that is used to carry the impression material to the mouth, to confine the material in apposition to the surface to be recorded, and to control the impression material while it sets to form the impression." (CCDT)

A *cast* is defined as "a positive likeness of some desired form." (CCDT) For our purposes a cast is a positive reproduction of a dental arch or a portion of a dental arch.

A *die* is "the positive reproduction of the form of a prepared tooth in any suitable hard substance usually in metal or specially prepared (improved) artificial stone." (CCDT) By definition a die is a cast of a single prepared tooth, that is, a tooth prepared by the dentist to receive an inlay or crown.

IMPRESSION MATERIALS

Impression materials are used to register or record the form and the relationship of the teeth and soft tissues of the oral cavity. There are three types of impression materials: rigid, thermoplastic, and elastic. All exhibit flow in their "working" state, and then by chemical or physical action they set to either a rigid or a resilient state.

Rigid Materials

Impression plaster and metallic oxide impression pastes are the most commonly used rigid impression materials. They set, by chemical reaction, to a solid consistency. Impression plaster is basically plaster of paris to which modifiers have been added to control its properties. Accelerators are added to speed setting time, and some brands of plaster contain potato starch to make the impression soluble in hot water, to facilitate recovery of the cast. In restorative procedures the use of impression plaster is usually restricted to registering relationships of castings that must be splinted or combined to form a bridge. Interocclusal relationships may be recorded in plaster.

A separating medium such as varnish, petroleum jelly, soap, or similar commercial preparations must be applied to plaster impressions before a cast is poured. Otherwise the gypsum cast material bonds to the impression plaster, making separation impossible and the cast unusable. Plaster is the only impression material that requires the use of a separating medium.

Metallic oxide impression pastes are often used to make impressions of edentulous arches. In fixed restorative techniques these impression pastes are used like impression plaster to record the relationships of crowns to one another and to the opposing arch. They are also used to record jaw relationships, such as centric occlusion, centric relation, and protrusive and lateral interocclusal records.

Thermoplastic Materials

Thermoplastic impression materials become soft on heating and harden to a rigid consistency when cooled. Impression compounds (modeling plastic) and impression waxes are examples. Impression compounds have been used for recording individually prepared teeth. Impression waxes are not widely used in fixed restorative techniques, but similar waxes are used to record the relationships of crowns to adjacent structures and to the opposing arch. Reversible hydrocolloid could be classified as a thermoplastic material, but it is usually included with the elastic impression materials.

Elastic Materials

Elastic impression materials flow when first prepared but set in the mouth to an elastic state. Accordingly they offer the distinct advantage of "flexing" to permit removal from undercuts. Only elastic materials can provide a truly accurate duplication of the dental arches. They return to their original shape after being distorted during removal from the mouth. Except for reversible hydrocolloid, which is soft when heated and sets to an elastic state when chilled, elastic impression materials set by chemical reaction. Currently used elastic impression materials are reversible hydrocolloids (agar), irreversible hydrocolloid (alginate), and rubber-base materials (polysulfides, condensation and addition reaction silicones, and polyethers). All remain elastic after setting. Common-usage terminology for impressions made with these materials is as follows:

Hydrocolloid Materials
Reversible: hydrocolloid impression
Irreversible: alginate impression

Rubber-base Materials
Polysulfide rubber: rubber impression
Condensation silicone: regular silicone impression
Addition silicone: polyvinylsiloaxane impression
Polyether: polyether impression

Storage is not as great a problem for the rubber-base impression materials as it is for hydrocolloid, both reversible and irreversible. Care must be exercised with all types of impressions, particularly those made of an elastic material, as distortion may occur if the impression materials are mishandled. Elastic materials must be protected from excessive changes in temperature. Hydrocolloid and alginate impressions are very sensitive to the loss or absorption of water; they must be carefully stored in a humidor to maintain 100 percent humidity. Rubber-base materials are subject to flow under load and must therefore be handled and stored without placing any continued force on the impression. All elastic impression materials are placed in rigid containers, but even so the impression may be deformed if not stored and handled correctly.

Summary

Compound and rubber impression materials are sometimes used in copper band containers to record the individual tooth. Rubber-base materials and hydrocolloid are used for tray impressions involving one or more prepared teeth. Alginate, plaster, wax, and metallic oxide pastes are used for relationship and opposing arch impressions. Alginate is universally used for study cast impressions.

IMPRESSION TRAYS

An impression tray is a container used to hold impression material in apposition to the tissues being recorded. Impression trays may be purchased (stock trays) or custom-made (custom tray) for an individual patient.

There are many types of stock trays available from dental manufacturers. The form of the tray depends in part on the material to be used in

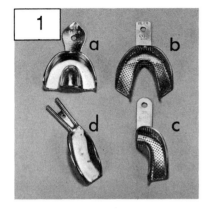

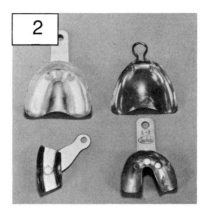

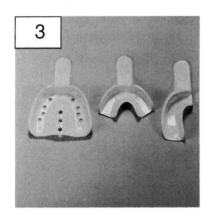

the tray: modeling compound, plaster, alginate, and so forth. Trays designed to be used with alginate have provisions—either perforations or mechanical undercuts—for mechanically retaining the impression material. Trays for plaster and compound impressions have no retentive devices. Trays designed for use with hydrocolloid have tubes attached that permit the tray to be cooled by circulating water. Stock trays are made of metal or resin and may be reused after sterilization. Trays used with elastic impression materials must be rigid.

Stock trays designed for use with hydrocolloid materials are retentive and are shown in **Figure** 1. Examples **a**, **b**, and **c** are used with irreversible alginate; **d** is a water-cooled tray designed for use with reversible hydrocolloid. Impression compound and plaster are used in the trays shown in **Figure 2**. These trays have no retentive mechanism. Rigid trays made of resin are shown in **Figure 3**. These trays are used to make impressions with rubber-base impression materials and must be

coated with special adhesives to retain the particular type of material.

Custom trays are made of resin and used for one individual, then discarded. The technique for constructing them is illustrated later in this section.

MATERIALS FOR CASTS AND DIES

The materials used to make dies and casts from dental impressions are plaster, stone, casting investment, electrodeposited silver and copper, low-fusing alloys, resins, and special die materials. The selection of a specific material is determined by the particular impression material used and by the purpose for which the die or cast is to be used.

Certain die or cast materials cannot be used with some impression materials, either because of their incompatibility or because of specific technical problems. The purpose for which a cast or die is made determines which material is used. The amount of time necessary to construct a particular die, and the materials that must be manipulated on the cast or die, are other factors to be considered in the selection of proper materials.

Gypsum products—plaster, dental stone, and die stone—are most commonly used to make casts and dies from dental impressions. Plaster and dental stone may be used for study casts. Casts of dental stone are also used for opposing arch casts and as the base portion of casts containing removable dies. Die stones are a specifically prepared gypsum product used for dies. They may also be used for casts. The primary advantage of the die stones is their hardness and resistance to abrasion during the waxing procedure.

All gypsum products, especially die stones, should be carefully handled according to the manufacturer's directions. The specified water/powder ratio and spatulation time should be followed. Most gypsum products may be safely separated from the impression within an hour after pouring. For safe strength a die or cast should set for 24 hours before being used. The use of stone dies is described in detail in later sections.

Some technicians and dentists use copper or silver to electroplate impressions made of impression compound or rubber-base materials. After a thin layer of metal is deposited, the impression is poured in die stone. The advantages of electroplating are the accuracy, strength, and abrasion resistance of the die surface that is produced. The disadvantage is the time involved and the cost of the equipment.

The advent of accurate and easy-to-use impression and die materials has made the development of castings by direct techniques essentially obsolete. Today virtually all castings are made indirectly on dies developed from elastic impression materials.

IMPRESSION TECHNIQUES FOR FIXED RESTORATIVE PROCEDURES

A dental laboratory technician competent in fixed restorative techniques must be able to handle four types of impressions: (1) impressions for study casts, (2) impressions of an individual tooth preparation, (3) transfer impressions used to establish the relationship of dies of prepared teeth to one another and to adjacent structures, and (4) tray impressions of one or more prepared teeth and their adjacent structures.

Preoperative or *study casts* are routinely made from alginate impressions. *Opposing casts*—casts of the arch that opposes the one in which restorations are being developed—are also usually made from alginate impressions.

In fixed restorative techniques, casts that contain dies on which restorations are to be made are referred to as *working casts*. An impression of the entire dental arch, or a portion thereof, is categorically referred to as a *tray impression*. These impressions are made with an elastic material (hydrocolloid or one of the rubber-base materials).

Impressions of individual teeth are made in copper bands (also called tubes) and are referred to as *band* or *tube impressions*. Bands for these impressions are available in different sizes; the dentist shapes the band to fit the prepared tooth. A copper tube is actually a miniature impression tray. Most band or tube impressions are made with modeling plastic (impression compound) or of one of the rubber-base impression materials. A band impression records only the prepared tooth—no adjacent structures.

The function of a *transfer impression* is to reproduce the exact relationship of one or more prepared teeth to each other and to adjacent structures in the same dental arch. When a tray impression is used to register the prepared tooth or teeth, all necessary intra-arch relationships are recorded. But when band impressions are used, no relationships are recorded. By some means the necessary relationships must be "transferred" from the mouth to the laboratory such that an individual die may be incorporated into a working cast in proper relation to other prepared teeth and/or adjacent structures. This is the purpose of a transfer impression. The working cast that is developed from such an impression is termed a *transfer cast*. Accuracy in making and handling transfer casts is essential for successful development of many restorations—especially large, multiabutment bridges.

The term *transfer* comes from the original procedure for constructing fixed bridges, in which the retainer patterns were developed by the direct or direct-indirect waxing technique. The resulting cast gold retainers were then seated on their respective abutment teeth, and an impression (usually plaster) was made over them. The castings were taken from the mouth, seated in the impression, and a cast poured that established the same positional relationship between the retainers as was present in the mouth. Thus the castings were "transferred" from the mouth to a cast in accurate relationship.

Instead of using completed retainers, many dentists use *copings* to make transfer impressions and casts. A coping is a "thin metal covering or cap over the prepared tooth." (CCDT) The primary purposes of transfer copings are to permit the accurate seating of a die in a transfer impression and to check the accuracy of a die. When a coping is used, it is seated on the prepared tooth and checked to see that it fits accurately at all points. If the coping was made to fit the die accurately and inspection shows that it accurately fits the tooth, the accuracy of the die is verified. A transfer impression, usually in plaster, is then made. The impression is removed from the mouth, and the transfer copings are removed from the prepared teeth. The transfer copings are then placed in the impression with their respective dies, and a cast is poured. This *coping transfer impression* provides a cast with the prepared teeth in accurate relationship to one another.

The final portions of this section demonstrate the pouring of impressions for preoperative study casts and the development of custom trays. The development of dies and working casts is covered in later sections.

POURING IMPRESSIONS FOR STUDY CASTS

Most study and opposing casts are made from alginate impressions. Study casts are commonly made before any restorative treatment is initiated. They are used to help the dentist plan proper treatment and

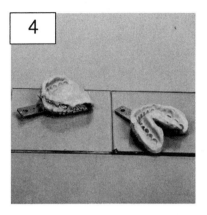 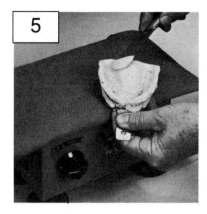 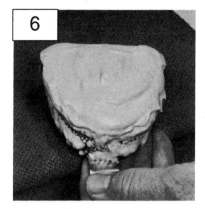 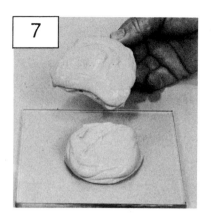

to explain the plan to the patient. Opposing casts, made in a similar manner, are used to help produce the correct occlusion in dental restorations.

The following procedures for producing casts from alginate impressions are basic to all phases of dental laboratory technology. Alginate impressions should be poured immediately after they are made, particularly if a dental appliance is to be made on the resulting cast. If delay is required the impressions should be stored in a humidor to maintain 100 percent humidity.

Figure 4   The impressions are prepared for pouring by washing away all the saliva that may remain in the impression. Saliva is easily removed by rinsing the impression with a slurry of water and plaster or dental stone. Excess water should be removed by shaking the impression; the surface should be damp, not dry.

Figure 5   A thick, creamy mix of dental stone is made by using the proper water/powder proportion. Ideally the mix should be mechanically spatulated under vacuum. The next best procedure is mechanical spatulation on a vibrator. Hand spatulation should be accomplished by "rubbing" the mix against the walls of the mixing bowl until completely smooth and then vibrating thoroughly. The pour is made by placing a small amount of the mix in one corner of the impression, placing it on a vibrator, and tipping it so the mix flows into the recesses within the impression.

Figure 6   Stone mix is added in increments to avoid trapping air bubbles, and the impression is progressively filled to the level of the tray flanges.

At this point one of three approaches may be taken to develop the base of the cast. First, the tray can be placed on its base so that it is not supported by alginate material that extends beyond the tray. Additional stone may be "stacked" to form an adequate base dimension—about one-half inch. With a properly thick mix of stone this is easy to do for upper impressions. However, with lower impressions something must be done to block out the tongue space if this approach is used. This can be easily done with a folded wet paper towel.

A second approach is to pour the impression up to flange height and let this stone set with the tray properly supported on the lab bench or suspended horizontally by its handle. Additional stone can subsequently be added to form an adequate base by inverting the cast onto a quantity of stone on a glass or plastic slab (see **Figure 7**). If the first pour has dried, its base should be rewetted before it is inverted. Again, an adequately thick mix of stone that will stack is imperative. The borders of the base and tongue-space areas of lower casts can then be shaped and smoothed. This is the most accurate method of pouring casts but obviously has the disadvantage of requiring more time to complete two mixes and pours.

A third approach is to pour the impression to flange height with a mix of stone that stacks well (one should be able to invert the mixing bowl for several seconds without the stone running or slumping). Place an appropriate quantity of stone (about $\frac{1}{2}$ inch thick) on a slab. Then directly, or after waiting for some setting to occur (depending on consistency of stone), invert the impression onto the stone (**Figure 8**). Although this is the most commonly used technique, it is dangerous in that the stone in the impression may slump when the impression is inverted and thus result in a distorted cast. This technique is only safe

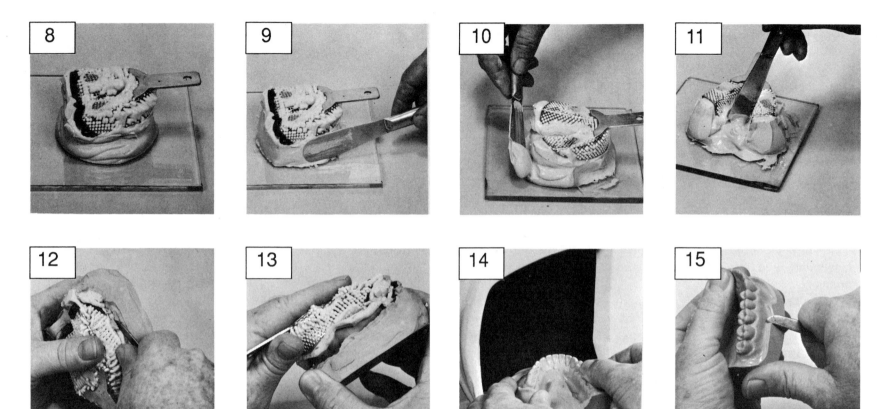

when the consistency of the mix and timing of the inversions are properly controlled.

Figure 9   The stone may be smoothed around the impression. *Avoid locking the impression tray into the cast.* Note that the stone is of a consistency that "stands" by itself and does not flow on the slab. Pouring impressions properly requires a firm mix of stone.

Figures 10 and 11   The same procedures are followed with a mandibular impression. The stone should not be allowed to build up on the lingual portion of the impression, as this will lock the impression tray into the cast. A plaster spatula is used to smooth away any excess from the tongue space to a level even with the bottom of the impression tray.

Figures 12 and 13   The stone is allowed to set for a minimum of 30

minutes. Any stone that lies above the edge of the impression tray is carefully trimmed away. The impression is then removed from the cast in the direction of the long axis of the anterior teeth, to avoid breakage.

Figure 14   The cast is trimmed on a model trimmer. The anatomic landmarks on the cast should be preserved. To prevent adherence of powder from the slurry water, casts should be thoroughly wet or dipped in detergent solution *before* trimming.

Figure 15   Any excess stone is removed from the land area with a knife.

Figures 16 and 17   The occlusal surfaces of the teeth are carefully inspected and any blebs (positive or raised defects) are removed. Note that the bases of the maxillary and mandibular casts are essentially

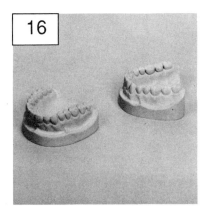
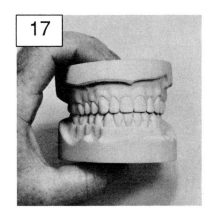
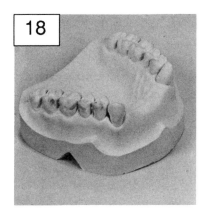
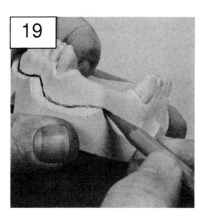

parallel when the casts are occluded. This usually occurs naturally when impressions are poured with a thick mix of stone and the top of the impression tray is kept level when inverted. Some trimming of the bases may be necessary.

CUSTOM TRAYS

Many dentists make tray impressions for fixed restorations in custom trays. Such trays offer the potential advantage of a uniform layer of impression material around the prepared teeth, making the impressions more accurate. Occasionally custom impression trays are made for only a portion of the arch.

One of the uses of study casts is to produce custom impression trays. The study casts are commonly used for other purposes before the custom tray is made, but may be used exclusively for the production of the custom tray. Custom trays are ordinarily made of modified methyl methacrylate resins, which, when mixed, are dead soft, which permits them to be accurately adapted.

The following technique is one accepted method for making custom trays.

Figure 18   The cast is ready for the construction of a custom tray.

Figure 19   The outline for the tray is drawn on the cast. This should be done by the dentist.

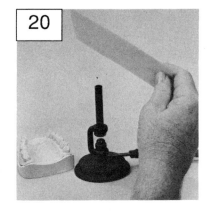
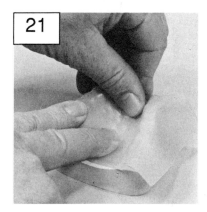

Figure 20   A wax spacer is used to provide room for the impression material within the tray. The spacer, or "shim," is made of baseplate wax, which is warmed before adaptation.

Figure 21   The baseplate wax is adapted uniformly on all surfaces of the cast. The dentist should prescribe the number of layers of baseplate wax to be used to form the shim. Two layers are normally used.

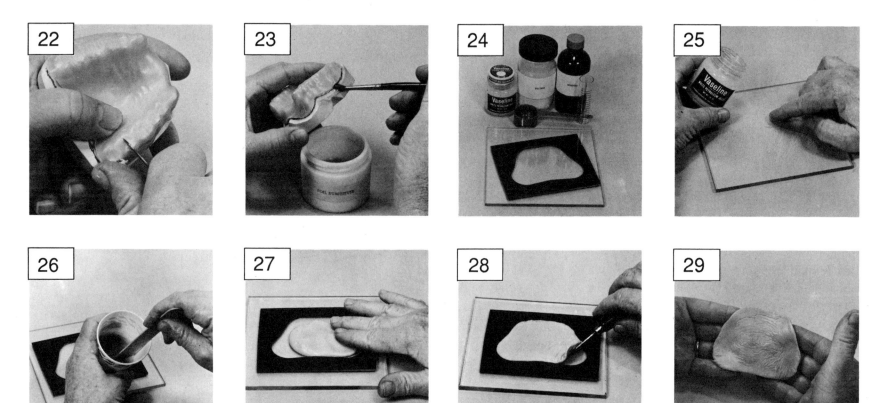

Figure 22　The baseplate wax is then trimmed to the outline for the tray. "Stops" may be provided by cutting holes in the wax spacer over three or four teeth *not* involved in the fixed restorative procedures. These stops should be spaced about the arch to provide a stable index for proper positioning of the tray.

Figure 23　Tinfoil substitute is applied to the exposed surfaces of the cast and over the wax shim if desired. Note how the shim has been trimmed to the outline for the tray.

Figure 24　The materials required for making trays are a glass plate, a template, petroleum jelly, and the monomer and polymer of the resin tray material.

Figure 25　Petroleum jelly is applied to the glass, and the template is positioned.

Figure 26　The tray material is mixed according to the manufacturer's instructions. This is commonly done in a paper cup, using a tongue blade as a spatula.

Figure 27　The tray material is placed in the template and is patted until a sheet of uniform thickness is formed. Rollers are also used to form the wafer.

Figure 28　The tray material is sticky when first mixed but soon becomes easy to handle. When the material becomes doughy and non-sticky, it is removed from the template by first lifting one corner with an instrument. A little petroleum jelly will facilitate handling these materials.

Figure 29　The sheet of tray material is lifted free of the template.

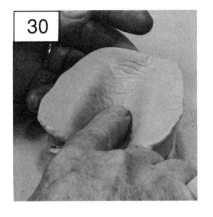
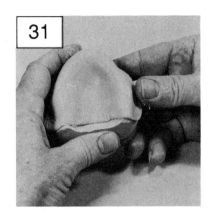
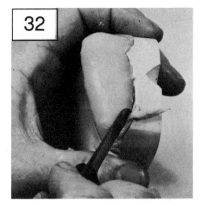
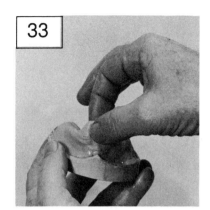

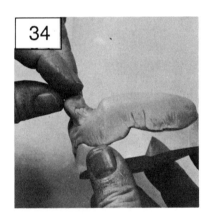
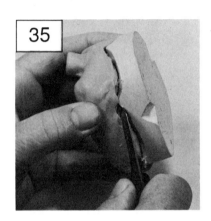
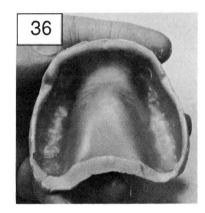
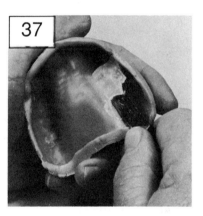

Figure 30 The tray material is centered on the cast over the wax spacer.

Figure 31 The palate is formed first. Then the borders of the tray are adapted, using light pressure so as not to cause thin spots in the wafer.

Figure 32 Excess tray material is trimmed from the cast with a knife.

Figure 33 Some excess material is molded into a handle and is attached to the tray by first moistening the area with monomer.

Figure 34 The handle is shaped into the desired form. Most dentists prefer a handle that is small and easy to grasp and is positioned to offer the least interference with the lip and opposing teeth.

Figure 35 The cast is set aside until the resin material sets. Heat will be given off during the reaction, which somewhat softens the wax. When the tray begins to cool, it may be removed from the cast. The wax will still be somewhat soft.

Figure 36 The tray as it appears after removal from the cast.

Figure 37 The wax spacer is removed from the tray. Complete removal of the wax may be ensured by stoning or abrading the surface with a large bur. Wax removal can be facilitated by chilling the wax in cold water after the tray has cured. However, the simplest means of ensuring complete wax removal is to prevent its contact with the tray by placing a piece of cellophane or polyethelene over the wax shim before adapting the resin.

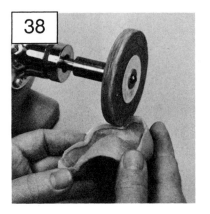 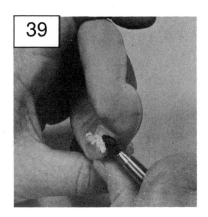 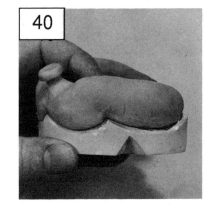 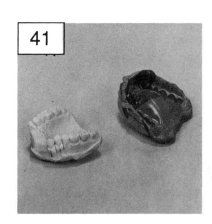

Figure 38   The excess tray material is removed with a coarse stone on a lathe. The borders are trimmed to the predetermined outline as identified by the ridge left by the edge of the wax spacer.

Figure 39   The handle may be improved by trimming with suitable instruments.

Figure 40   The tray is complete and ready for delivery.

Another popular technique for placement of the resin material is the "sprinkle method." This involves applying alternate increments of monomer and polymer until desired thickness and extension are established. Establishing a tray of uniform thickness is difficult with this technique.

Figure 41   A rubber impression has been made in the tray. The cast, containing removable dies, is also shown. The technique for making this type of cast is presented in Section 5.

REVIEW QUESTIONS

1. Define impression, cast, and die.
2. Name two rigid impression materials and their uses.
3. Name two groups of elastic impression materials and, for each material, describe the precautions to be observed when storing the impression.
4. Name some materials most commonly used for the construction of dies.
5. Name the four types of impressions that a competent fixed restorative technician must be able to handle.
6. What is the advantage of using a custom tray for an impression?

SECTION 5

Developing Working Casts from Tray Impressions

The dentist uses tray impressions for fixed restorative techniques in order to record the prepared teeth, adjacent teeth, and associated structures. Tray impressions are used routinely for onlay and crown restorations. Impressions for extensive fixed restorations require great skill, as all preparations must be completely and accurately recorded. This is particularly difficult with full crown preparations that have extensive subgingival margins.

Tray impressions may be made of hydrocolloid (**Figure 1**), rubber impression material (**Figure 2**), silicone impression material (**Figure 3**), or polyether impression material. The techniques for handling these impression materials are basically the same. However, hydrocolloid impressions should be poured immediately or stored during any waiting period in 100 percent humidity (in a humidor) to prevent distortion. Rubber-base impressions are relatively distortion-free if stored dry at a reasonable temperature for short periods (2 to 6 hours). These materials must be stored so that they are fully supported by the tray and are not subjected to any load. For example, material extending beyond the end of a tray will slowly deform if the tray is placed on the bench such that it rests on the impression.

There are many methods of pouring tray impressions and obtaining casts suitable for the construction of restorations. Several techniques are described in this section most of which result in a cast that has removable dies.

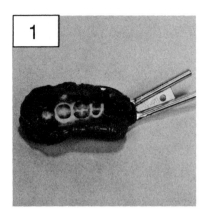
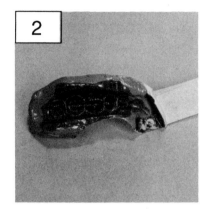
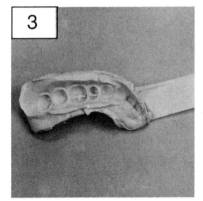
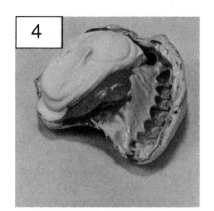

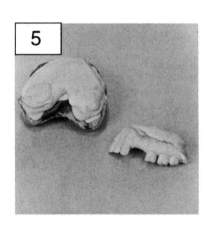
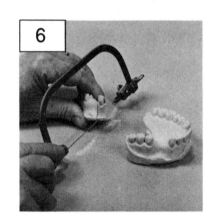
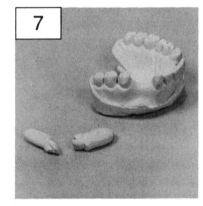
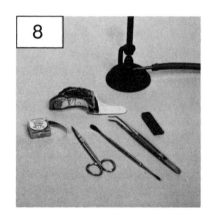

SOLID CAST AND INDIVIDUAL DIES

A simple method of obtaining a working cast from an elastic impression is to make two pours. The first is used to make a cast with individual dies; the second produces a cast used for establishing relationships.

Figure 4   The section of the impression containing the prepared teeth is poured with die stone. The base is poured to sufficient thickness so that the cast may be grasped and removed from the impression when the die stone sets.

Figure 5   After the first pour has set and been removed, the entire impression is poured with die stone.

Figure 6   The first cast is sectioned with a fine-bladed saw to provide an individual die of each prepared tooth. Each die will have an adequate length of stone root form to provide a handle.

The second cast is removed from the impression and trimmed.

Figure 7   The individual dies are prepared for waxing as described in Section 7. The marginal areas about the prepared teeth on the second cast (full arch) are exposed by trimming excess stone with a knife or bur.

If necessary the solid cast may be trimmed, preferably with a knife. Precautions must be taken when any cast containing dies of prepared teeth is trimmed on a model trimmer. The dies must be protected from

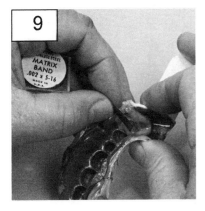 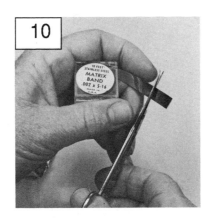 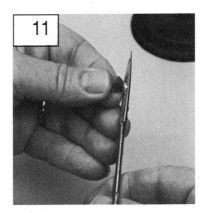 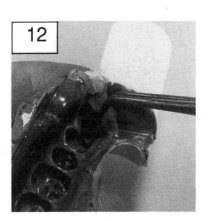

excessive water as their surface may become etched by the washing effect, with consequent inaccuracies. Also, stone dust particles from the slurry water tend to adhere to the surface of the dies. This residue must be thoroughly removed before any waxing is done; otherwise the dust will become incorporated in the wax pattern and contaminate the mold and subsequent casting.

The result of this technique is a solid cast that maintains the relationship between prepared and unprepared teeth, and separate individual dies of the prepared teeth. During construction the patterns are transferred between dies and cast. The solid cast is used to establish relationships between adjacent and opposing structures; then the individual dies are used to perfect the margins.

This technique has some disadvantages: distortion may occur when transferring wax patterns between die and cast; accurate seating of the castings on the cast may be awkward and uncertain; and it is not suitable for extensive restorations, particularly when a large bridge framework must be waxed and cast in one piece. The technique is most suitable for small fixed bridges or individual restorations.

WORKING CASTS WITH REMOVABLE DIES FROM TRAY IMPRESSIONS

Most dental laboratory technicians prefer working with a cast that contains removable dies. In this case only one die is involved in establishing a given pattern. Thus there is no necessity for transferring wax patterns from one die to another. The technique for making a cast with

removable dies is a little more complex than the one just described. However, the time saved and accuracy achieved in subsequent steps more than make up for the extra effort.

There are several techniques for making a working cast with removable dies. Three basic types are described in this section: (1) the stripping technique, (2) the double pour section technique, and (3) the precision dowel pin and die technique.

STRIPPING TECHNIQUE

The stripping technique may be used for both rubber-base and reversible hydrocolloid impressions. Single or double strips can be used for preparing removable dies.

Stripping the Rubber-base Impression

Figure 8 Instruments and materials required to strip a rubber-base impression: a sharp pair of scissors, a wax spatula, a pair of tweezers, utility wax, .002-inch steel matrix band material, and a Bunsen burner. The matrix material should be 5/16 wide, or 7/16 inches trimmed to about 5/16 inches wide.

Figure 9 The approximate length and contour of a strip of matrix material required to bridge the space between the facial and lingual surfaces of the impression is judged.

Figures 10 and 11 A length is cut from the matrix band material and is

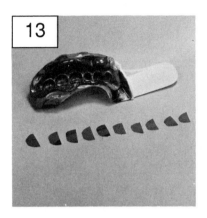

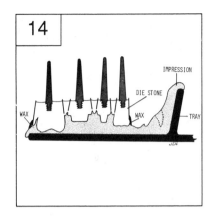

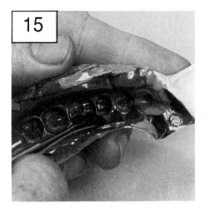

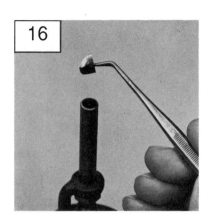

contoured, by trial and error, to fit between the sides of the impression.

Figure 12 The contoured piece of matrix material is tried in place. It should be just shy of the sides of the impression and be approximately 0.5 millimeter short of contacting the gingival margins in the impression.

Figure 13 In the double stripping technique two pieces of matrix band material are required for each movable die. This impression contains three prepared teeth. Ordinarily the unprepared teeth adjacent to each prepared tooth are also made removable; this permits easier removal of the die of the prepared tooth and permits the technician to establish proximal contact areas more accurately. Hence in this impression five removable dies are required, and ten strips are cut. Note that the pieces of matrix material have been contoured to fit each interproximal space and have been arranged in proper sequence.

In the single stripping technique, one strip instead of two is cut for each interproximal space; thus in this example, with five removable dies, six strips are prepared instead of ten.

Figure 14 This cross section shows the proper position of the metal strips in the impression for the double strip technique. Note that the pieces of strip material for each die diverge occlusally and converge apically. Two strips of metal material have been placed for each die to assure occlusal divergence of each die form. Note also that the strip material does not touch the impression in the area of the gingival margins of the prepared tooth. The two end pieces of the strip material are sealed to the impression with wax, to form a dam that walls off the segment of the impression to be poured with the die stone.

When single strips are used, only one interproximal strip is placed between each removable die. Each interproximal strip except the two end strips, which diverge occlusally, should be parallel to the long axis of the die and dowel pin. The sides of each removable die may have to be tapered later with a bur so that each die can be removed and reseated independently of each adjacent die.

Figure 15 A rib of utility wax is flowed on both the facial and lingual walls of the rubber impression opposite each interproximal area to be stripped. Care must be exercised to prevent the wax from flowing into the tooth impression or onto a prepared tooth margin.

Figure 16 The appropriate piece of matrix material is gently warmed in the Bunsen burner flame.

Figure 17 The warm matrix strips are then carefully positioned and held in place until the wax cools.

Figure 18 The strips for each die are placed so that they diverge occlusally in relation to the impression; or, said another way, they converge slightly toward one another at their exposed edges. The resulting die will be narrower mesiodistally at its apical end than at the gingival margin level (see **Figure 14**). This is essential, to ensure that the dies can be removed from the cast. The dies will be moved occlusally to remove them from the cast.

Figure 19 The appropriate pieces of matrix material have been placed for the first four teeth that are to become removable dies. Only the two strips for the second molar remain to be placed.

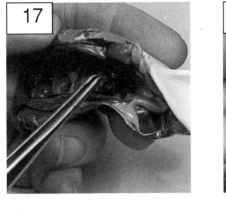
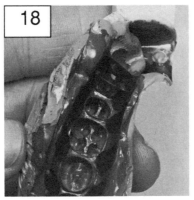
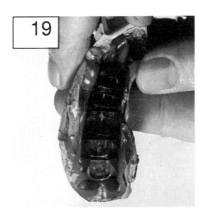
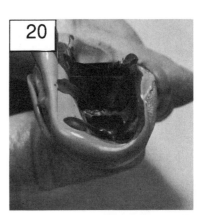

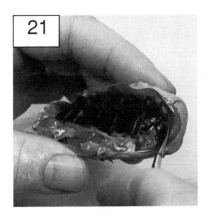
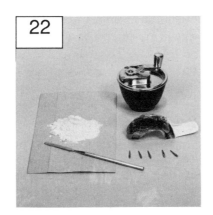
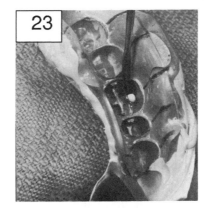
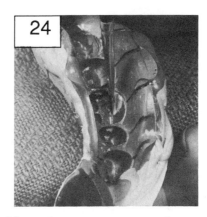

Figure 20 Utmost care must be taken to ensure that the occlusal edge of the strips does not touch the impression material that records the gingival margin of the prepared tooth. (This is also illustrated in **Figure 55**.)

Figure 21 The last pieces of matrix material are placed in position. The matrix material on either end of the impression (forming the external surface of the die of the unprepared tooth at each end) is sealed to provide a dam that will confine the die stone. Additional wax may be added in the angles between the strips and the impression to ensure stability.

Figure 22 One of the improved die stones is used to pour this segment of the impression. It is proportioned according to the manufacturer's directions. The powder is added to the water in the mixing bowl and hand-spatulated until thoroughly wetted. The mix is completed by mechanical spatulation—preferably under vacuum—to produce a denser stone mix. Note that five dowel pins, one for each removable die, have been set aside on the bench ready for immediate placement.

Figures 23 and 24 The die stone is placed in small increments on one wall of the tooth surface, using either an instrument (**Figure 23**) or a brush (**Figure 24**). (To facilitate showing the proper position of the instruments in relation to the impression, the impressions shown in these illustrations are not stripped.)

Figure 25 The impression is held on a vibrator, causing the stone to flow into the remote recesses of the occlusal surface. Slight teasing and wiping with a brush while vibrating may be desirable, to ensure that no air is trapped in a remote angle of the impression. As soon as the tooth surface is covered, a slightly larger instrument may be used, and larger increments of stone are progressively added. One quickly learns to keep the "pour" progressing by adding an increment of stone in a

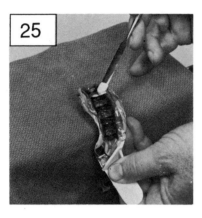 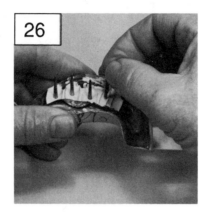 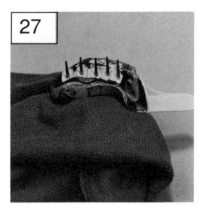 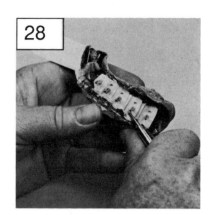

second die while the first is being vibrated, and so forth, as the working time for some of the die stones is limited. Where impression material is thin, as sometimes occurs in a gingival crevice, die stone should be placed on each side, so that equal pressure is maintained on the thin material and it is not pushed to one side or the other, causing the die to become distorted.

Figure 26 Each die is filled as previously described until the die stone is about 1 millimeter below the edge of the matrix strips. A tapered dowel pin is then quickly positioned in each die. The pin is placed in the center of the die with a slight pumping motion to the depth that just covers all the knurled end, leaving the shoulder of the pin flush with the stone surface. When all dowel pins are seated, they should be aligned so that they are parallel and will permit ready withdrawal of the dies individually or as a group. Whether parallel with each other or not, the dowel pins must be aligned within the "path of draw" of the dies as dictated by the position of the matrix separating strips.

Figure 27 The impression is set aside and stabilized so that the dowel pins do not move while the die stone is setting.

Figure 28 After the die stone has set, dimples or slots may be made in the base of each die to less than one-half the depth of a number 6 or 8 round bur. This is an optional step that provides an additional index to ensure accurate position of the die.

Figure 29 When stripping impressions for fixed bridges, care must be taken to provide for accurate duplication of the edentulous ridge be-

tween the abutment teeth. The strips adjacent to the edentulous ridge should be placed as close to the abutment margins as is safe (0.5 millimeter). They should be sealed at their occlusal edge (the deep surface of the impression) just like other "terminal" strips. It is important to use a minimum of wax against the surface of the edentulous ridge, as heavier application will cause a defect in the cast. After the dies are poured and have set, but before the base is poured, the wax along the occlusal margin of the strips adjacent to the edentulous area may be removed. This eliminates any defect in the edentulous ridge of the cast. (Many technicians prefer that the edentulous ridge area be made as a removable die when tissue-contacting pontics are being fabricated. In that case it is not necessary to seal the end strips in the edentulous space as done for each "terminal" end strip.)

Before the base is poured, any die stone that may have spilled or leaked into the impression and occlusal edge of the strips or into the adjacent unstripped teeth or edentulous ridge areas should be flicked out with a suitable instrument.

Figure 30 The impression may be surrounded with a strip of boxing wax to facilitate pouring the base.

Figure 31 A suitable separating medium is applied to the exposed stone surfaces. This should be a commercial gypsum separator, soap, or sodium silicate. Thick separating media such as petroleum jelly or waxes must not be used, as they destroy the positive seating of the die in the base.

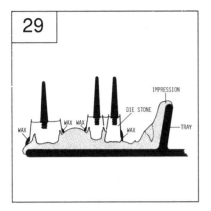
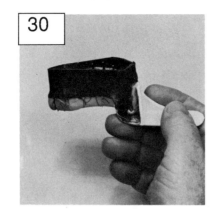
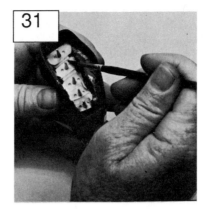
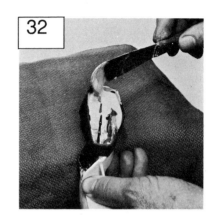

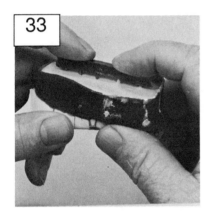
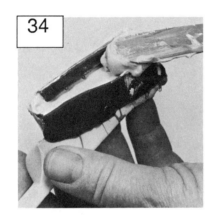
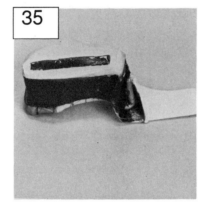
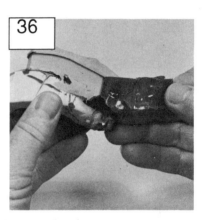

Figure 32 The base pour of the impression is made with regular dental stone. Care should be taken that air is not trapped in the remaining tooth impressions, especially the teeth immediately adjacent to any prepared teeth. The base must have sufficient thickness for strength, but the ends of the dowel pins must never be completely covered with stone.

Figure 33 If the cast is to be mounted on an articulator, it is desirable to leave the base pour ⅛ inch below the end of the dowel pins. If the cast is not to be mounted, it is best to carry the base slightly above the level of the pins. Then the stone immediately over the end of the dowel pins is wiped away with a fingertip or instrument. As illustrated in this photograph another means of accomplishing this neatly is to press a rope of utility wax lightly onto the tips of the dowel pins before the base pour is completed.

Figures 34 and 35 The base pour is finished flush with the surface of the rope of utility wax and is allowed to set.

Figure 36 The boxing wax is removed from the cast and impression.

Figure 37 The cast is separated from the impression by pulling them apart. Even though this removal may require some force, there is usually little danger of breakage if the two are pulled straight apart and the stone has completely set (18 to 24 hours after pouring is desirable). However, if the dies are long and thin (particularly mandibular incisors), breakage is possible. In such situations it may be best to section the impression tray with a separating disc and peel the rubber from the cast.

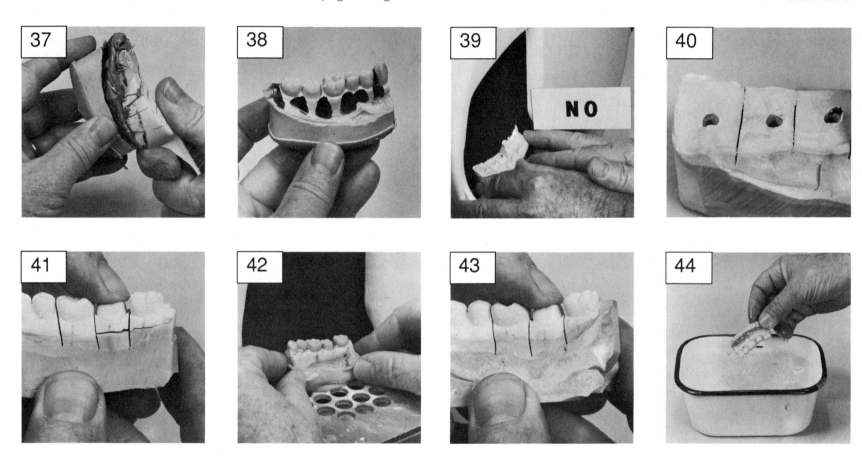

Figure 38 The cast is shown immediately after recovery from the impression. Gross trimming of the cast should be unnecessary, as the impression was boxed before pouring. Preferably, any necessary trimming should be done with a knife. However, if reduction on a model trimmer is required, it should be done *before* the dies and strips and the wax that seals them are removed from the cast. All trimming should be done dry, to avoid dissolution or washing of the die surface.

Figure 39 *Never trim a working cast on a model trimmer with the dies removed!*

Figures 40 and 41 This demonstrates what happens when a cast is trimmed with the dies removed. Stone dust from the air or from the slurry water accumulates on the surface of the die seat and in the dowel pin holes and is virtually impossible to remove. The debris in the dowel

pin holes prevents the die from completely reseating, thus destroying the accurate relationship between die and base. It is especially crucial to avoid this problem in working casts on which bridges or splints are to be made.

Figure 42 Contouring on a model trimmer must be accomplished with dies in place.

Figure 43 When the cast is trimmed with dies sealed in position, the accuracy of their seating is not disturbed. Note the perfect juncture between dies and base.

Figure 44 Should it be necessary to reduce a working cast with a "wet" model trimmer, the adherence of the slurry can be minimized if the cast is dipped in a solution of detergent before trimming.

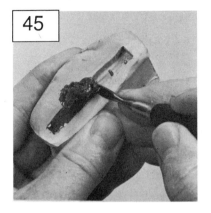

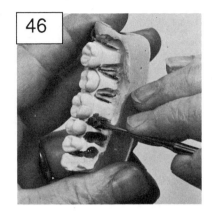

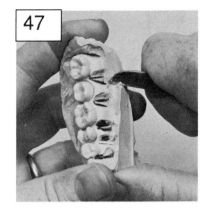

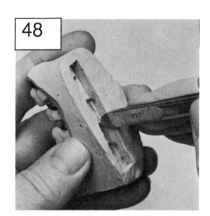

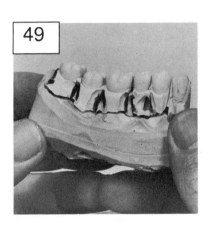

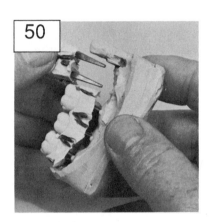

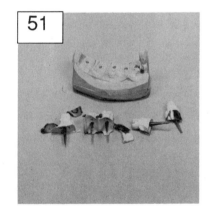

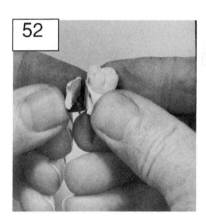

Figures 45 and 46 Wax is removed from the trough in the base of the cast and from between the dies. Having the tips of the dowel pins within a trough in the base of the cast permits the dies to remain completely seated when the cast is set on the bench top.

Figure 47 Any sharp or rough margins of stone remaining are removed with a knife. Be careful not to scar any of the dies.

Figure 48 The dies are removed from the impression by pushing or gently tapping the end of each dowel pin with an instrument such as the handle of a knife or plaster spatula.

Figure 49 The dies have been loosened from the base.

Figure 50 Once loosened, the dies should be removed by hand.

Figure 51 The dies, strips, and interseptal pieces of stone immediately after removal.

Figure 52 The separating strips and segments of interseptal stone are peeled from the dies and discarded.

Figure 53 *Before the dies are reseated, the dies and base are carefully inspected for any debris or friable edges of stone.* Any debris is removed, and sharp edges that may break away in use are blunted, so that no loose material will fall into the dowel pin holes.

The cast is now ready for the dies to be trimmed in preparation for waxing and other construction procedures. Preparation of dies is covered in Section 7.

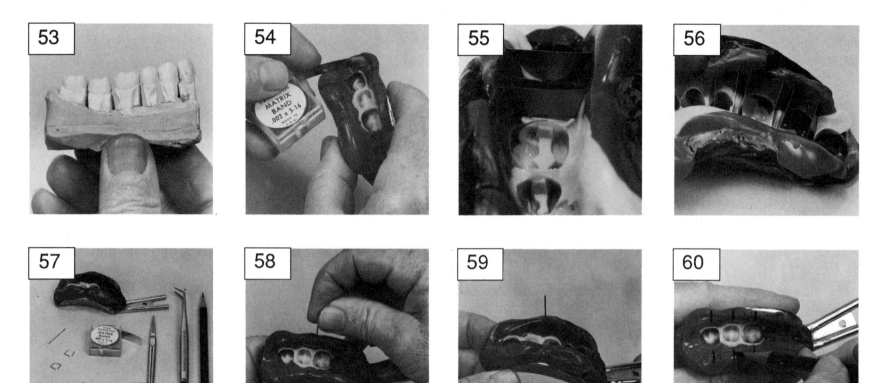

Stripping the Hydrocolloid Impression

Figure 54   The objectives of stripping a hydrocolloid impression are the same as for the rubber impression. Execution is simpler. The strips are cut a bit longer than the interflange width and are positioned by letting them slice into the soft gel material. No waxing is necessary.

Figure 55   Care must be taken to insert the strips cleanly, straight into the impression material, so that they do not touch the margins of the preparations. There should be a clearance of 0.5 millimeter between the strips and the margin of the impression. If the strips are too wide occlusogingivally, they may be narrowed before insertion or even removed, cut, and then reinserted. The strips should extend no more than ⅛ inch above the flange of the impression.

Figure 56   The stripping of the hydrocolloid impression has been completed. The terminal (outside) strips that are not adjacent to prepared margins can be seated until they contact or penetrate the occlusal surface of the impression. This dams off the area of the impression to be poured with die stone.

The impression is poured and dowel pins are positioned in the same way as with the rubber-base impression. Remember that reversible hydrocolloid impressions distort rapidly upon the absorption or loss of water. They must be poured as promptly as possible with a minimum of working time and should be stored in a humidor during all waiting periods.

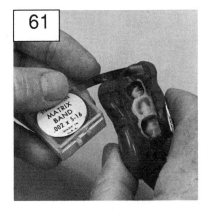

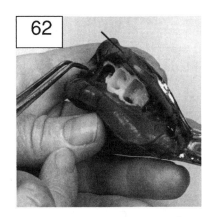

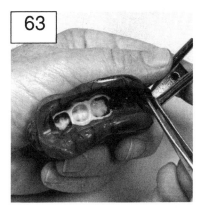

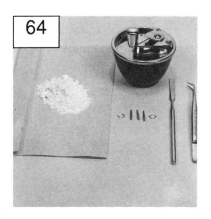

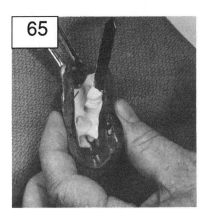

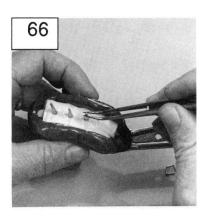

DOUBLE POUR SECTION TECHNIQUE

A second basic approach to obtaining a working cast is a double pour technique in which the dies to be removable are separated with a small, thin-bladed saw.

Figure 57 The impression selected to demonstrate this technique is a hydrocolloid impression for a single crown. In this impression, the three molar teeth (the prepared tooth, and one tooth on either side) are to be made removable. The instruments and material for this technique include an indelible pencil, tweezers, scissors, steel matrix band material, dowel pins, a straight pin, and bent wire loops.

Figures 58 and 59 The straight pin is positioned in the facial flange of

the impression so that it is parallel to the desired path of draw for the dies.

Figure 60 The mesiodistal center of each tooth to be made as a removable die is marked on the facial and lingual flange of the impression with a marker. These lines will be used to orient the dowel pins.

Figure 61 Strips of matrix material are cut for either end of the impression. Only two pieces are required.

Figures 62 and 63 The terminal strips to confine the die stone are inserted into the impression material. (In a rubber impression these strips would be placed and sealed with utility wax as previously described.)

Figure 64 Die stone is mixed according to the manufacturer's directions.

Figure 65 After the die stone is teased into all recesses using a spatula or brush, it is built to a reasonable thickness above all margins but below the edge of flanges.

Figure 66 Dowel pins are inserted between the marks on the flanges and made parallel to the guide pin (see **Figures 58 and 59**).

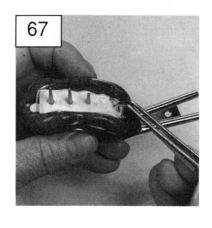

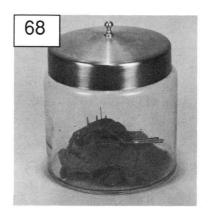

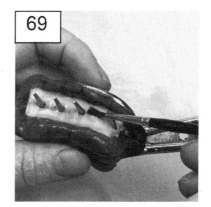

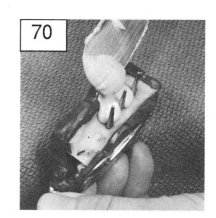

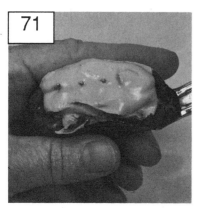

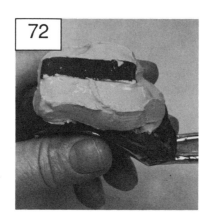

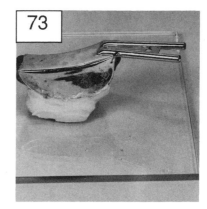

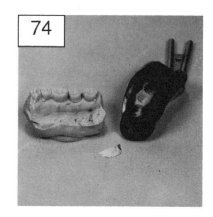

Figure 67   Bent wire retention loops are half-embedded in the areas that are *not* to be removable. The number and size of wire loops required varies depending on the impression.

Figure 68   The impression is stored in a humidor while the die stone sets.

Figure 69   Gypsum separator is applied to the set die stone. Any die stone that has extended beyond the terminal strips is carefully removed.

Figure 70   The base pour is made with regular dental stone.

Figures 71 and 72   A strip of wax is laid across the ends of the dowel pins. The stone addition is completed as previously described.

Figure 73   The impression may be inverted to form a flat base on the cast.

Figure 74   After the base pour has set, the cast is removed from the impression.

Figure 75   If the cast is to be shaped on a model trimmer, that should be done before any dies or wax are removed. The utility wax is removed from the cast base.

Figure 76   At this point the critical procedure of sawing out the dies must be accomplished. Using a spiral jigsaw, or preferably the flat-blade type of die saw, cuts are made that extend completely through the first pour of die stone on either side of each tooth to be removed. When adequate space exists between the margin of the prepared tooth and the

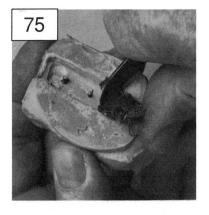

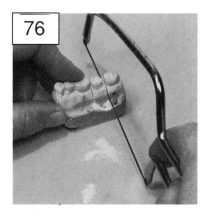

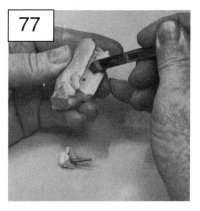

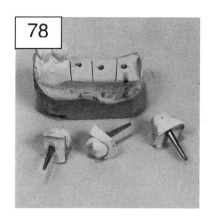

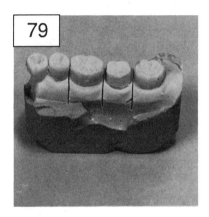

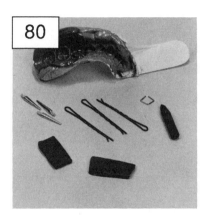

adjacent tooth, this procedure is relatively simple. However, when the prepared margin is very close to the adjacent tooth or, even more critical, when the margins on two adjacent prepared teeth are very close together, it is difficult to insert the saw blade between the dies without touching the margins. In extreme situations it is best to remove the block of dies from the cast and saw from the gingival (base) side to a point just below the margins of the prepared teeth. Dies thus sawed can usually be separated by applying pressure between the dowel pins to cause a fracture between the margins.

Figure 77   All dust and debris on the cast is thoroughly removed by air blast. The dies are removed by pressing or tapping on the ends of the dowel pins.

Figure 78   The dies have been removed from the casts. No debris must

be allowed to collect on the base of the dies, the base portion of the cast, or in the dowel pin holes.

Figure 79   The removable dies are reinserted into the base and are now ready to be prepared for waxing (Section 7).

Paralleling Dowel Pins before Pouring

Having all the dowel pins parallel is a distinct advantage when working with removable dies; when multiple-unit restorations are to be waxed and cast in one piece, it is essential. Commercial devices are available that will set dowel pins parallel to one another and hold them in position before the dies are poured. There are also a number of laboratory techniques for arbitrarily positioning dowel pins before the dies are poured. One very simple, effective technique is shown here. No equipment other than a few bobby pins is required.

Figure 80   The armamentarium for this technique includes a dowel pin and bobby pin for each die, bent wire loops, sticky wax, and strips of boxing wax.

Figure 81   The dowel pin is placed in the bobby pin as shown.

Figure 82   The bobby pin is positioned across the flanges of the impression such that the dowel is centered over the tooth. Sticky wax is used to secure the bobby pin in position.

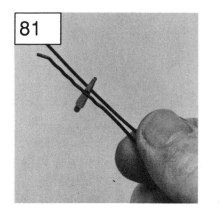
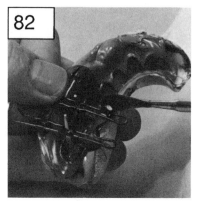
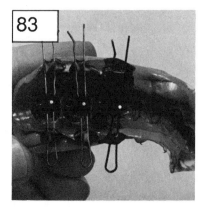
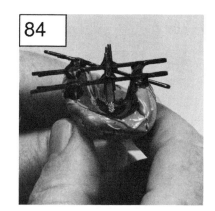
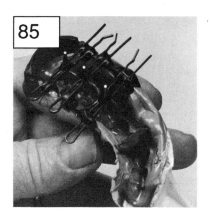
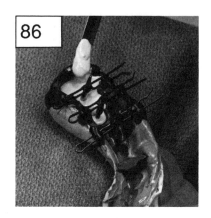
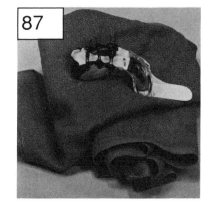
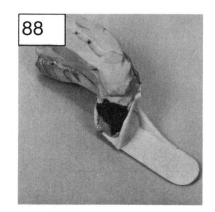

Figure 83　The dowel pin is adjusted in vertical position by sliding it up or down within the bobby pin.

Figure 84　When all bobby pins are in position, the dowel pins are paralleled by eye and their position fixed with sticky wax.

Figure 85　Metal or wax strips are positioned to form a dam at either end of the area to be poured.

Figure 86　Die stone is mixed and poured to a level that encompasses the knurled end to the dowel pins.

Figure 87　Bent wire loops are half-embedded in the areas that are *not* to be removed, and this first pour is allowed to set.

Figure 88　After the die stone has set, the bobby pins and sticky wax are removed from the impression, and the gypsum separator is applied. The base of the cast is poured with dental stone and allowed to set. Note that the ends of the dowel pins have been left uncovered without using a strip of utility wax as was done in previous examples. If the mix of stone used for this step is thick enough, it stands by itself and can be shaped as desired.

Figure 89　The cast and impression are separated. Any trimming of the cast is done before the dies are separated.

Figure 90　The dies are separated by sawing through the first pour of stone. All debris is removed.

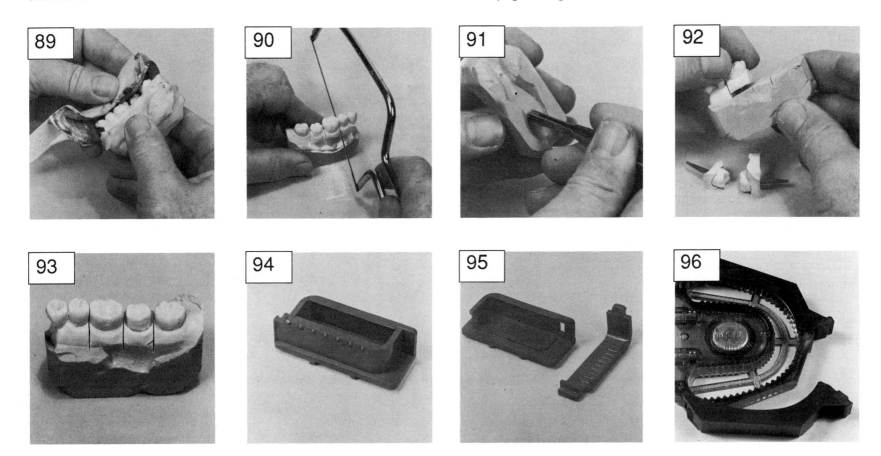

Figures 91 and 92 Dies are removed by first tapping or pushing against the dowel pins and then drawing them out with the fingers. After disassembling, all debris and weak edges are removed so that the dies may be accurately returned to position.

Figure 93 The dies are reassembled in the cast.

Di-Lok Tray and Similar Techniques

The Di-Lok tray and similar techniques are another modification of the double pour section technique. The Di-Lok tray is made so that one side and end are removable (**Figures 94 and 95**). Procedures for using the tray provide for removable dies without the necessity of placing dowel pins. Relationship of the dies to one another is established by the tray. The Accutrac tray system is similar in design and use (**Figure 96**).

Figure 97 The margins of the dies of prepared teeth are trimmed as described in Section 7. The cast is reassembled in the tray using the fracture lines and saw grooves to position the parts accurately.

Figure 98 The tray has been reassembled until the dies lock into position.

One disadvantage of these tray techniques is the time consumed assembling, disassembling, and reassembling the dies during the waxing procedures. Accuracy of these techniques is suitable for individual restorations, but questionable for splinted units or bridge construction.

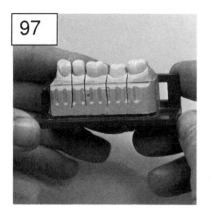

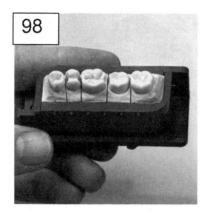

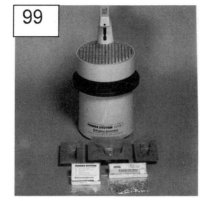

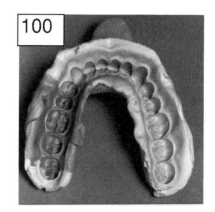

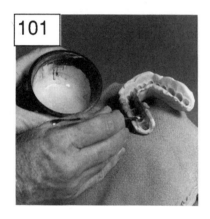

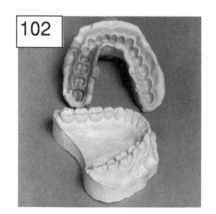

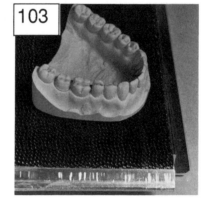

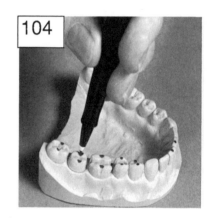

PRECISION DOWEL PIN AND DIE TECHNIQUE

Pindex System

The Pindex System (**Figure 99**) is a sophisticated technique that provides an accurate reproduction of an original master model with removable dies and sections, which permits a repeatable and precise procedure.

Figure 100 A full mandibular arch impression is shown with three prepared teeth on the patient's right side: a premolar onlay, a molar onlay, and a molar full crown.

Figure 101 The master cast is poured with die stone in small increments to avoid air entrapment, with a controlled amount of vibration on a towel-covered vibrator to aid the stone to flow better.

Figure 102 The master cast is removed from the impression. A solid, bubble-free cast is an absolute necessity for accuracy.

Figure 103 The cast is trimmed first on a model trimmer. Then the base is further refined against a flat-surface grinder of the Pindex equipment to provide a perfectly flat surface before drilling the holes for the removable dies and sections. The base should be about 15 millimeters high from the bottom of the base to the gingival margin of the prepared teeth.

Figure 104 Each hole to be drilled is located and marked with a pencil or felt-tip pen on the occlusal surface of the teeth in the master cast. Care must be exercised to provide a maximum interdistance between the facial and lingual pin holes so that the pins and sleeves can be placed in this space without interference. Care must also be exercised

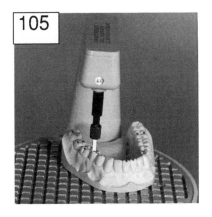

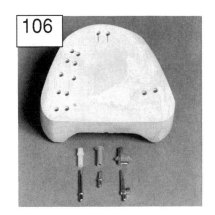

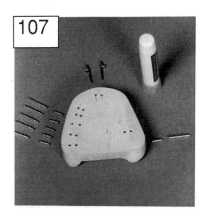

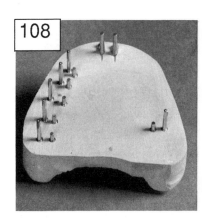

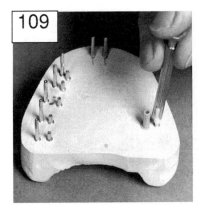

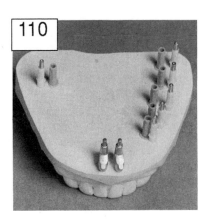

to plan the type of pin holes to be drilled according to the size of the teeth. In this example, premolars and molars have two holes, incisors have one hole.

Figure 105 The cast is placed on the work table of the Pindex unit. The switch on the unit is turned on, as indicated by the glowing of the red pilot light on the front surface of the unit's arm. The beam pointer is focused and adjusted until the smallest and brightest illuminated dot is obtained. The marks on each tooth are aligned with the illuminated dots (**Figure 105**). The model is gripped with both hands—thumbs on the model and the other fingers in the hand ring—and the work table is slowly pressed downward with gradual, even pressure until the end stop is reached and the illuminated dot automatically switches off. Sequentially, all the holes are drilled to full depth in the cast base, using a slow movement that allows the drill to do the cutting. The model should be

slightly damp—neither bone dry nor soaking wet. *Clean any debris from holes* with compressed air after drilling is completed.

Figure 106 The bottom side of the cast, with all the holes drilled and the types of index pins and sleeves to be used in each hole. The index pins are identified as follows in order from left to right. The long pin with the white sleeve is placed in the facial hole of the two holes in premolars and molars. The short pin with the gray sleeve is used in the lingual pin hole of the premolars and molars. The dual pin and metal sleeve are used for narrow anterior teeth and small cast sections.

Figure 107 Cast complete with index pins ready to be cemented into place with a cyanoacrylate cement. The cement is placed on the short end of each pin, which is then placed in the pin hole. As a matter of convenience and access, the short pins are cemented first, then the long pins in sequence.

Figure 108 Pins have been cemented into place, ready for the placement of the sleeves.

Figure 109 A sleeve holder is used to place the sleeves on the index pins. The white sleeves are placed on the long pins, and the gray sleeves on the short pins. The sleeves should be positioned so that their flat portions face each other between the pins.

Figure 110 The pins and sleeves have been placed. Note the incisor pins and metal sleeves.

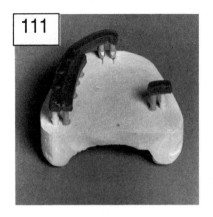

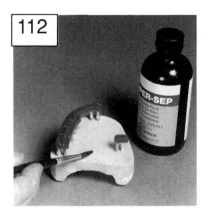

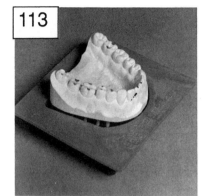

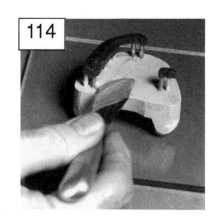

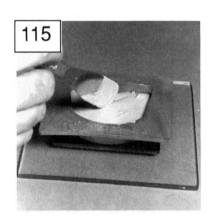

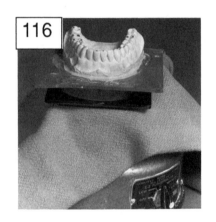

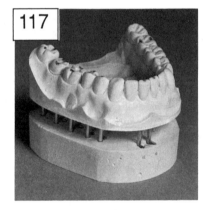

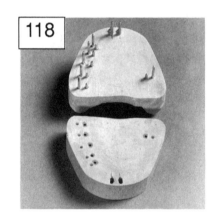

Figure 111   A strip of rope wax or carding wax is placed over the long pins and over the open ends of the gray sleeves of the short index pins.

Figure 112   Separating medium is placed on the bottom of the base of the master cast.

Figure 113   The placement of the master cast in the rubber mold is carefully checked before adding the additional stone to the base.

Figure 114   Stone is carefully placed between the pins under the wax on the master cast.

Figure 115   The rubber mold is partially filled with stone.

Figure 116   The master cast is placed into the rubber mold until it is

seated, using gentle vibration either on a vibrator or by hand. Care should be taken that stone fills any voids.

Figure 117   When the stone base has set, the master cast is removed from the mold and the base is trimmed as needed. The completed master cast with the pins can be removed from the cast base in one piece.

Figure 118   The master cast with pins in place and the sleeves in the base, prior to sectioning. The sectioning of the dies is made from the underside of the master cast.

Figure 119   The dies and sections are numbered before they are cut apart, so that they can be identified and replaced easily.

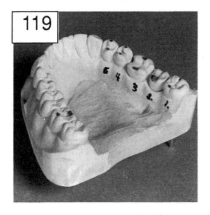
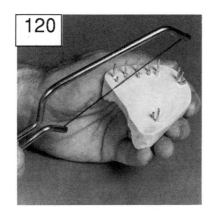
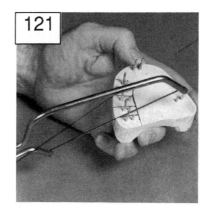
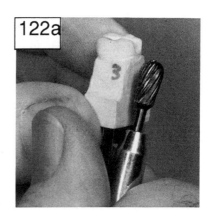

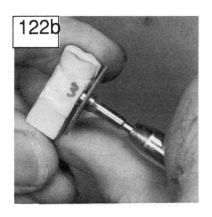
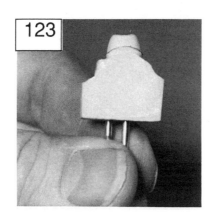
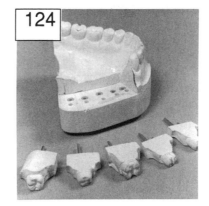
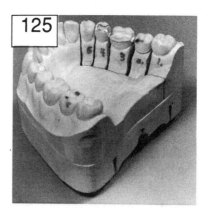

Figure 120 The sections may be cut from the underside of the cast with either a hand saw or a band saw.

Figure 121 The individual dies are cut from the underside to within 2 to 3 millimeters of the prepared tooth margin so that, when squeezed together, the dies will break apart without damage to the die margins.

Figure 122 Each die of section is placed against a tapered grinding bur (a) or a Carborundum wheel (b) to remove the excess stone and to obtain a slight taper toward the base of the die and dowel pin, so that the dies will not interfere with each other when seated in and removed from the cast base. A grinding wheel mounted on a lathe may be used in place of the bur or wheel.

Figure 123 The margins of the prepared teeth (dies) are identified and

trimmed in the conventional manner, as described in Section 7.

Figure 124 The master cast with dies trimmed and ready to be placed in the cast base. The dies, cast, and pin holes have been cleaned so that no debris will interfere with the proper seating of sections or dies in the base.

Figure 125 The master cast completely assembled and ready for use.

Figure 126 The completed master cast, ready to be mounted on an articulator.

The Pindex System permits casts to be mounted in a precise method on an articulator, so that they can be removed from the articulator

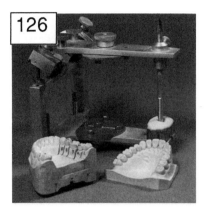 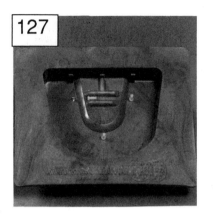 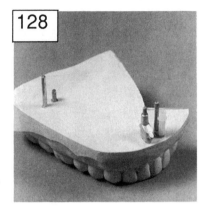 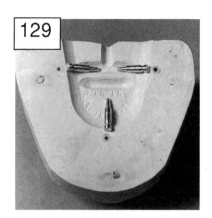

during waxing and finishing procedures. Casts may also be removed and shipped independently of the articulator.

Mounting on an articulator may be achieved in several ways according to individual preference and cast. When the rubber mold (**Figure 127**) is used initially to pour the model base, a template containing metal pins may be inserted beneath the rubber mold. The pins project through the bottom of the mold, and the short white self-articulating sleeves are placed over them.

The base is added to the master cast as illustrated in **Figures 115 and 116**. When the master cast and base are ready to be mounted to an articulator, the self-articulating pins are placed into the sleeves (**Figure 130**) and the master cast and base are mounted on the articulator in the conventional manner.

When short index pins and dual pins are used in constructing a master cast, various types of sleeves may be used with articulating pins that are placed where they would be located most advantageously, in a triangular configuration as far apart from each other as is convenient. **Figure 128** illustrates a metal dual-pin sleeve that has been replaced by a long white pin sleeve. **Figure 129** shows a cast where the gray sleeves have been utilized on the short pins before placing the wax strip and pouring the remainder of the cast base. In either instance, the articulating pins shown in **Figure 129** are placed in the sleeves before the cast is mounted on an articulator.

Figure 130 A maxillary cast that has been prepared for mounting using the self-articulating pins and short white articulating sleeves. The self-articulating pin and sleeve system can be added to any cast base at any time, by drilling three pin holes in a triangular configuration

with the Pindex System drill and fixing the self-articulating white pin sleeves into place with cyanoacrylate cement. The self-articulating pins can then be placed in the sleeves and the articulator mountings made in the conventional manner.

Figure 131 Casts ready to be reassembled in the articulator.

Figure 132 The cast mounted on the articulator, which has been adjusted for further procedures necessary to complete the case.

SUMMARY

The techniques described in this section are examples of sound procedures for developing casts and dies from tray impressions. Which technique should be employed depends in every case upon the type of prosthesis material, the types of restorations to be made, and the preferences of the technician and dentist. Each technique produces good results, and each may be slightly varied to meet the individual needs of a given situation.

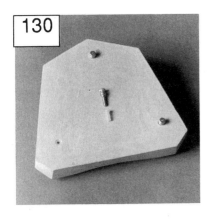
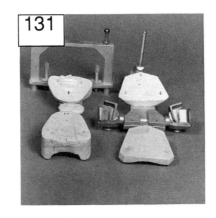
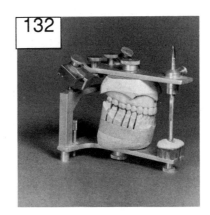

REVIEW QUESTIONS

1. Name the four types of elastic impression material that may be encountered in tray impressions.
2. What precaution is necessary when the impression material extends beyond the end of a tray?
3. Describe three basic techniques for making a working cast with removable dies.
4. In the double stripping technique of an impression for removable dies, how (in what directions) should the pieces of metal material for each die section diverge and converge?
5. How should die stone be placed when a very thin portion of impression material is present around a prepared tooth?
6. If it is necessary to trim a cast with removable dies on a model trimmer, when should the cast be trimmed?

SECTION 6

Developing Dies from Band Impressions

A second method of recording teeth prepared for full crowns is the band impression. Band impressions are used to record an individually prepared tooth. Fixed restorations involving multiple preparations require a band impression for each prepared tooth. The choice of a band or a tray impression is determined by the dentist after consideration of the amount of preparation that lies below the crest of the gingiva and the number of teeth that are involved.

Band impressions may be made of impression compound or one of the rubber-base impression materials. The bands are copper, either annealed or hardened, and come in a variety of sizes. To develop an impression the band is contoured to fit the prepared tooth, filled with the desired impression material, and seated on the preparation until the impression material is set. As with tray impressions, when an elastic material is used for a band impression, the container must be rigid. Thus the copper bands that are to be used for rubber impressions are usually reinforced after adaptation with a low-fusing paste solder. Because compound is not elastic when "set," bands used for compound impressions need not be rigid.

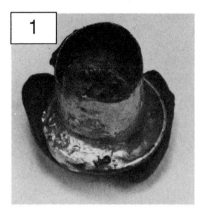
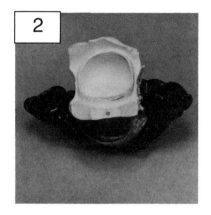
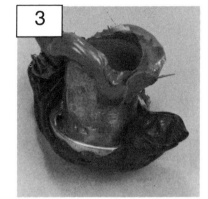
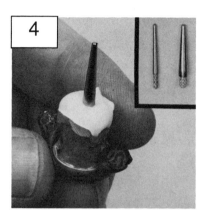

Figure 1 shows a band impression of a lower molar crown preparation, made with impression compound. **Figure 2** shows a band impression made with silicone rubber-base impression material. **Figure 3** shows a band impression made with a polysulfide rubber-base impression material. These materials have been discussed in Section 4, along with the materials used to make dies.

POURING A STONE DIE IN THE BAND IMPRESSION

Two objectives must be kept in mind when making a stone die from a band impression: (1) to cause no distortion of the impression and (2) to develop a strong, accurate die.

Figure 4 It is relatively easy to produce a die from an impression in which all the margins are recorded within the confines of the band (see **Figure 3**). The impression is merely handled carefully to avoid distortion and is poured to excess with die stone in a conventional manner. A dowel pin of appropriate size (**Figure 4**) is placed in the die stone, and the impression is set aside until the stone has set.

Figure 5 It is more difficult to pour a band impression in which a portion of the margin is recorded in rubber that extends beyond the end of the band. Rubber that is not supported by the band can be distorted by the weight of the stone used to pour the die. This free, usually thin edge of rubber would be displaced outward by the weight of the stone if the impression were poured in the manner just described (see **Figure 4**).

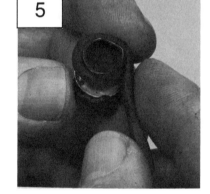
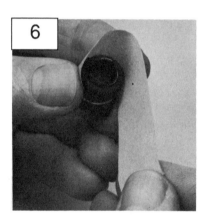

These "free-standing" marginal edges of rubber are instead handled as they are in tray impressions. The stone is allowed to flow freely on both sides of the free edges so that the rubber "floats" in a state of equilibrium. To accomplish this, an outer wall must be present to contain the stone. Such walls are readily provided in a tray impression by the terminal metal separating strips that are placed before the dies are poured. For a band impression, the outer wall is made by wrapping a thin strip of wax or masking tape around the circumference of the band. Extreme care must be taken to ensure that the wax or tape does not touch the "free-standing" edge of rubber.

Figure 5 shows a thin rope of utility wax being placed *on the band*; this is similar to the first step for boxing edentulous impressions. The rope of wax provides a height of contour about which tape or wax may be wrapped so as to stand away from the marginal free flange of rubber.

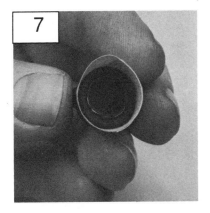
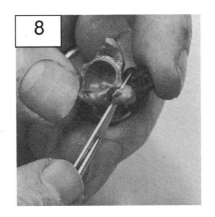
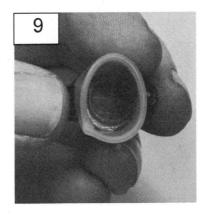
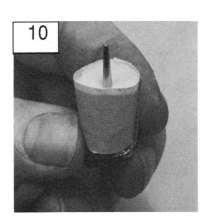

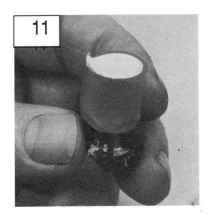
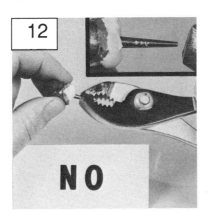

not necessary for all impressions, is an excellent routine procedure, as it provides ample stone root form to facilitate handling of the die.

Figure 10   The impression is poured by adding stone in successive small increments, to avoid trapping air bubbles. High-frequency vibration is necessary. A dowel pin is usually incorporated in the stone.

Figure 11   This impression, wrapped with soft wax, has been poured without incorporating a dowel pin. Correct trimming of the completed root form can provide an index to position such a die in a working cast without a dowel pin.

The same techniques are used to make dies from either rubber-base impressions or impressions made with impression compound. When wax is used to prepare the impression it should be soft wax that does not require heating, as heat may distort an impression made from impression compound.

Figure 6   A piece of masking tape or thin gauge wax is wrapped around the impression to form a wall that stands away from the free edge of the impression material.

Figure 7   The band impression is ready to be poured.

Figure 8   Often the excess rubber material on the outside of the band may be trimmed with a very sharp instrument to leave a collar about which the tape or wax may be wrapped.

Figure 9   This impression, prepared by trimming the excess impression material, is ready to be poured. It has been wrapped with a layer of thin wax (the one shown in **Figure 7** was wrapped with masking tape). Preparing the band impression with masking tape or soft wax, though

RECOVERY OF THE DIE FROM THE BAND IMPRESSION

Figure 12   The simplest means of removing a die from a rubber-base copper band impression is to hold the root form or dowel pin and pull the die from the impression. This is commonly done by grasping the dowel pin with pliers. However, grasping the dowel pin directly with

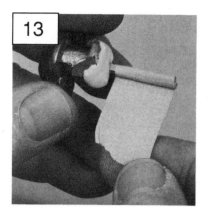

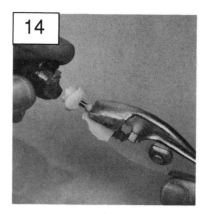

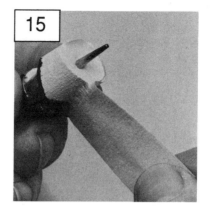

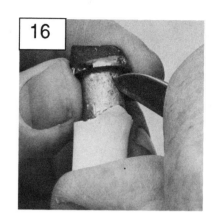

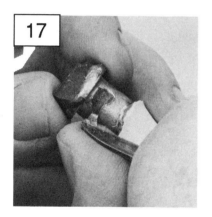

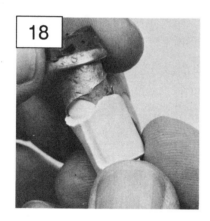

the pliers will scar the dowel pin, jeopardizing its use as a positive index in a working cast.

Figure 13   If pliers are used to remove a die from a rubber-base impression, the dowel pin should be wrapped with masking tape or a similar cushioning material.

Figure 14   The die is removed by pulling it straight from the impression.

This method of removing dies from rubber-base band impressions should only be used when the die has smooth surfaces and a large cross-sectional dimension. Long, narrow dies and those with undercuts may easily break when separated in this manner.

Impressions made of impression compound are safely removed in a similar manner after first warming the compound in hot water.

Figure 15   If masking tape or soft wax has been used to pour the impression, it is removed before the die and impression are separated.

Figure 16   The second and safest way of removing a die from a rubber-base band impression is to peel the copper band from the impression and the die. This method must be used when the die is long, has a thin cross-sectional area, or has marked undercuts or surface roughness. The first step in peeling the band is to penetrate the band with a knife near the occlusal end, where there is a known thickness of rubber separating the band and die. The knife tip should slit the band just enough to permit grasping a free edge.

Figure 17   The band is peeled from the impression material in a spiral fashion, working toward the gingival margin.

Figures 18 and 19   The impression is easily removed from the die when a sufficient amount of the copper band has been peeled away.

This method of separating the die from the band rubber impression is recommended for routine use. It must be used if recovery of all dies without breakage is to be assured.

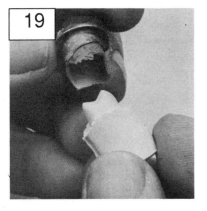 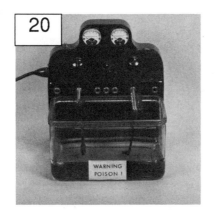 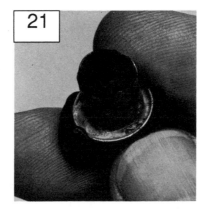 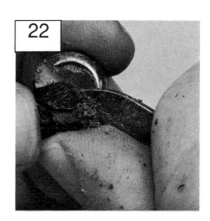

ELECTROFORMED DIES

Electroformed dies are made by plating the surface of a compound impression with copper, or a rubber impression with silver. The body of the die is then poured with die stone or resin. If a tray impression has been plated, the dies and cast are poured according to the double pour section technique.

Electroformed or plated dies are accurate and have a tough, strong surface that is pleasant to handle. Low-voltage direct current is needed for electroplating. The plating equipment consists of a transformer to reduce the voltage of the power supply, and a rectifier to convert the alternating current to direct current.

Figure 20   This commercial plating device contains a transformer and rectifier with a variable resistor to regulate the current. The amount of current determines the rate at which metal is deposited on the impression. A milliammeter indicates the amount of current passing through the plating bath. This bath is a chemical solution necessary for plating. The solution differs depending upon the metal used. Directions are supplied by the manufacturers of the plating equipment.

Normally an acid solution of copper sulfate is used for copper plating and a silver cyanide solution is used for silver plating. The electrolytically pure metal plate, copper or silver, is immersed into the plating solution so that the immersed area is equal to that of the impression to be plated. The direct current causes dissolution of the metal, and the pure metallic ions flow from this anode (positive pole) to the surface of the impression, which is the cathode (negative pole) of the system.

Copper Plating

In copper plating the plating bath is commonly an acid solution of copper sulfate, and the anode is pure copper. The manufacturer of the plating equipment will distribute the plating solution or provide the exact formula. Some homemade plating devices work satisfactorily.

Figure 21   Compound impressions are most easily copper-plated. Rubber-base impressions can be copper-plated, but not with great consistency.

Figure 22   The closed end of the copper band impression is scraped clean to expose the metal surface. This permits good metal-to-metal contact with a cathode holder.

Figure 23   The clean band impression is placed on the cathode platform.

Figure 24   The band impression is attached to the cathode platform with utility wax. Care must be taken not to let any wax flow between the band and the platform. Contact between the band and the platform is necessary to conduct the electrical current.

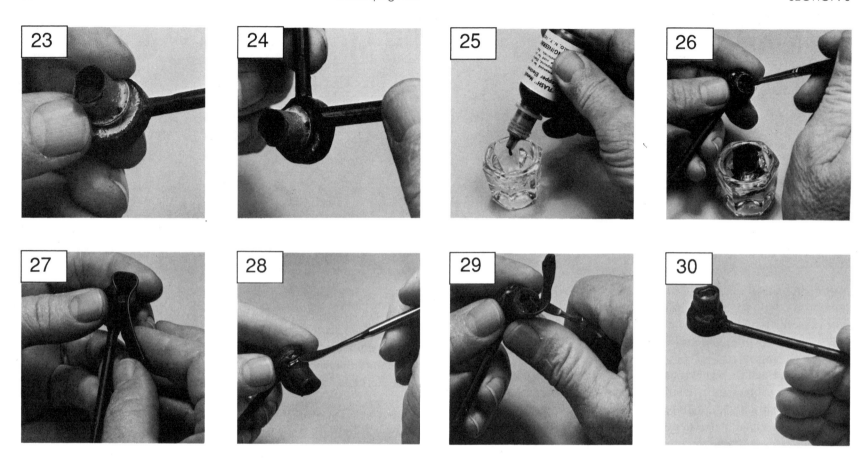

Figure 25   A metalizing agent, usually composed of colloidal graphite and copper powder, is used to coat the surface of the impression. A small amount is placed in a glass dish with a drop of water and mixed with a brush.

Figure 26   The metalizing solution is brushed evenly over the surface of the impression and over the edge of the copper band. The impression is air-dried, and any excess metalizing agent is removed with a dry brush and compressed air. The impression should have a thin, uniform coating of the metalizing agent. Uncoated areas should be repainted and the impression dried again. Because metalizing agent deteriorates rapidly, any excess is best discarded.

Some operators prefer to add the metalizing agent *after* the wax extension has been placed on the impression, as shown in **Figures 27 through 29**.

Figures 27 and 28   A piece of 28-gauge gauge wax is wrapped around the impression and carefully sealed in place.

Figures 29 and 30   The wax is cut back to produce an extension that projects 2 millimeters beyond the cervical end of the band. If the margin of the prepared tooth in the impression is near the end of the band, this extension must be placed before the metalizing agent is used. The wax extension is not necessary if the entire margin is 2 millimeters or more within the band. The purpose of the wax extension is to insure an adequate amount of copper for trimming the die correctly.

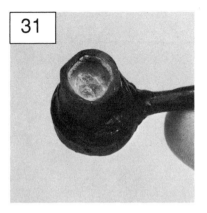 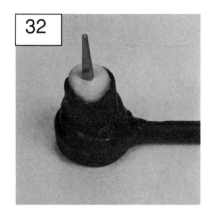 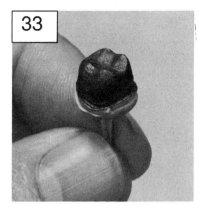 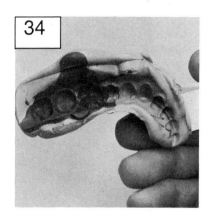

Before immersion, the copper band impression is filled with electroplating solution with a medicine dropper, to ensure that air bubbles will not be trapped inside. The impression and cathode platform are then immersed in the plating bath. The end of the cathode holder is attached to the proper plating terminal (**Figure 20**). The open end of the impression band must face the anode (copper plate). The copper anode is placed in the bath at least six inches from the impression, so that the immersed area is equal to or slightly greater than the area of the impression to be plated.

The current is turned on and adjusted according to the manufacturer's suggestions. Usually 15 milliamperes is suitable to start plating a single impression. After 20 minutes the cathode holder is removed from the bath and the impression is inspected to be sure that an even coating of copper is covering it. Plating should not occur too rapidly, or a poor surface will result and the deeper portions of the impression will not be covered. The impression is refilled with the medicine dropper and immersed in the plating bath. Plating usually requires 12 to 15 hours.

Figure 31 When plating is completed, the impression is removed from the solution, washed, and removed from the cathode holder if desired. Some technicians prefer to leave it attached to the cathode holder, as this becomes a convenient handle.

Figure 32 The plated impression is poured with stone or resin. Soft wax or masking tape may be used to produce a root form, or a dowel pin may be used, as illustrated in this photograph. The technique is the same as that for any band impression.

Figure 33 The copper die after it has been removed from the impression, which was accomplished in the same manner as a die made completely of die stone.

Silver Plating

Silver plating has been used to make dies since the inception of rubber-base impression materials, as it produces more consistent results with these materials than copper plating does. Silver plating cannot be used with impressions made from impression compound, because the alkaline silver-plating bath softens this material.

Silver plating involves essentially the same process as copper plating. The same equipment is used, but with a lower current. A pure silver anode is used in a silver cyanide plating bath. Silver cyanide solution is extremely poisonous and must be handled with care. Hands, clothing, and the work bench area must not be contaminated, as any acid that comes into contact with the solution produces hydrogen cyanide gas, which is also extremely poisonous. The plating bath should be covered at all times and should be placed in a well-ventilated area. The mixing and care of silver-plating solution should be executed as directed by the manufacturer of the plating equipment.

Silver plating is easier with the polysulfide rubber-base impression materials than it is with a silicone rubber-base impression material. Some of the silicone materials appear to be more readily copper-plated than silver-plated.

The silver-plating technique described here utilizes a tray impression of polysulfide rubber-base material. A band impression made with the same material can be silver-plated following the same general instructions given for copper plating.

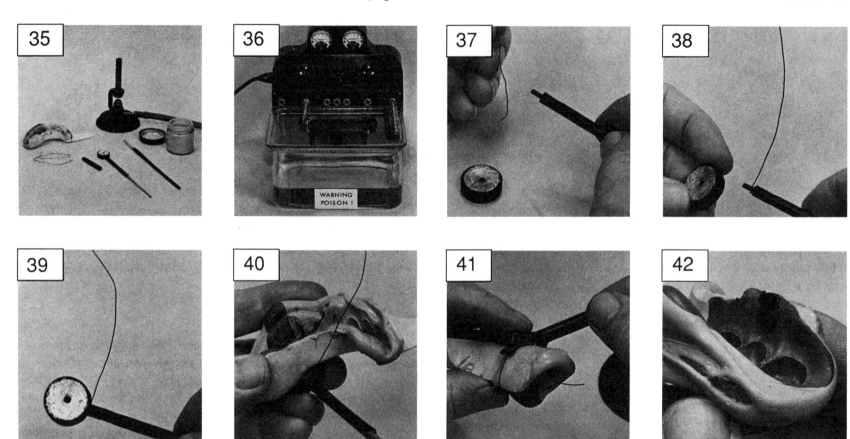

Figure 34   The polysulfide rubber-base impression.

Figure 35   The materials required to prepare the impression for silver plating: a metalizing agent, a brush, a cathode holder, sticky wax, copper wire, and the impression.

Figure 36   The same type of equipment is used as for copper plating.

Figure 37   There are several methods of attaching the tray to the cathode portion of the plating equipment. The method shown produces good results. The handle of the cathode holder is removed from the platform.

Figure 38   A piece of copper wire is wrapped around the handle.

Figure 39   The cathode holder is reassembled.

Figures 40 and 41   The cathode holder is placed on the resin impression tray and is fixed in place with sticky wax. The copper wire is bent to lie against the inside surface of the impression flange.

Figure 42   Sticky wax is placed so that it covers the wire except for the 2 millimeters nearest the prepared tooth.

Figure 43   Silver metalizing powder is applied to the prepared tooth areas. It is placed approximately 2 millimeters beyond the prepared areas of the tooth and is extended to cover the end of the exposed copper wire. The excess powder is removed with a stream of air.

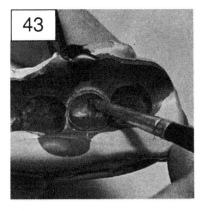
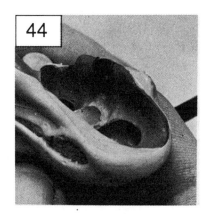
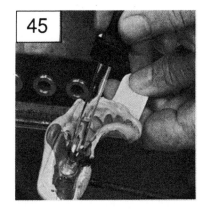
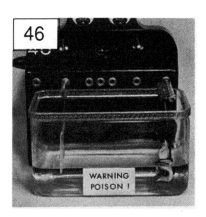

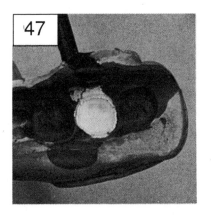
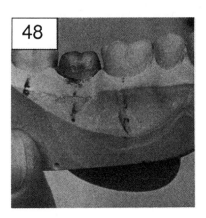

Figure 44   The impression is now ready to be placed in the plating solution.

Figure 45   The impression is attached to the plating device. The impression is filled with electrolyte solution using a medicine dropper, to prevent the inclusion of air bubbles. Care should be taken not to touch the impression with the end of the medicine dropper.

Figure 46   The impression is placed in the plating solution so that it faces the silver anode. The immersed area of the silver anode is adjusted to approximate that of the impression area being plated. Specific instructions for the adjustment of the machine are available from the manufacturer. Usually, the current is adjusted to 5 milliamperes for a single tooth impression and 10 milliamperes per tooth for larger im-

pressions. This current is maintained for approximately 30 minutes to 1 hour, until a thin layer of silver is deposited over the entire impression.

The impression is then removed from the plating solution and carefully washed and dried. It is checked to make sure there is a proper coating of silver. Soft green wax should be flowed over any silver deposit in the interproximal soft tissue areas where a heavy deposit of silver is not needed. Do not flow molten wax into the tooth areas.

The impression is refilled with electrolyte, to prevent air bubbles, and returned to the plating bath. Do not trap air bubbles. The current is usually adjusted to 15 to 20 milliamperes for each tooth in the impression. Normally 10 to 12 hours of plating produces a suitable thickness of silver. The time may vary with equipment and a particular impression.

Figure 47   The plated impression is removed from the plating bath, washed with water, and dried. The plating is carefully checked.

Figure 48   The die and working cast are prepared according to one of the methods shown in Section 5. If multiple units have been plated, the double pour section technique is best employed, as the metal surface will have to be sectioned between adjacent dies.

REVIEW QUESTIONS

1. Name two methods of recording teeth prepared for fixed restorations.
2. What type of material is used for the band when a band impression is made?
3. What is the simplest means of removing a die from a rubber-base band impression? What precautions are necessary if a brass dowel is used?
4. What is the safest way to remove a die from a rubber-base band impression?
5. What two metals are commonly used to make electroplated dies? With which type of impression materials is each metal used?

SECTION 7

Preparation of Dies

The preceding sections have described techniques for developing suitable dies from tray and band impressions. Further preparation of these dies is necessary before they can be effectively used to develop restorations. Before patterns can be waxed, excess root form must be trimmed, access to margins must be established, and undercuts in prepared surfaces must be eliminated. Proper preparation of dies has a significant and direct influence on the quality of the final restoration.

The preparation of dies proceeds in three steps: (1) trimming the root portion of the die, (2) establishing access to the margin, and (3) preparation of the die surface.

The *principles* stated here relate to all dies; but the *techniques* described are for stone dies and may or may not relate to dies made from other materials.

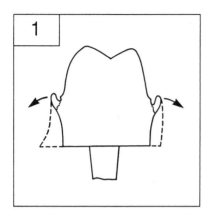
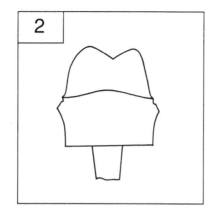
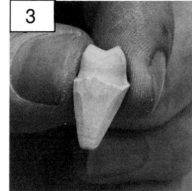
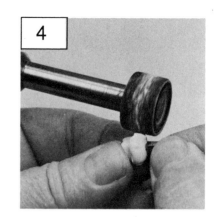
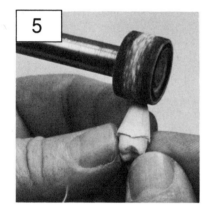
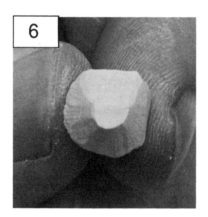

TRIMMING THE ROOT PORTION OF THE DIE

Figure 1   Trimming the root portion of the die (commonly referred to simply as *trimming the die*) means removal of any excess stone from the axial surface of the root portion of the die to permit convenient handling and access to the marginal area. Dies made from tray impressions and individual dies that will *not* be incorporated in any type of working cast require only gross trimming to permit access to the marginal area.

Figure 2   Individual dies that *will* be incorporated in a working cast must be trimmed and their root form shaped to present a smooth taper that will permit their withdrawal from the cast to be poured about them.

Figure 3   If the die has been developed completely in stone (no dowel pin), flat surfaces or shallow grooves must be placed on the tapered root form to provide positive indexing of the die in the working cast.

Figures 4 through 6   The arbor band on a lathe provides a convenient mechanism for gross trimming. The arbor band can also be used to shape and taper a stone root form. Utmost care must be taken to prevent abrasion of the margin. Not as obvious, but very important, is to avoid scarring of dowel pins if present. Final trimming (or all, if desired) is accomplished with separating discs, mounted stones, or tungsten carbide trimmers in the handpiece or lathe. Carbide trimmers in the straight handpiece are especially useful and are preferred by many for the entire trimming process.

Careful technicians purposely avoid trimming any of the base of a die developed in a tray impression—especially on the facial surface. The untrimmed base serves as a readily evident index to the fully seated position of the die and is essential for stability of the die in the working cast (see **Section 5, Figure 43**). Should it be necessary to trim the facial portion of the die base all the way to the model, this should be done by forming a right-angle butt joint so that an index of absolute seating is maintained (see **Figure 1**).

Figure 7   Preliminary access to the margin is usually best obtained by using a strong knife blade to "grasp" the collar of stone surrounding the margin and break it away from the die. This ensures good visibility and access for completion of the trimming and establishing access to the margin. Some fear this approach, but if the impression recorded tooth surface beyond the margin and the base portion of the die has been properly trimmed, the margin cannot be broken by pulling away the edge of stone that surrounds it (see **Figure 1**).

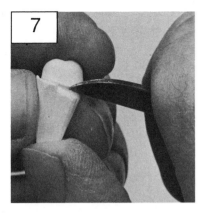

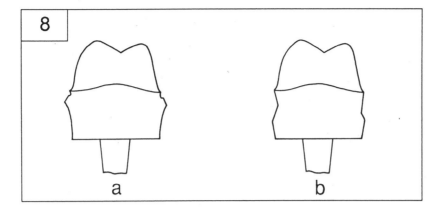

ACCESS TO THE MARGIN

The significant step in die preparation is establishing access to the margin. Accurate marginal adaptation of the casting to the tooth is probably the most important single factor in success or failure of a cast restoration. Such accuracy is difficult to achieve unless the margin is well defined in each phase of development—in the preparation, impression, die, wax pattern, and finally the casting. Of these, accuracy and definition of the margin on the die is most important. The only purpose of the impression is to provide an accurate die. The only means of obtaining an accurate margin in the pattern and casting is to develop them on an accurate die. Thus in a sense the die is the objective of all steps that precede it, and it is the basis for accuracy of adaptation in all procedures that follow its development.

Accuracy of a die is not created; it is only maintained. An accurate die results from correct pouring of an accurate impression. Once the die is developed, no changes can make it more accurate. There are, however, changes that can often facilitate the use of the die to develop an accurate wax pattern. The most significant of these is determining and establishing proper access to the cavosurface angle of the margin. This is commonly referred to as *ditching the die*.

Ditching a die is accomplished by altering the contour of the root portion of the die so that the cavosurface angle of the gingival margin stands distinct. Only gingival margins are ditched, usually for certain areas of full crown or partial crown dies. Less frequently the gingival margins of inlay dies require ditching.

Ideally the impression and hence the die duplicate a portion of the unprepared tooth surface beyond the margin. When and where it is present, this band of unprepared tooth surface may serve both to define the cavosurface angle of the margin and to indicate the contour of the wax pattern in the marginal area. This natural contour should be maintained. The marginal area exposed by just breaking away the excess stone in **Figure 7** is an excellent example of this situation.

Unfortunately access to some submarginal areas of many crown preparation dies is either inadequate or inappropriate to define proper *cut-off angle* for carving the margin of the wax pattern. This contour of the marginal region of restorations that extend subgingivally is referred to as the *emergence angle* because this is the portion of the restoration that emerges from beneath the gingival tissue. Specifically, two conditions may exist that warrant modification of the submarginal contour of the die to establish proper access for carving the margin.

Figure 8   First, the impression may not have recorded, or may have torn during removal so that it does not provide a record of adequate dimension of tooth surface beyond the margin in some areas. Clearly some dimension of tooth surface beyond the cavosurface angle of the margin must be recorded for this angle to be identified. However this dimension may be as little as 0.1 or 0.2 millimeter (**Figure 8a**)—not enough to provide a guiding surface for carving a wax margin. In such cases the recorded contour should be maintained as best possible but extended to provide sufficient access for the margin carving instrument (**Figure 8b**).

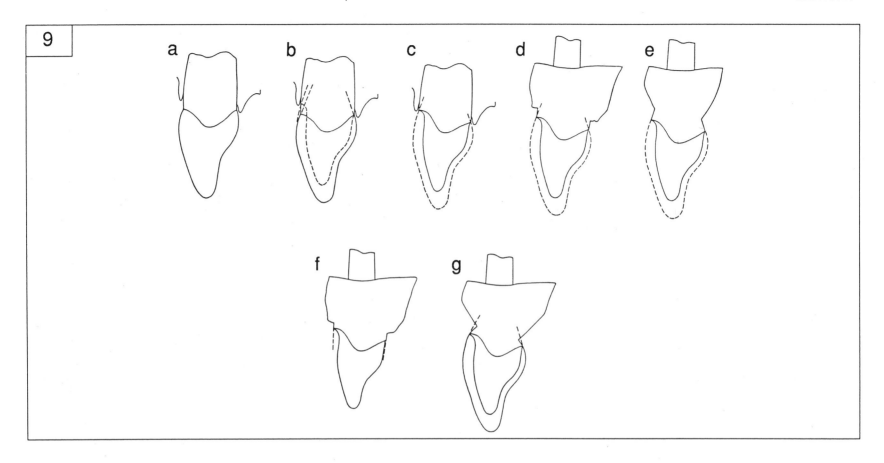

Figure 9 The second condition is created by margins that are prepared at or just apical to the cervical line of the tooth. Recession of facial gingival tissue on maxillary anterior teeth (**Figure 9a**) frequently requires that margins be extended onto the root surface and that the height of contour of crown restorations be "relocated" for esthetic reasons (**Figure 9b**). In addition margins frequently fall at or just below the cervical line (**Figure 9b, lingual**). *In neither case will the contour of the tooth beyond the margin identify correct emergence angle contour for the wax pattern* (**Figure 9c**). Accordingly, in such cases the die that results from a completely adequate impression will not identify the correct contour for the margin of the wax pattern (**Figure 9d**). The die must be modified (*ditched*) to permit access for a carving instrument to create the proper emergence angle for the pattern (**Figure 9e**). Though this procedure seems quite simple and obvious when the outline of the natural or desired tooth form is superimposed, as in these drawings, the correct contour is nebulous and difficult to identify on the bare die

(**Figure 9f**). In fact it must be "found" while developing the axial contours of the wax pattern. In such areas the most adequate procedure is to "overditch" the die so that access is available to carve the desired contour as best it can be determined (**Figure 9g**).

Figure 10 Though not related to restorations covered in this manual, a third situation that many believe warrants modification of the die deserves mention here. When developing porcelain-fused-to-metal restorations, a very narrow marginal collar of metal is commonly used on the esthetically critical facial surface. Processing and contouring the porcelain veneer normally requires some surfacing of this metal in addition to the final polishing. Many operators thus prefer to have a few more degrees of emergence angle in the pattern and casting to compensate for the loss of metal in processing. The die must be modified accordingly to allow access for appropriate cut-off or emergence angle.

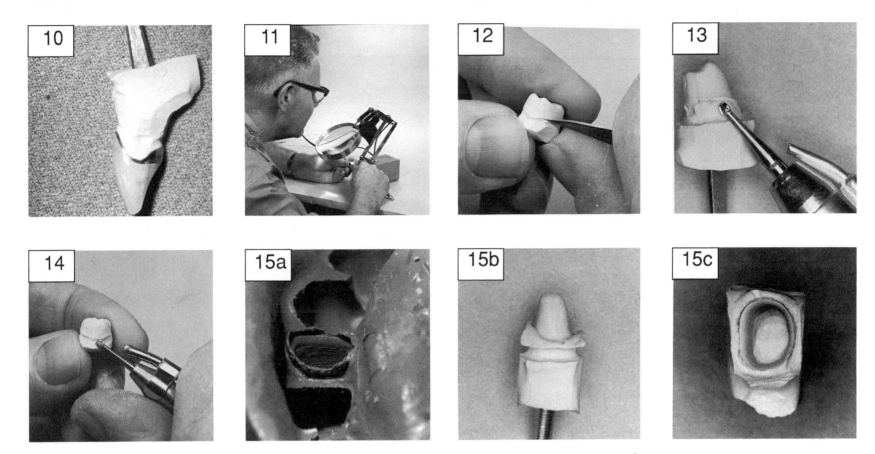

Figure 11   Two methods of ditching are common: the use of a very sharp hand instrument (usually a scalpel), or of a rotary instrument (usually a round bur in a straight handpiece). Whatever instrument is used for removal of the stone, the most important requisite for accurate ditching is excellent visibility (good light and magnification).

Figure 12   Of the hand instruments the Bard-Parker scalpel with a number 11 blade is most commonly used. The blade edge is placed just beneath the margin, and excess stone is shaved away from the margin so that an appropriately angled surface is created.

Figures 13 and 14   The rotary instrument of choice is usually the number 4 or number 6 round carbide bur. It is best used on a completely dry die with an air tip on the handpiece to keep debris blown away thus maintaining clear visibility. The shank of the bur should be held approximately perpendicular to the margin—not parallel, as that might

well permit the rotating bur to "crawl" toward the margin. A palm-and-thumb grasp of the handpiece is employed to provide maximum stability while the die surface is recontoured. Steel burs may be used, but they have a short life when cutting stone. Tungsten carbide burs last indefinitely.

Figure 15 is a sequence representing a simple, normal example of die preparation for a full crown.

Figure 15a   A well-defined chamfer margin and a generous zone of unprepared surface subjacent to the margin have been recorded in the impression, except for one area where the impression tore just beneath the cavosurface angle of the margin.

Figure 15b   The die has been poured and grooved with a round bur just beneath the terminal extension of the impression. A similar result could

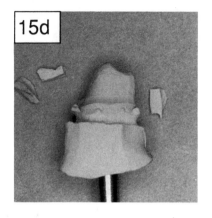

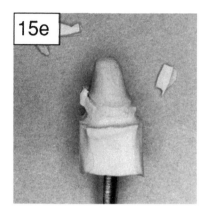

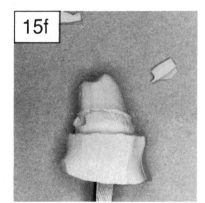

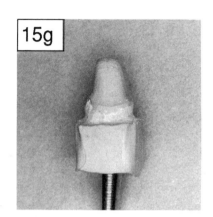

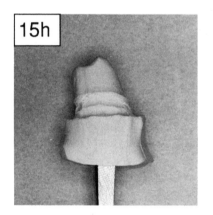

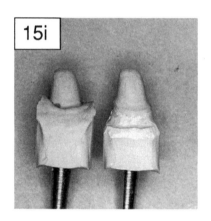

have been obtained using a pear-shaped acrylic bur and reducing the axial surfaces of the die up to the same level. Such trimming should not reduce the dimension of the base of the die, as this may impair stability.

Figure 15c   Determining where to locate the groove or termination of axial surface trimming is readily done by repeated observations from an occlusal perspective. Note the space that extends beyond the marginal cavosurface angle, except in the region where the impression tore on the proximal (bottom of photo). (The lingual access cannot be seen due to angle of the photograph).

Figure 15d   Once the dimension of the supporting stone has been reduced by the groove or by surface trimming (see **Figure 1**), the flange of stone can be grasped with a stout knife blade and easily broken away (see also **Figure 7**). Access to the mesial margin is now clearly avail-

able. Note also the angulation of the recorded unprepared surface on the facial and lingual of the die. Obviously these margins are located above (occlusal to) the cervical line.

Figure 15e   With excess stone broken away from the facial, the cavo-surface angle of the margin in the area of the torn impression can be clearly seen. Though attachment of the excess stone is quite close, it is still safe to grasp the top edge of the stone and break it away, as there is clear separation of the excess from the cavosurface angle of the margin. To be safer still, the groove could be extended up closer to the margin.

Figure 15f   The gross excess stone was broken away without extension of the groove. All areas of the margin are now exposed. However, access to carve the margin of the wax pattern on this proximal is restricted by the proximity of remaining excess stone.

Figure 15g   Viewed from the facial, the restriction to carving access is even more evident. Additional trimming to smooth away the remaining rough edges of excess stone has been completed in all areas except the critical proximal surface.

Figure 15h   The excess stone on the critical proximal surface has been trimmed away, leaving the slight border of recorded unprepared tooth surface that was present just beneath the margin. This last procedure could be referred to as ditching the die. However, it was in fact simply a critical trimming procedure, as an unprepared surface at an appropriate angle to establish cut-off length and emergence angle of the wax pattern was available, though limited. True ditching is necessary when no

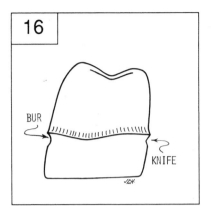

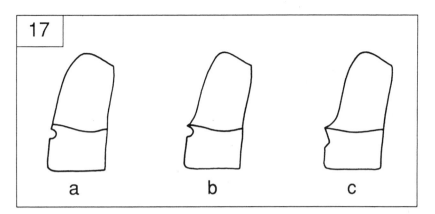

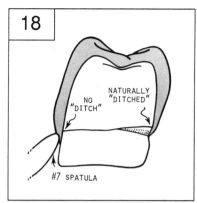

unprepared surface is available or when the contour of the unprepared surface will not facilitate carving a proper emergence angle for the wax pattern.

Figure 15i　The unprepared and prepared die. (The unprepared die was obviously made by a second pour of the impression. Note that a portion of the marginal area of the impression has torn away and remains embedded in the die. This frequently happens on the first pour and recovery, making a second pour fruitless.)

Figure 16　Regardless of method, the objective of ditching a die is to provide access to the cavosurface angle of the margin so that the wax pattern can be terminated precisely along this angle with proper marginal contour.

Figure 17a　Dies are often incorrectly ditched just "close to" the margin, and not exactly to the cavosurface angle. If subsequent waxing and carving of the margin of the pattern are accomplished using this ditch as a guide, the result is a margin that is overextended. Thus if ditching is necessary, it should be accomplished so that the cavosurface angle of the margin is clearly distinct.

Figure 17b　On the other extreme, ditching should not be so pronounced as to leave the margin undermined.

Figure 17c　The contour of the prepared margin is significant in this regard. Heavy chamfer and shoulder margins are easily undermined by ditching. Because the prominence of the cavosurface angle of these

margins makes them very easy to locate when carving the wax pattern, ditching for the purpose of definition is not indicated. However, as these margins offer no more guidance to contour than any other margin, light ditching may be indicated to establish a guiding surface if one is not naturally present. Conversely, ditching of a slice or light chamfer margin is much less likely to undermine the cavosurface angle and is usually necessary to establish sufficient definition of the marginal angle to facilitate locating the margin of the pattern (see **Figure 18**).

When properly executed, the ditch should serve to protect the cavosurface angle of the margin; not weaken it. The pattern margin should *not* be carved with a sharp, cold instrument that might abrade the marginal angle on the die, but should be wipe-carved with a smooth, warm instrument. The surface of the ditch adjacent to the margin should serve as a guide for the carving instrument to "cut off" the wax at the exact correct length (see **Figure 20**). By having a guiding surface at a distinct angle to the prepared surface of the die, the "cut-off" length of the wax pattern can be easily determined without chasing an edge of wax up and down the die surface in the hope of having it terminate along the marginal line.

Figure 18　Carving to a line on an essentially flat surface is impossible, because the line is hidden until the wax is carved back to expose it.

Figure 19　This immediately means that the wax is overcarved and short of the margin. Attempts to correct this are but repeats of the same blind dilemma.

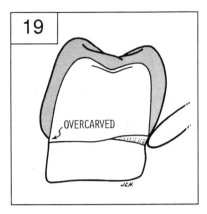
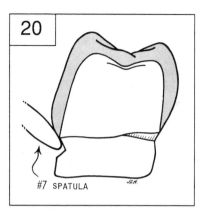

Figure 20 Only by having a guiding surface at a distinct angle to the prepared die surface can the exact length of the pattern be precisely established. Fortunately such an angle is often naturally present, thereby eliminating the necessity for artificially creating it (see **Figures 18 through 20, lingual**).

The smallest diameter or circumference of the crown of a natural tooth occurs at the cervical line. This means that when the margin of a preparation is created occlusal to the cervical line, the tooth surface just apical to the prepared margin will be curving inward (that is, a definite angle will exist between the unprepared submarginal surface and the prepared supramarginal surface). When such unprepared surface at a definite angle to the prepared surface is naturally present, it is usually a valid indication of the correct contour for the marginal region of the pattern (see **Figure 20, lingual**). When no angulation exists, (that is, the surface of the tooth and hence the die is essentially straight or flat), this cannot be interpreted as a true indication of contour for the marginal region of the pattern. Such a flat surface means that the prepared margin is at or below the cervical line of the tooth (see **Figure 19, facial**). Supracervical contour must be reestablished arbitrarily in such situations as the natural guiding surface is not indicative of normal anatomic contour (**Figure 20**).

The location and amount of this supracervical contour is dependent upon its relationship to, and the contour of the adjacent soft tissue. However, evidence of *normal* soft tissue contour *cannot* be provided on *any* die that presents a subgingivally positioned margin. Therefore, *the technician has no possibility for accurate guidance to marginal contour unless such is provided by the unprepared tooth surface just gingival to the margin.* When this tooth guidance is either not present or not valid, the only safe alternative is to provide an adequate thickness in the pattern margin to insure a sound casting, adequate contour for support, and protection of soft tissue. This approach tends to result in overcontouring. The only controls for establishing this contour are a thorough knowledge of dental anatomy and possibly the contour of adjacent teeth. The final decision can be made only by the dentist when the casting is positioned in the mouth and is surrounded by the investing soft tissues in a normal state of health. Obviously it is much easier to correct positive contour errors (overcontour) by surfacing than it is to correct negative errors (undercontour) by a soldered addition or remaking the casting.

PREPARATION OF THE DIE SURFACE

Preparation of the die surface may involve nothing more than the proper application of a die lubricant. Frequently undercuts may be present in the die as a result of excavation of decay or old filling material during preparation of the tooth. Such excavations are often "based out" by the dentist before the impression is made. If not, the undercut areas in the die must be "blocked out" with undercut wax or spackling compound *before the die is lubricated*, because the lubricant will prevent adhesion of the block-out material.

Lubricant should not be applied to the die until all trimming and block-out is completed, as the lubricant tends to retain stone dust on the die surface. If such debris is incorporated in the wax pattern, it may remain in the investment mold and contaminate the casting.

The instruments, materials, and environment for lubricating and blocking out the die are common to the waxing procedure. This phase of die preparation is demonstrated in Section 12.

SUMMARY

Meticulous preparation of dies is an important phase of the entire process of constructing restorations, because the die is the foundation on which the technician builds.

After gross trimming, each die should be carefully examined to evaluate definition of, and access to, the margin. Contour of the pattern margin may sometimes be indicated by the recorded, unprepared tooth surface adjacent to the margin. The validity of this indication depends primarily upon its relation to the cervical line of the tooth. If the "indicating" surface is coronal to the cervical line, it is usually valid; if apical to the cervical line, it probably is invalid. When there is no valid tooth surface indication, only knowledge of dental anatomy and the contour of adjacent teeth can guide the technician to an acceptable marginal contour, as soft tissue contour is not recorded on a die.

Carving of the wax pattern margin is facilitated by a distinct angle of the submarginal die surface with the prepared surface of the die. When this angulation does not occur naturally, it is established by ditching the die. *If there is any question as to the exact location of the cavosurface angle of margin at any point on a die, the entire die should be examined by the dentist.* Ideally the dentist should examine and ditch, where indicated, every die.

Development of a reasonably contoured, accurately fitting margin is the most important challenge facing the technician involved in developing dental castings. Proper preparation of the die is a significant, indeed indispensible, aid to the success of developing an excellent wax pattern.

REVIEW QUESTIONS

1. List the three steps for the preparation of dies.
2. Describe how preliminary access to the margin of a die is usually best obtained.
3. What is the most significant step in the preparation of a die?
4. Discuss the statement that "accuracy of a die is not created; it is only maintained."
5. What is the purpose(s) of ditching a die?

SECTION 8

Developing Working Casts from Transfer Impressions

Individual dies of prepared teeth obtained from band impressions are of no real value as such. Until relationships with adjacent and opposing teeth are established, little progress can be made toward developing the pattern for a restoration. Relationships for a single restoration can be established by the dentist's carving the contour of the wax pattern directly in the mouth, then transferring the pattern to the individual die for completion of margins. This is termed the *direct-indirect technique* for developing a wax pattern. Now that accurate elastic materials and techniques for tray impressions are widely available, it is rarely used.

If the wax patterns are to be made by the technician (indirect technique), some type of working cast must be developed. There are a number of ways that anatomic relationships may be recorded in the mouth and transferred to the laboratory for conversion into a working cast. These procedures are known as *transfer techniques*, and the resultant working cast is often termed a *transfer cast*. Because so many different transfer techniques are used, identification of each is impractical. This section gives an explanation of the general principles involved, and representative examples.

TRAY IMPRESSIONS

The most straightforward and accurate approach to transferring oral relations to the laboratory for indirect construction of onlays, crowns, or bridges is the tray impression using hydrocolloid or rubber impression material. Such impressions, when complete and developed from quality material properly handled, provide accurate duplication of pre-pared teeth and adjacent structures. Thus the tray impression provides all the relations needed for laboratory construction of a restoration, except occlusion. Why, then, is any other approach to duplication of oral structures ever used? The answer is simple. Tray impressions, especially of full crown preparations, may be difficult and on occasion (for all practical purposes) impossible to accomplish. In such cases copper band impressions are used, resulting in individual dies.

TRANSFER IMPRESSIONS

When band impressions are used to register individual preparations, some additional impression is needed to record anatomic relationships and transfer them to the laboratory. Several types of impressions are used to provide such a duplication of oral relationships; as a group they are referred to as *transfer* or *relationship impressions*. They provide a means of transferring from the mouth to a working cast the relationship of prepared teeth to one another and to the adjacent unprepared teeth in the arch.

SEMIACCURATE TRANSFER IMPRESSIONS

The most simple means for transfer in single crown situations is the semiaccurate transfer impression: a tray impression of the supragingival portion of prepared teeth and adjacent structures, which can be

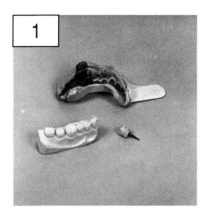
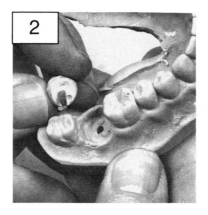
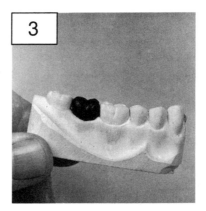
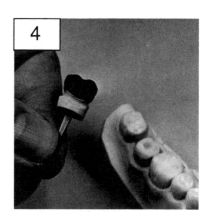

made with a wide variety of materials—wax, compound, plaster, zinc oxide pastes, rubber, alginate, hydrocolloid, and others. These impressions are intended to serve as a mechanism of transferring oral relationships into a working cast without the requirement of recording preparation margins.

They may be used in any of three ways: poured as a solid cast, poured as a cast with removable dies, or individual dies may be seated in the impression and the cast poured about them. The objective of such impressions is not to record margins but to provide a reasonably accurate transfer of intra-arch relationships.

Figures 1 through 4   Impressions taken with elastic materials are usually used by pouring a solid cast (**Figure 1**) or a cast with removable dies (**Figure 2**). When a solid cast is poured, stone representing soft tissue contours about the preparation is removed, providing access to all accurately reproduced surfaces of the preparation. A pattern can then be grossly established on this cast using the relationships provided (**Figure 3**). Obviously this technique is restricted by poor access, especially in the interproximal areas. Nevertheless a gross pattern thus developed can be transferred to an individual die for completion of contour and development of the final margin (**Figure 4**).

Probably the best technique for handling an elastic impression is to treat it just like an accurate tray impression. It can be poured so as to provide a working cast with a removable die, using either the stripping or double pour section technique. When this is done, the dies are removed and trimmed to their terminal point of accuracy. The wax pattern can then be developed on this working cast and transferred to

the individual die for completion of the margin. If duplication of the axial walls of the preparation is limited, the sequence might be changed so that the pattern is initiated on the individual die, then transferred to the working cast for completion of gross contour, then repositioned on the individual die for completion of the margin.

Obviously a significant portion of the preparation must be common and accurate to both the working cast die and the individual die if such transfers are to be completed accurately. The dentist must be acutely aware of this in terms of cement bases which might be present in the preparation. Often these may become dislodged when one of the impressions is taken and thus absent when the other impression is accomplished. The result is dies with different configurations, which makes transfer of a pattern very tedious or impossible.

Impressions made with rigid materials are usually used by seating the individual dies in the impression and pouring the cast about them. Relationships between the die and adjacent structures are thus established, and the wax pattern can be developed.

In either case, the probable errors incorporated in such techniques must be compensated. Crown patterns should be developed with slightly heavy contacts and possibly should be slightly high in occlusion, depending upon the type of occlusal record employed. If such an approach must be used for a bridge situation, at least one joint (connector) is left open to compensate for possible error in the relationship of the two dies. A final, accurate record of relationship is taken directly in the patient's mouth at the time the castings are trial-seated. This record, usually a plaster index, can then be used to relate the pieces accurately for soldering of the final joint.

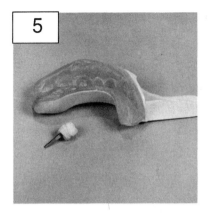

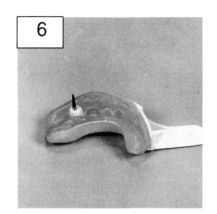

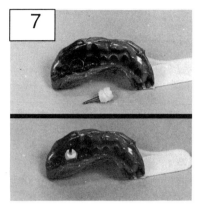

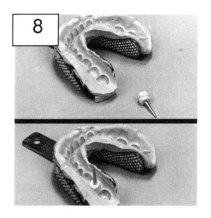

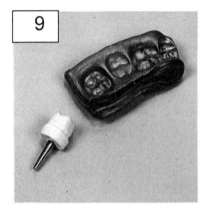

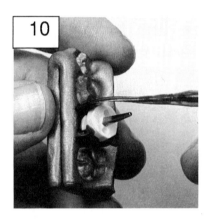

Figures 5 and 6   The critical factor in incorporating a die into a transfer impression (**Figure 5**) is finesse in seating the die into whatever impression material is being used.

Seating a die into a wax impression requires firm, positive pressure directing the die exactly into the void without rocking or tipping it. The greatest error in this technique occurs when sharp occlusoaxial angles on the die drag or scrape wax from the walls of the impression and force this wax ahead of the die into the impression. To ensure that such wax remnants do not prevent its complete seating the die should be almost completely seated, then removed and the impression carefully inspected for any displaced wax. After removal of any wax debris this procedure can be repeated until a positive seat of the die is obtained (see **Figure 6**).

Seating a die into a compound or plaster impression is much more

positive, but these impression materials are seldom used as it is difficult to remove them from the undercut areas presented by unprepared teeth in the mouth.

Figures 7 and 8   Seating a die into a flexible material is most uncertain. Because of their elasticity, rubber and alginate impressions provide an unstable index for the die. However, dies can be seated properly into these materials by gently "feeling" them into position. Once placed, dies can be maintained in position by sealing them to the impression with the wax that is used to block out the undercuts in root portions of the die. After the application of a suitable separating medium, the cast can be poured, using a minimum of vibration to avoid displacement of the die. Though this technique may yield a perfectly accurate working cast, the result is always uncertain.

Another commonly used semiaccurate transfer mechanism is the interocclusal record made with wax, zinc oxide paste, or impression material. The example described here is a procedure that uses a wax record.

Figure 9   Using a suitable thickness (probably ¼ to ⅜ inch) of an appropriately softened bite wax, a centric occlusion record is obtained in the quadrant involved. When chilled and removed, this wax record provides an occlusal index of the prepared and adjacent teeth in the involved quadrant, and an index of the occlusal surfaces of the opposing teeth related in centric occlusion.

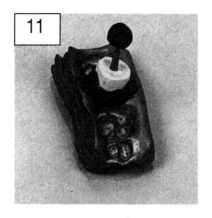

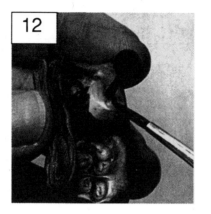

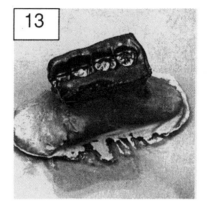

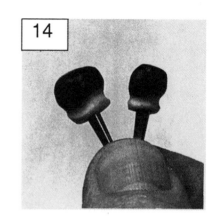

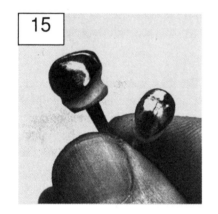

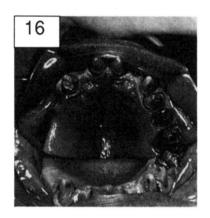

Figures 10 and 11   As described previously for the wax tray impression, the die is carefully seated into its index in the wax bite. This position is sealed by flowing wax about the undercut areas of the root portion of the die, being careful not to get wax in the record of adjacent teeth. Utility wax has been added to the end of the dowel, in this case, to facilitate maintenance of access to the dowel pin when the cast is poured.

Figures 12 and 13   Separating medium is applied to the exposed stone root surface. A strip of boxing wax or masking tape may be placed about the periphery of the wax impression. Stone is poured into the impression, duplicating the contours of the adjacent teeth and surrounding the die. When this stone has set, the impression and cast thus poured can be inverted and the wax bite wrapped again so as to box the opposing side of the impression. A stone pour is made to provide the

opposing cast. The result is a quadrant working cast and opposing cast related in centric occlusion. Before this assembly is separated, it is mounted in a suitable hinge articulator such that the occlusal relationship of the working cast and its opposing cast is maintained. Procedures for developing and relating opposing casts are covered in Section 10.

COPING TRANSFER IMPRESSIONS

Cast Metal Coping/Plaster Impression Transfer

The most accurate transfer impression technique when full crowns are involved is the cast metal coping/plaster transfer impression.

Figure 14   Copings are made by developing thimble-like wax patterns on the individual dies.

Figure 15   The patterns are invested and cast of any suitable alloy. The less expensive nonprecious alloys are commonly used.

Figure 16   A coping is made for each die to be incorporated in the working cast. Usually a plaster impression is used when all or most remaining teeth in the arch are prepared. Each tooth is coped for the transfer impression.

The copings are seated on the prepared teeth, and a plaster impression is made to record the copings and any edentulous ridge and/or adjacent teeth that may be necessary.

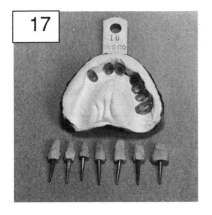

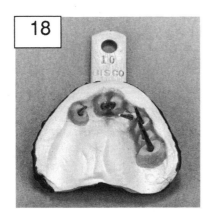

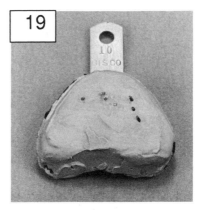

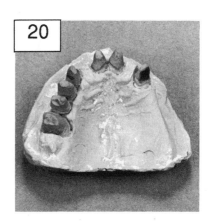

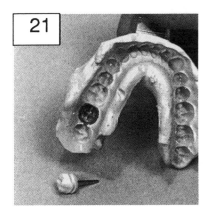

Figure 20 The result is a working cast with removable dies that are accurately related to one another and to other pertinent structures.

The purpose of the copings becomes apparent. They serve as an intermediate index to receive the die with definite relationship, and provide an appropriately contoured surface to ensure accurate indexing and seating in the plaster impression. To seat dies directly into a plaster impression without the intermediate coping index is often difficult and uncertain, as their form, size, and surface texture may well be unsuitable.

Figure 17 The impression is removed from the mouth. It may be necessary to remove the impression tray and then remove the plaster impression in segments. When this occurs, the segments (if large and not critical in terms of coping placement) can be carefully repositioned in the tray like a jigsaw puzzle. The segments are affixed to the tray with sticky wax, and the copings are accurately seated in the impression.

Figure 18 The dies are carefully seated in the copings and are sealed in place with wax, which also serves to block out undercuts. The base of the die must be kept clean, to permit establishing a stable seat between the die and the transfer cast.

Figure 19 A separating medium is applied to the plaster impression and all exposed portions of the dies. The cast is poured in stone.

Coping/Elastic Impression Transfer

The problem inherent in removing the rigid plaster impression from the mouth when unprepared teeth and/or bony undercuts are present has led to coping transfer techniques that use elastic impression materials. Two basic approaches are recognized.

Figure 21 The elastic impression of isolated copings transfer technique is similar to the semiaccurate procedure of seating an individual die directly into an elastic impression. The procedure can be made more certain by interposing a coping, especially when dies of badly broken down or small teeth are involved. Both cast copings and copings made of pattern resin (Duralay) are used.

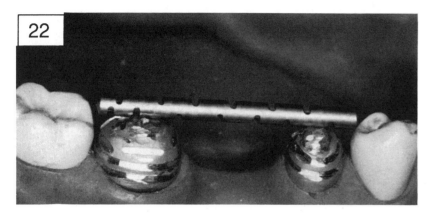

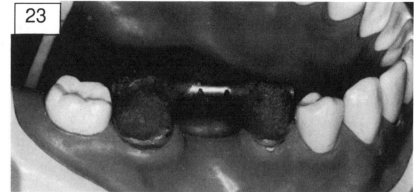

Figures 22 and 23   Elastic impression of connected copings. Although a slight error in relationship between multiple preparations to receive individual crowns might be manageable, an error in relation between multiple abutments for a rigid prosthesis can be irreparable. Most operators thus prefer in such cases to interconnect copings rigidly when transfer impressions are to be made with elastic impression material. Both cast copings and resin copings may be used for such procedures. Regardless of type of coping, the interconnection of copings is done with pattern resin. Edentulous spaces are connected via rigid metal bars. These bars are commonly made from straight handpiece bur shanks, cut to proper length. Multiple small notches are cut along the length of the rod to ensure that it will be locked absolutely into the resin (**Figure 22**).

Once all copings are placed and checked for accurate seating and appropriate retention, resin is added by brush-bead technique, either to tie adjacent copings together or to affix an interconnecting bar (**Figure 23**). If cast metal copings are being used, their surfaces must be made retentive by cutting notches and/or grooves prior to placement of the resin (**Figure 22**). Retention of the coping complex on the teeth must be carefully evaluated and, if necessary, adjusted so that the complex is stable but can be readily removed.

Once the transfer impression is accurately formed, the techniques for developing the working cast are essentially the same for all types of impressions.

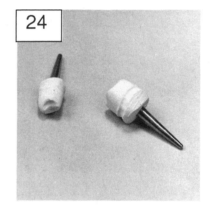

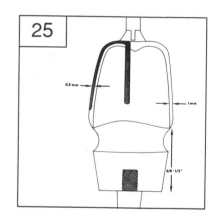

TECHNIQUES FOR COPING TRANSFER IMPRESSIONS

Development of Copings

Whichever type of impression material is used (plaster or elastic), the basic technical procedures are the same for a coping transfer.

Figure 24   Preparation for such an impression begins with development of the individual dies. They should be completely prepared: trimmed, ditched, and blocked out if indicated. If cast copings are to be used, wax patterns must be carefully developed with two particular considerations in mind.

First, *the patterns must be accurate in both gross and marginal adaptation*. Although marginal adaptation of the coping is not neces-

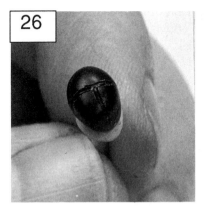

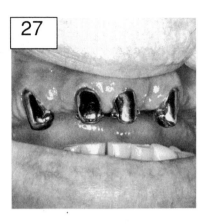

sary to accomplish an accurate transfer impression and subsequent working cast, it is necessary if advantage is to be taken of this opportunity to verify accuracy of the die. Other than providing an accurate means of transfer, the greatest value of the cast coping transfer technique is that it provides the opportunity to verify die accuracy by seating a casting accurate to the die on the corresponding prepared tooth for inspection. Failure to develop the transfer coping with accurate margins means loss of this important advantage.

Secondly, *the accuracy in adaptation of the pattern must be accomplished without damage to the die*. This concern is focused primarily on the marginal area. Abrasion of the die margin while carving the coping pattern will obviously render it inaccurate for development of the final wax pattern.

Figure 25 The coping pattern should be developed as a thimble of uniform thickness (between 0.5 and 1.0 millimeters). No "tooth-like" contouring is necessary or desirable, merely a uniform thimble-like cover. Patterns of this nature are most conducive to accurate casting. Another reason for maintaining minimum contour in the coping is that these patterns are developed on individual dies with no knowledge of proximal relationships. When the thickness of metal exceeds the 1.0-millimeter range, conflict between copings and adjacent teeth or between adjacent copings is easily possible (see **Figure 17**). Time and effort are saved by minimizing the possible necessity of grinding away interfering contour.

Figure 26 If the preparation does not cause a distinctly angular form in the external contour of the coping pattern, some alteration will be necessary to ensure accurate indexing of the coping in the impression. The simplest, most effective indexing for plaster impressions is by means of shallow longitudinal V-shaped grooves running one-half to two-thirds the length of the pattern, but not involving the marginal one-third. Unlikely as it may seem, copings have sometimes been erroneously seated in the impression (rotated 180°) when two or four symmetrically positioned grooves were used. To prevent this possibility, three grooves—involving three of the four axial surfaces—should be aligned with the long axis of the coping. *Do not develop undercuts that would later lock copings into plaster impressions.*

Figure 27 Two mechanisms are used for indexing copings in elastic impressions. Some operators prefer to coat the copings with appropriate adhesive, so that they will be "bonded" to the impression. Others prefer to develop one or two smoothly rounded blebs on the coping surface, so that they can be accurately reseated should they be removed inadvertently or intentionally.

When the wax patterns are complete, they should be invested and cast with the same care that a full gold crown casting would be given (see Sections 12 and 13). Keep in mind that the dies will be seated in these castings, and that the accuracy of the dies must not be altered.

Inspection of the coping casting also requires the same care that a restoration casting would receive. Careful inspection is imperative if the die is not to be damaged by blebs, fins, or other irregularities when the casting is seated. In this regard, if a *marginal drag* is evident as the casting is placed on the die, it may be wise lightly to burnish *out* the marginal edge of the coping. The die must not be scarred while developing the transfer cast, lest it be rendered useless for the final restoration.

Marginal accuracy must be checked when the coping is seated on the tooth. Polishing the coping is not necessary, only smoothing through the rubber wheel (Burlew) stage (see Section 15).

When the casting is completed (cleaned, smoothed, thoroughly inspected, and corrected if necessary) it should be carefully seated on its respective die. The fit must be absolutely definite, but placement must be accomplished with no scuffing or abrasion of the die, especially in the marginal area. When all copings are ready, the intraoral procedures involved in taking the transfer impression can be accomplished.

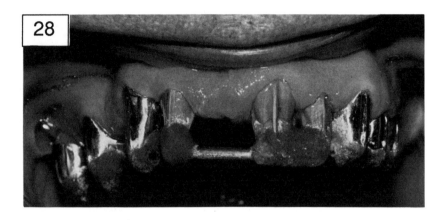

Taking the Impression

A full understanding of the coping transfer concept requires some consideration of the basic intraoral procedures involved. The first chairside procedure is removal of the temporary restoration(s) and careful debridement of the tooth (see **Figure 16**). The copings are then seated one at a time on their respective teeth and critically evaluated for marginal adaptation and complete seating. Some dentists desire an *inspection port* (a hole or slot at an appropriate area on the incisal or occlusal) to facilitate determination of complete seating. It is somewhat difficult to cut such a hole in the casting without creating some deformation—bending, burring, or dragging—of the metal surrounding the breakthrough. By whatever method, it must be assured that each and every coping is accurately seated and stable in its position.

When all copings are properly seated, the impression is made. If all teeth in the arch are prepared and coped, a straight plaster impression may be indicated unless marked soft tissue and bony undercuts are present and cannot be blocked out. The plaster impression may be taken in any sort of rigid, non-undercut tray. The conventional aluminum plaster impression trays are usually used. A tray that would lock the plaster within it is never used, as it might be necessary to remove the tray and section the plaster in order to execute its removal from the mouth. Such sectioning does not necessarily destroy the usefulness of the impression. If the segments are large and not too numerous, they can be reassembled accurately in the tray and maintained by appropriate application of sticky wax (see **Figure 17**).

If unprepared teeth remain in the arch or significant bony undercuts are present, an elastic impression is probably indicated. These impres-

sions are usually made with a rubber-base impression material. As mentioned, they may involve isolated copings or interconnected copings. These may be bonded to the impression with adhesive or indexed or locked by contour. When all copings are securely seated, the impression is made—usually by injecting material about the gingival regions and between copings and then carrying a tray filled with material into place so that the entire coping assembly as well as adjacent teeth and soft tissue are recorded (see **Figure 28**).

Assembly and Pouring of the Impression

If the impression was removed intact with all copings in place, the next step is to ensure their accurate seating and prepare to seat the dies in their respective copings. If the impression was of plaster and removed in segments, these must be carefully repositioned in the tray and maintained as indicated with sticky wax (see **Figure 17**). All loose particles must be blown away, and the pieces tediously repositioned in proper sequence. Copings that are pulled with the impression but partially displaced should be completely removed and repositioned after meticulous inspection and cleaning. Copings that were separated from the impression during its removal should be handled in like fashion. *All loose fragments of plaster must be removed from both coping and impression before any attempt is made to seat the coping.*

If the impression is an elastic material, it is important to make sure that the copings are firmly seated and that no tags of impression material are present about the margins that might interfere with seating the dies. If the copings have separated from the impression, any edges of material that might interfere with reseating them must be removed.

Two approaches to seating copings and dies are available: the copings may be seated and then the dies seated in the copings; or the copings can be placed on the dies and the combination seated in the impression. Which technique is best depends on individual preference and the coping-die, coping-impression relationships. The latter method is generally preferred. At times further trimming of the root portions of the dies may be necessary to prevent conflict between dies as they are seated (see **Figure 18**). The root portions of the dies must be trimmed so as to *draw*: they should be ground to taper in the same directions as their dowel pins if this has not already been adequately accomplished.

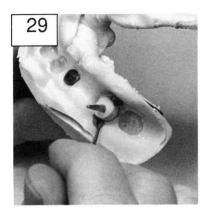
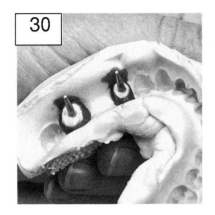
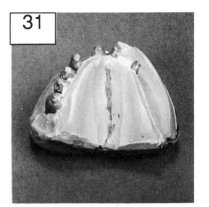
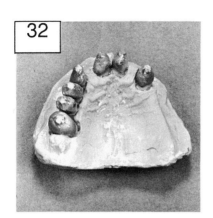

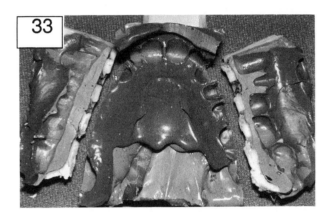

Dies with stone root forms (no dowel pins) must be tapered and flats or grooves created to index their position in the working cast.

Figure 29   Instability of the die and coping in the impression may be readily resolved by anchoring the coping and die to the impressions with sticky wax.

Figure 30   When seating of all units (dies and copings) is complete and verified, this relation is fixed and undercuts about the root portion of the dies are blocked out by flowing wax between the dies and copings. Utility wax or baseplate wax may be used as preferred. A suitable gypsum separator is applied to exposed portions of the dies and to all exposed plaster. A mix of stone sufficient to pour the cast is made. Pouring should be accomplished carefully to avoid air bubbles, *but using a minimum of vibration to avoid displacement of a die or coping.*

Removing the Working Cast from the Impression

After the stone is completely set, the cast and impression must be separated. This is a critical procedure, as it is very easy to break dies during separation of the cast and impression. Only one *sure* technique is available.

Figures 31, 32, 33   First, the impression tray is removed from the impression. This should be readily accomplished, as no undercuts are present in the tray. Next, the plaster is scored along the crest (occlusal portion) of the arch form with a suitable knife. This groove should be deepened progressively until the occlusal portion of all copings is exposed. For maxillary plaster impressions an additional groove should be cut through the plaster in the center of the palatal portion of the impression. Lateral scores are developed through the facial wall of plaster and joined with the occlusal score, thus isolating segments of the plaster impression. Each segment may be removed with moderate prying pressure directed so as to break it away from the coping(s) and die(s). This procedure is repeated progressively about the arch facially and then lingually, until all plaster is removed.

A similar approach may well be appropriate for coping/elastic impressions—especially when anterior or fragile posterior dies are involved. Assuming that a plastic impression tray has been used, the tray itself can be sectioned by carefully cutting with a disk or bur in the same manner described for sectioning the plaster impression. Segments of

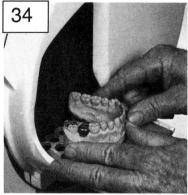
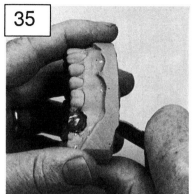
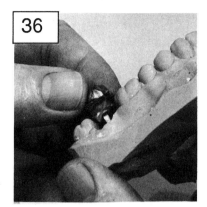
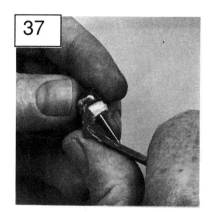

the tray can be removed from the elastic impression material. The impression material can then be removed in segments or in entirety as desired.

Figure 34 If the cast needs to be trimmed on a model trimmer, this must be done *now*, before any dies (and preferably before any copings) are removed.

Figures 35 and 36 When all of the impression plaster is cleared, the dies (with copings) are removed. If necessary, any wax that is present may be softened with warm water or preferably by placing the cast on top of a burnout oven (or in some other warm environment) before removing the dies.

Figure 37 All wax and debris is cleaned away from cast and dies.

Figure 38 Any rough flanges of stone from the cast are trimmed off. A final inspection should make sure that no debris is present on the die or cast, especially in the dowel pin hole.

Figure 39 (also 20) Each die is carefully seated in place. An accurate working cast is now complete.

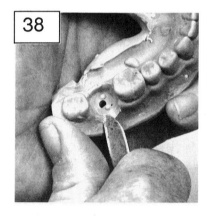
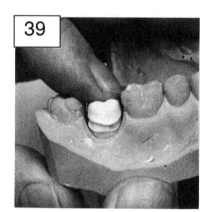

REVIEW QUESTIONS

1. What is the most accurate way to transfer oral relations to the laboratory for indirect restorative procedures?
2. Tray impressions provide all the relationships necessary for laboratory procedures except one. Name and discuss.
3. What are copings, and what purpose do they serve?
4. Discuss the reason for the removal of fragments of plaster from the coping and impression before seating the copings in the impression prior to pouring the impression.
5. Discuss the procedure for separating the working cast from the impression when plaster is used in the coping transfer technique.

SECTION 9

Occlusion

Webster's Unabridged Dictionary defines *occlusion* relating to dentistry as "the bringing of the opposing surfaces of the teeth of the two jaws into contact; also, the relation between the surfaces when in contact." Ramfjord and Ash's textbook *Occlusion* defines occlusion as "the closure of the dental arches and the various functional movements with maxillary and mandibular teeth making contact." Implied in this definition is the interrelationship between "the anatomic alignment of the teeth and the rest of the masticatory system."

An ideal occlusion consists of an essentially perfect anatomic arrangement and alignment of teeth resulting in: (1) stable vertical relationship of the jaws in centric, (2) harmony of contact of the teeth in the functioning segments of the arches, and (3) absence of contact between teeth in the nonfunctioning segments of the arches during eccentric excursions.

The nature of tooth contacts that occur in centric closure and during eccentric movement of the lower jaw have been demonstrated to have a profound effect on the health of the periodontium, muscles, and temporomandibular joints (TMJs). Obviously the ideal contact patterns of teeth occurring in centric and during jaw movement must be thoroughly understood before one can develop restorations that preserve the health of these structures.

MORPHOLOGIC OCCLUSION

A review of the anatomic characteristics of occlusion is appropriate, as these relationships are the basis for functional occlusion.

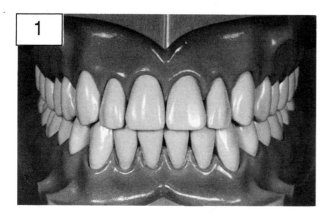

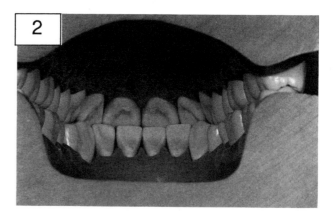

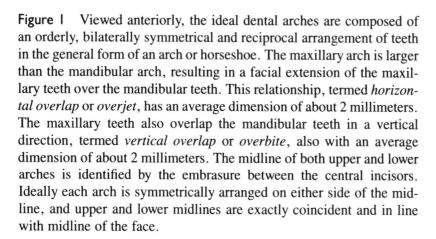

Figure 1 Viewed anteriorly, the ideal dental arches are composed of an orderly, bilaterally symmetrical and reciprocal arrangement of teeth in the general form of an arch or horseshoe. The maxillary arch is larger than the mandibular arch, resulting in a facial extension of the maxillary teeth over the mandibular teeth. This relationship, termed *horizontal overlap* or *overjet*, has an average dimension of about 2 millimeters. The maxillary teeth also overlap the mandibular teeth in a vertical direction, termed *vertical overlap* or *overbite*, also with an average dimension of about 2 millimeters. The midline of both upper and lower arches is identified by the embrasure between the central incisors. Ideally each arch is symmetrically arranged on either side of the midline, and upper and lower midlines are exactly coincident and in line with midline of the face.

Figure 2 Viewed from the lingual, the reciprocal overlap relationship is apparent: the mandibular teeth overlap the maxillary teeth both horizontally and vertically. The functional significance of overlap is described later under the heading Factors That Influence the Articulation of Natural Teeth.

Figure 3 Viewing one-half of the arches, the specifically ordered occlusal arrangement of the teeth is evident. Detailed evaluation of these relationships is the next subject for consideration, but some of the general features should be recognized here as morphologic landmarks. The mandibular teeth are mesial to corresponding maxillary teeth. This general relation is classically exampled at two points.

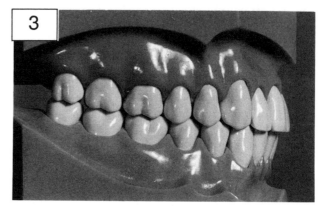

The mesiofacial cusp of the maxillary first molar occludes with the occlusofacial groove of the mandibular first molar. The mandibular canine occludes on the mesial half of the lingual surface of the maxillary canine. Thus the mandibular teeth are ideally one-half cusp-width mesial to the corresponding maxillary tooth. This arrangement results in each tooth occluding with two opponents, with two exceptions: the mandibular central incisor and the maxillary third molar. This classic pattern is termed a "tooth-to-two-tooth" occlusion. Variations to both the distal and mesial occur as Class II or III malocclusions. One must become quite familiar with the ideal morphologic characteristics of occlusion, so that variations and their functional implications can be readily recognized.

FUNCTIONAL OCCLUSION

The term *morphologic occlusion* relates to the static anatomic arrangement and relationship of teeth. The term *functional occlusion* refers to the dynamics of occlusion. There are two aspects or implications of functional occlusion: the activity of the muscles and joints that produces mandibular movement, and the contact relationships of teeth and the factors that influence or determine these relationships. For obvious reasons, the focus here is on the latter.

There are three basic criteria for a successful functional occlusion: (1) stable centric occlusion, (2) appropriate functional occlusion, and (3) adequate nonfunctional disclusion. Understanding the rationale and specifics of these criteria is essential, as they are inherently important to all occlusal contact relationships.

INTERRELATIONSHIP OF MORPHOLOGIC AND FUNCTIONAL OCCLUSION

From the discussion above, one can quickly determine that an "ideal" occlusion is one that presents an ideal morphologic arrangement of teeth that are so related as to satisfy all three fundamental requirements for a successful functional occlusion. The interrelationship between the morphologic arrangement of teeth and their functional potential is so precise that any variation in ideal morphology will affect functional occlusion. However, many of these variations are not sufficiently significant to cause the functional occlusion to be unsuccessful. Frequently a nonideal morphologic occlusion can be functionally successful due to the capacity of the muscles and TMJs to accommodate or adapt to dysfunctional circumstances under the control of the proprioceptive mechanism—the same neuromuscular control that allows you to close your eyes and still be able to move your arm so precisely that you can touch the tip of your nose. In the strict sense, any occlusion that is not morphologically correct or does not satisfy each requirement of a successful functional occlusion is not "ideal." However, since this is the usual circumstance for the overwhelming majority of the population, most such occlusions must be recognized as "normal."

Variations from ideal that often result in normal occlusions include:

1. CR/CO discrepancy: tooth-dictated skid from CR to CO.
2. Malaligned teeth: rotated, tipped, supra- or infraerupted, resulting in altered horizontal and vertical overlap relations.
3. Noncompensated occlusal plane: cusp steepness, Curve of Spee and/or Wilson in excess of combined influence of anterior and posterior guidance.
4. Inadequate anterior guidance: although the result of malaligned teeth or jaws or excess wear, inadequate anterior guidance is so significant in impaired functional occlusion that it should bear independent recognition. The relative adequacy of anterior guidance is the key to the potential functional success of an occlusion. The importance of adequate anterior guidance is readily observable as one views the morphologic relationship of anterior teeth.

To understand these basic factors and be able to evaluate, adjust, or restore occlusion, one must develop an organized knowledge of mandibular movement, the patterns of tooth contact associated with mandibular motion, and the factors that influence these contact relationships of teeth. These are the subjects that are covered in this section.

CENTRIC OCCLUSION

The starting point for understanding occlusion is centric occlusion. *Centric occlusion* is the position of the lower jaw that results in maximum interdigitation of the teeth. *Centric relation* is the position of the lower jaw that occurs when the condyles are in their most physiologic fully seated position in the glenoid fossae. Closure of the jaw in a position of centric relation to the point of initial tooth contact results in centric occlusion (maximum interdigitation of the teeth) in only about 10 percent of the population. In most people the lower jaw will skid (from initial contact of the teeth in centric relation) forward and probably to one side or the other over a distance of 0.5 to 1.5 millimeters to centric occlusion. This is commonly referred to as a *CR/CO skid*.

A CR/CO skid has a profound effect on the stable vertical relationship of the jaws and is one of the most important and controversial aspects of the subject of occlusion. For the moment, however, let us bypass this condition and focus on what constitutes a stable vertical

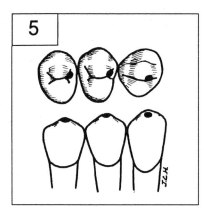

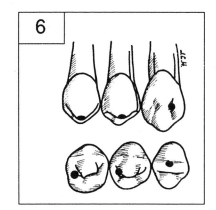

relationship of the *teeth* when they are in maximum interdigitation—that is, the specific positional and contact relationships of the ideal centric occlusion as it might exist in one of the 10 percent of people who have no CR/CO discrepancy. This focus will eventually bring us back to the nature and significance of the CR/CO skid.

The importance of centric occlusion is the stability of the vertical relationship of the jaws that results from the maximum interdigitated relationship of opposed teeth. Thus the most important question is the direction of forces that results from any given pattern of contact. Teeth are strongest and most stable when forces are directed along their long axes. Hence the basic positional aspects of centric interdigitation and their variations are the first factors to consider.

Faciolingual Interdigitation

As noted in the morphologic overview of occlusion, the maxillary arch of teeth is normally larger than the mandibular arch and overlaps it both horizontally and vertically. As a result, the lower incisors contact on the lingual inclines of the maxillary incisors. The facial cusps of the lower posterior teeth contact in the central groove zone of the upper posteriors. The lingual cusps of upper posterior teeth contact in the central groove zone of the lower posterior teeth. Thus in the posterior segments *the lower facial and upper lingual cusps are centric holding cusps*. When these cusps come into ideal contact in the faciolingual center of the opposing tooth, *the forces of vertical closure of the lower jaw are transmitted along the long axes of the opposed teeth*. However, if faciolingual interdigitation is slightly off, so that these cusps come into contact on inclines, the opposed teeth will tend to be tipped and displaced. Thus from the faciolingual aspect, ideal posterior centric

contact exists when the centric holding cusps (lower facial and upper lingual) are in stable contact in the faciolingual center (central groove zone) of the opposing tooth, resulting in axially oriented forces.

Figure 4 The *cusp tips* that are involved in centric contacts are the *lower incisal edges and the facial cusps of mandibular posterior teeth and the lingual cusps of maxillary posterior teeth*. Faciolingually there are two ranges of centric contact for each posterior tooth: a cusp tip contact and a fossa or marginal ridge contact. When speaking of the posterior teeth collectively these two areas are referred to as the *facial and lingual ranges of centric contact*. Anterior teeth have only one range of centric contact.

Figure 5 The *facial range* of centric contact occurs where the lower incisal edges contact the lingual of the maxillary incisors and the mandibular facial cusps contact in the central groove region of the opposing maxillary teeth. The example shown here, involving canines and premolars, identifies the lower facial centric holding cusp tips and the approximate location of their contact in the central zone of the corresponding upper teeth.

Figure 6 The *lingual range* of centric contact exists only in the posterior segment, as it is established by the maxillary lingual cusp tips contacting in the central zone of the opposing mandibular teeth. Illustrated here are the centric holding maxillary lingual cusp tips and the approximate location of their contact in the central zone of the corresponding lower tooth.

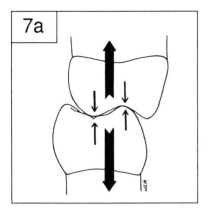

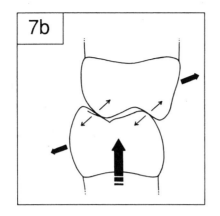

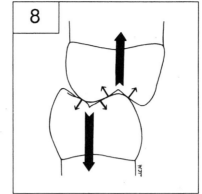

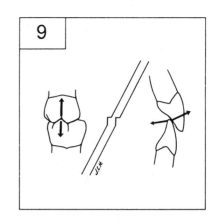

Note that in each figure centric contact is illustrated on the canines. Does this mean that there are two ranges of centric contact on the canines? Obviously the dual range of centric contact is only possible on the multicusp posterior teeth. Closer observation should reveal that the canine centric contact is in line with the facial range of centric contacts. The unique position of the canine as the "cornerstone" of the arch results in anatomic and functional characteristics that are transitional between the anterior and posterior teeth. As related to centric occlusion, the canine is like the anterior teeth, having only one range of contact that occurs on the incisal edge of the lower and lingual surface of the upper. Because these are inclined surfaces, anterior centric contacts are not vertically stable.

Figure 7a   Having two zones of contact on the posterior teeth helps to ensure that the *forces of centric closure will be directed along the long axis of the tooth*.

Figure 7b   Obviously very little variation in the faciolingual location of centric contacts could occur and still result in axially oriented forces, as such shifting would place the contacts on inclines. The simplest, most effective, and surest way to impose an axially oriented force between two bodies is to load a very convex surface against a flat surface. Thus a relatively convex cusp tip loaded against a relatively horizontal opposing tooth surface will impose a force in line with the path of closure.

Figure 8   Frequently the surface against which the cusp tip closes is not horizontal. Contact on such an incline will tend to tip the teeth.

However, if the incline contact is balanced by equal contact on an opposing incline, this wedge-like contact might well be resolved to an axial orientation. At the same time that we visualize this, it might be well to realize that the farther up the inclines these contacts occur, the more difficult it will be to time and equate them to result in an axially oriented force.

Figure 9   This direction of force along their long axis is the primary reason that posterior teeth are better able to withstand the force of vertical closure and hence maintain occlusal vertical dimension than are the anterior teeth. Normally the forces on anterior teeth are so tangential that if posterior support is lost, the anterior teeth will be pushed out of position by the force of closure. Because the lower anterior teeth form an arch inside the curvature of the upper arch, the forces imposed by closure push them together to produce a buttressing effect. In contrast, the upper anterior teeth are forced facially and apart from one another. The resultant "flaring out" of the upper anteriors is recognized as one of the cardinal signs of *posterior bite collapse*.

Obviously this could occur as a result of loss of all posterior teeth. But it can also occur due to the loss of just one or two posterior teeth, which permits the remaining teeth to tip or supererupt out of position. This "united we stand, divided we fall" principle has many examples in the stability of occlusion.

Variations in Faciolingual Interdigitation

As with all aspects of occlusion, variations from ideal faciolingual

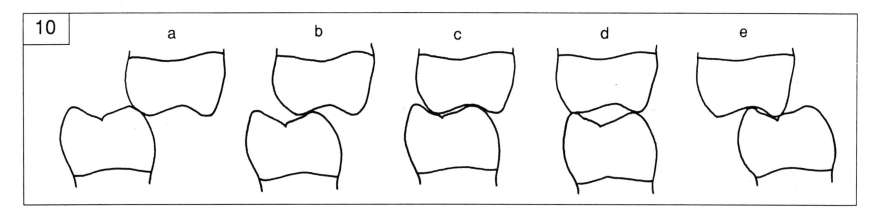

10   a   b   c   d   e

interdigitation (**Figure 10c**) are fairly common. Obviously such discrepancies may occur in one of two directions—toward the facial or toward the lingual. They may result from malalignment of one or both members of a pair of opponents, or from a general discrepancy in size and position of the arches. Because the maxillary arch is static and the mandibular arch is the mover, positional relationships are usually spoken of in terms of the location of the lower tooth in relation to its maxillary opponent.

Linguoversion   Any discrepancy toward the lingual will result in the lower facial cusp opposing the upper lingual cusp (**Figure 10b**). A one-half tooth-width discrepancy will result in opposition of the centric holding cusps. In extreme examples the lower tooth may close completely lingual to the maxillary opponent (**Figure 10a**). As stated, this may be due to malposition of a single opposed tooth or to a severe retrognathic (Class II) relation of the lower jaw, in which case one or more teeth on each side may be in complete linguoversion.

Facioversion   Discrepancy in the opposite direction (toward the facial) may result in the lower facial cusp opposing the upper facial cusp. Obviously this will also mean that the lower lingual cusp will be opposite the upper lingual cusp. This cusp-to-cusp relation is commonly referred to as an *end-on occlusion* (**Figure 10d**). More extreme facioversion may result in the lower facial cusps being completely facial to the upper facial cusps. This results in the upper facial cusps occluding in the central fossa of the lower opponent and the lower lingual cusps occluding in the central fossa of the upper. Thus the normally noncentric holding cusps become the centric holding cusps. This relation is known as a *crossbite*, and though abnormal it can have

adequate potential for centric stability (**Figure 10e**). This is in marked contrast to the obviously less stable "end-on" relationship.

As evidenced by these examples it becomes obvious that Class II (retrognathic) jaw relationships promote linguoversion and Class III (prognathic) relationships promote a facioversion of the lower teeth.

Mesiodistal Interdigitation

In the ideal morphologic and functional occlusal arrangement, the overlap of the maxillary arch would appear to mean that the maxillary teeth are anterior to their mandibular opponents. This is obviously true in the anterior segment where the maxillary incisors extend facial or anterior to their mandibular counterparts. However, close observation reveals that in the posterior segments the mandibular teeth are in fact anterior to their maxillary counterparts. *Key landmarks are the first molars, where the upper mesiofacial cusp occludes opposite the facial groove of the lower molar, and the canines, where the lower canine cusp tip occludes on the mesial aspect of the lingual surface of the upper canine.* Thus the lower posterior teeth are one-half cusp-width anterior to the upper posterior teeth, and yet the lower incisors are lingual or posterior to the upper incisors. The transition occurs at the canines and is obviously possible because the lower incisors are in fact so very much smaller mesiodistally than the maxillary incisors.

If it seems inconsistent to think of the lower posterior teeth being anterior to their maxillary counterparts and the lower anterior teeth being posterior to their counterparts, a simple solution is available: change the terminology. In fact all of the lower teeth are *mesial* to their upper counterparts by one-half cusp-width. Here again, it is possible

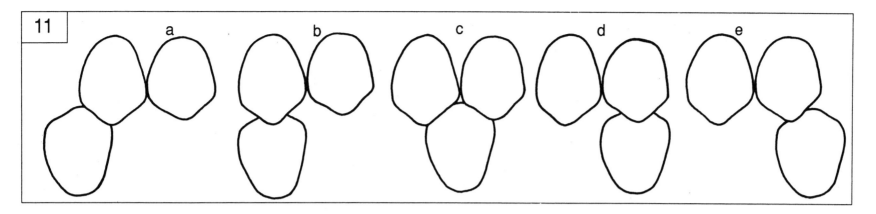

11   a   b   c   d   e

for the lower teeth to be mesial and yet lingual to the maxillary teeth, because of the smaller dimension of the lower arch. Further study of the normal mesiodistal interdigitation of teeth reveals that this arrangment results in each tooth occluding with two opponents, with two exceptions: the lower central incisors and the maxillary third molars (or if third molars are not present, the maxillary second molars). This is referred to as a *tooth-to-two-tooth occlusion* and is classically represented by the lower second premolar interdigitated between the upper first and second premolars (**Figure 11c**).

Referring back to **Figure 5**, one can now consider the mesiodistal location of these facial range contacts. The lower premolar cusp tips contact the opposing maxillary premolars in the area of the mesial marginal ridge. This pattern of centric contact means that during lateral function the lower cusp will pass through the embrasure to the mesial of the corresponding upper cusp. For example, the lower first premolar passes through the embrasure between the upper first premolar and canine. Stated generally, the lower posterior teeth normally interdigitate one-half cusp-width mesial to the corresponding upper tooth (**Figure 11c**).

The mesiodistal location of the lingual range centric contacts can be seen in **Figure 6**. Whereas the lower facial cusps contact the mesial aspect of the corresponding upper tooth, the centric-holding upper lingual cusps contact the distal aspect of the corresponding lower tooth. Thus there is one-half cusp-width difference in the mesiodistal location of the facial and lingual range centric contacts.

Variations in Mesiodistal Interdigitation

As with faciolingual interdigitation, a broad range of variations may occur in mesiodistal relations.

Distoversion As described in the discussion of faciolingual interdigitation, the lower jaw may be displaced distally in relation to the upper arch (Class II), resulting in the lower facial cusps occluding mesiodistally in line with the upper facial and lingual cusps (**Figure 11b**). This represents a half-cusp mesiodistal discrepancy and results in a *tooth-to-tooth occlusion* rather than the normal tooth-to-two-tooth occlusion. This discrepancy may be even more severe, causing closure of the lower posterior teeth with a full cusp-width (or more) distal displacement (**Figure 11a**). In the most extreme variation, the lower jaw may be so retrognathic that the lower teeth are all completely lingual to the teeth in the upper arch.

Mesioversion Variation may also occur with the lower jaw being displaced anteriorly or mesially (Class III). As described in the discussion of the faciolingual variations, this causes the lower arch to be larger or more prominent facially in relation to the upper arch, resulting in an end-on or even a crossbite relationship. Obviously in the end-on relation there is a half-cusp mesial displacement (**Figure 11d**); in the crossbite relation this discrepancy may be a full cusp-width or more (**Figure 11e**). Again the end-on Class III relationship (lower facial cusps opposing upper facial cusps and lower lingual cusps opposing upper lingual cusps) may also produce tooth-to-tooth rather than tooth-to-two-tooth interdigitation (**Figure 11d**).

Summary of Centric Interdigitation

Ideal occlusal interdigitation results in the centric holding cusps contacting in the central groove zone of their opponents and the lower incisors contacting the lingual surfaces of the upper incisors. Mesiodistally the lower teeth are mesial to their upper counterparts by one-half cusp-width resulting in a tooth-to-two-tooth occlusion.

Variations in faciolingual relationship may occur as a result of malposition of one or both members of an opposed tooth pair. They may also occur as a result of posterior (Class II) or anterior (Class III) displacement of the lower jaw. Faciolingual discrepancies may range from the lower tooth being completely lingual to the upper, to the lower facial cusp occluding with the upper lingual, through normal interdigitation, to an end-on relation, or finally to a full crossbite.

Except when teeth are missing, or spaced as a result of a tooth/arch size discrepancy, all mesiodistal variations are due to positional displacement (Class II or III) of the lower arch in relation to the upper arch. Mesiodistal variation may range from the lower teeth being a full cusp-width or more distal (Class II) through normal interdigitation, to an end-on occlusion, and finally more severe anterior displacements of the lower jaw, resulting in posterior and even anterior crossbite occlusion (Class III).

Clearly no specific pattern of centric interdigitation can be identified for all patients. Yet if good occlusion is to be part of the restorative result, every dentist and every technician involved in such treatment procedures must be able to recognize and generate a stable centric occlusion. In support of this understanding, knowledge of an ideal or classic pattern of contact is essential.

Centric Contacts

Knowing ideal interdigitation and having some appreciation for the range of variations that occur, consider now the specifics of centric contact. Suppose that you are a dentist faced with the challenge of achieving a full mouth reconstruction. All teeth have been previously covered with very poorly contoured crowns that have flat, ill-defined occlusal anatomy. The occlusion is so far off that the patient must close with the lower jaw forward and several millimeters to one side in order to find some sort of stable "bite." In other words, there is nothing to go by—all the normal or ideal dental (tooth) occlusion landmarks have been destroyed. It is your job to redesign this problem—to determine centric relation position of the jaw, to determine and achieve adequate anterior guidance, to decide what functional occlusal arrangement would be most appropriate, whether the occlusal vertical dimension is correct, and so on. Let us assume that all of these factors are determined and focus strictly on the question of how to arrange and contour the occlusal surfaces to provide a centric occlusion that will result in a stable vertical relationship of the jaws. Although the position of the teeth (roots) in such a case may not permit an ideal centric interdigitation, you will not know this unless you do in fact know *what is* an ideal centric contact pattern.

An ideal centric occlusion is one that provides:

1. *Location* of centric contacts such that forces of vertical closure are resolved along the long axes of the opposed teeth.
2. *Distribution* of these contacts to involve support from all teeth. (The incisors will be passive in relation to posterior teeth.)

3. *Timing* of contacts such that they occur simultaneously (within 10 microns).
4. *Relationship* of the opposed patterns of contact that establishes a physiologically acceptable position of the condyles in the temporomandibular joints.

Pattern of Centric Contact   As with all aspects of occlusion, numerous variations in the pattern of centric contacts occur. However, there are two basic pattern concepts—the natural and gnathologic. The focus here is on the natural pattern of centric contact and its variations, with some allusions to gnathologic concepts. Knowing the patterns of centric contacts requires a learned or memorized response like learning the ABCs or multiplication tables. Centric contacts are normally identified by describing the location of the contact made by the involved cusp. In the anterior quadrant the lower incisal edges are the "cusps" in centric and functional occlusal relations. The review given below covers each contact in sequence for one-half of the arches.

Natural Pattern of Centric Contact: Location of Contacts
Figure 12   Central Incisors   Incisogingivally the lower central incisor contacts the lingual surface of the maxillary central incisor, ideally in the middle one-third. This location may vary from the cingulum to the incisal edge. Mesiodistally the mesioincisal corner of the lower central contacts the mesial marginal ridge of the upper central, and the distoincisal third contacts at about the mesiodistal center of the upper lingual fossa. With wear there may be a continuous line of contact along the facioincisal angle of the lower central and the lingual surface of the upper central. This is a tooth-to-tooth relationship for the lower central incisors.

Figure 13   Lateral Incisors   Incisogingivally the lower lateral incisor ideally contacts the lingual surface of the maxillary central and lateral incisors in the middle one-third. This location may vary from the cingulum to the incisal edge. Mesiodistally the mesioincisal corner of the lower lateral incisor contacts the distal marginal ridge of the maxillary central incisor. The distal one-third of the incisal edge of the lower lateral incisor contacts the mesial marginal ridge of the maxillary lateral incisor. This is a tooth-to-two-tooth relationship.

Figure 14   Canines   Incisogingivally the lower canine ideally contacts the lingual surface of the maxillary lateral incisor and canine in the middle one-third. This location may vary from the cingulum to the incisal edge.

Mesiodistally the prominent mesioincisal corner of the lower canine contacts the distal marginal ridge of the upper lateral incisor, and the cusp tip or distal arm of the lower canine contacts the upper canine on its mesial half. This is a tooth-to-two-tooth relationship.

Figure 15   First Premolars   Faciolingually the lower first premolar interdigitates with its facial cusp in the central groove zone of the upper first premolar. The lingual cusp of the upper first premolar occludes in the central groove zone of the lower first premolar.

Mesiodistally, when viewed from the facial, the lower first premolar is positioned between the upper canine and first premolar, which characterizes the tooth-to-two-tooth occlusion. Ideally the facial cusp tip of the lower first premolar contacts the center of the mesial marginal ridge of the upper first premolar. Within normal limits this contact may vary from the distal marginal ridge of the upper canine to the mesial pit of the upper first premolar. The lingual cusp tip of the upper first premolar ideally contacts the center of the distal marginal ridge of the lower first premolar. Within normal limits this contact may vary from the distal pit of the lower first premolar to the mesial marginal ridge of the lower second premolar.

By virtue of their being the first multicusp teeth in the arch, the first premolars provide the potential for initiation of the lingual range of centric contacts. However, this is frequently not the case, as the marked lingual slope of the occlusal surface of the lower first premolar often precludes contact with the lingual cusp of the upper first premolar.

Figure 16   Second Premolars   Faciolingually the facial cusp of the lower second premolar interdigitates in the central groove zone of the upper second premolar. The lingual cusp of the upper second premolar occludes in the central groove zone of the lower second premolar. Mesiodistally, as viewed from the facial, the lower second premolar is positioned between the upper first and second premolars. This is the classic example of the tooth-to-two-tooth occlusion.

Ideally the facial cusp tip of the lower second premolar contacts the center of the mesial marginal ridge of the upper second premolar.

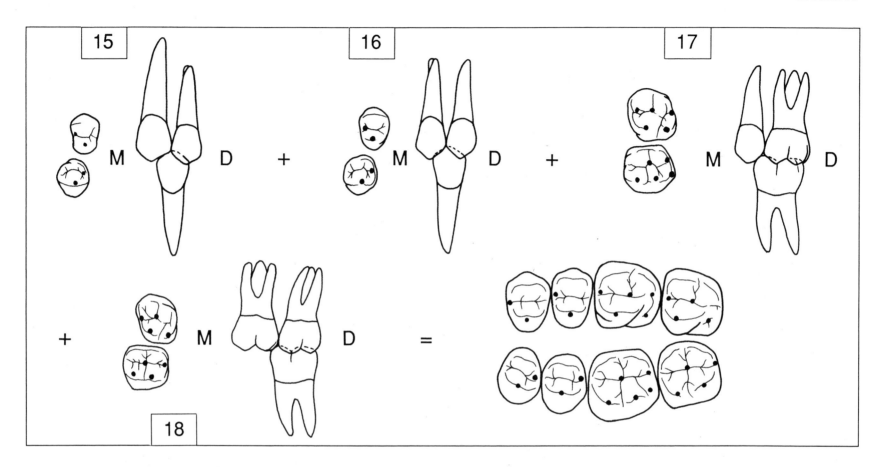

Within normal limits this contact may vary from the distal marginal ridge of the upper first premolar to the mesial pit of the upper second premolar. The lingual cusp of the upper second premolar contacts the center of the distal marginal ridge of the lower second premolar. Within normal limits this contact may vary from the distal pit of the lower second premolar to the mesial marginal ridge of the lower first molar.

It should also be noted that the tooth-to-two-tooth interdigitation makes it appear that the lower facial cusp tips contact in the opposed occlusal embrasure and that the cusp arms contact both of the adjacent marginal ridges in centric. Such "wedging" contact is undesirable, and stable contact must be provided directly by the cusp tip on one or the other of the marginal ridges—not in the embrasure.

Figure 17   First Molars   Faciolingually the facial cusps of the lower first molar contact in the central groove zone of the upper first molar.

The upper first molar lingual cusps contact in the central groove zone of the lower first molar. Mesiodistally the mesiofacial cusp of the lower first molar interdigitates positionally and functionally between the upper second premolar and first molar.

Ideally the lower mesiofacial cusp contacts the mesial marginal ridge of the upper first molar in centric. Within normal limits this contact may vary from the distal marginal ridge of the upper second premolar to the mesial pit of the upper first molar. Although lower facial cusps that interdigitate between adjacent upper teeth should contact one or the other of the marginal ridges in centric, the mesiofacial cusp of the lower first molar is the most likely exception. Because it is a very wide, blunt cusp, the mesiofacial cusp of the lower first molar may contact both the distal marginal ridge of the upper second premolar and the mesial marginal ridge of the upper first molar.

The distofacial cusp of the lower first molar contacts in the central fossa of the upper first molar and interdigitates functionally between the facial cusps of the upper molar. Within normal limits this contact may vary from the junction of the triangular ridges of the upper first molar mesial cusps to the oblique ridge.

The distal cusp of the lower first molar may or may not provide a centric contact. When it does, this contact will ideally occur on the distal marginal ridge of the upper first molar. Within normal limits this contact may vary between the distal pit of the upper first molar and the mesial marginal ridge of the upper second molar.

The mesiolingual cusp of the upper first molar contacts in the central fossa of the lower first molar and interdigitates between its lingual cusps. Within normal limits this contact may vary from the junction of the triangular ridges of the lower mesial cusps to the junction of the ridges of the distal and distolingual cusps.

The distolingual cusp of the upper first molar contacts the distal marginal ridge of the lower first molar. Within normal limits this contact may vary between the distal pit of the lower first molar and the mesial marginal ridge of the lower second molar.

In summary, there are potentially five centric holding contacts that occur between the first molars. Two of these occur from cusps occluding in the central fossa of the opposing molar: the upper mesiolingual cusp and the lower distofacial cusp. There are potentially three facial range contacts (from the three lower facial cusps) and two lingual range centric contacts.

The interdigitation of the upper mesiofacial cusp in the facial groove of the lower first molar is the posterior key or landmark in determining Angle's classification of occlusal relationship.

Figure 18 Second Molars Faciolingually the facial cusps of the lower second molar interdigitate in the central groove zone of the upper second molar. The lingual cusps of the upper second molar contact in the central groove zone of the lower second molar.

Mesiodistally the mesiofacial cusp of the lower second molar interdigitates between the upper first and second molars, providing the characteristic tooth-to-two-tooth relationship. Ideally the tip of the lower mesiofacial cusp contacts the mesial marginal ridge of the upper second molar in centric. Within normal limits this contact may vary from the distal marginal ridge of the upper first molar to the mesial pit of the upper second molar.

The distofacial cusp of the lower second molar contacts in the central fossa of the upper second molar. Within normal limits this contact may vary from the junction of the triangular ridges of the mesial cusps of the upper molar to its oblique ridge.

The mesiolingual cusp of the upper second molar contacts in the central fossa of the lower second molar. Within normal limits this contact may vary from the junction of the triangular ridges of the mesial cusps to the junction of the ridges of the distal cusps of the lower second molar.

The distolingual cusp of the upper second molar contacts the distal marginal ridge of the lower second molar. Within normal limits this contact may vary from the distal pit of the lower second molar to the mesial marginal ridge of the third molar if present.

In summary, there are four potential centric holding contacts between the second molars: two facial range and two lingual range. Although the lower second molar interdigitates mesiodistally in the usual tooth-to-two-tooth relationship, the upper second molar opposes only the lower second molar, leaving it in a tooth-to-tooth relation when third molars are not present.

Figure 19 Third Molars Contact relations for third molars are usually similar to the second molars. However anatomy of third molars is quite variable. The most common variations are three facial cusps on lower third molars and only one lingual cusp on upper third molars. **Figure 19** shows the complete pattern of ideal naturally occurring centric contacts. A perfect example of this ideal pattern probably does not exist in any human dentition, though some come very close.

Poded Centric Contacts
Figure 20 The simple point/surface (cusp tip/plateau) pattern of natural centric contact is often not possible when establishing contact in the central fossa of molar teeth. Unworn teeth with steep anatomy would require a spike cusp as sharp as an ice pick to create a single point contact in the central pit. Such a cusp point would obviously never occur naturally and would be dangerous if produced in a restoration—not to mention that it would probably interfere with excursive movements of the mandible. How, then, is centric contact support provided by such cusp/central fossa relationships?

Figure 21 Clearly the only possibility is that the slopes of the cusp tip contact the slopes forming the perimeter of the central pit. The classic example is the contact of the distofacial cusp of the lower first or second molar in the central fossa of the upper opponent. Three major inclines or slopes converge to form the central fossa of the upper molar: (1) the distal slope of the triangular ridge of the mesiofacial cusp, (2) the mesial slope of the triangular ridge of the distofacial cusp, and (3) the facial slope of the mesiolingual cusp. This topography lends itself to a wedging contact of the lower cusp between the three inclines—a *tri-poded contact*. The specific aspects of the lower cusp that form such a contact are the mesial arm, the distal arm, and the triangular ridge (lingual incline).

The number of inclines that converge to form the central pit deter-mines the number of "pods" in such contacts. For example, in the central fossa of the lower second molar four inclines converge to form the central pit. Accordingly the mesiolingual cusp of the upper second molar may form a "quadrapod" contact with this central fossa. Occa-sionally only two converging inclines are available to be contacted, and a bipod is formed. In any case the rationale for stability (resolution of force along long axis of teeth) in such contact relations is that contacts are "balanced" on opposed inclines—whether two, three, or four in number.

The disadvantage of such contact patterns is the difficulty in estab-lishing and maintaining stability. Although interdependent multiple contacts can readily be established on the wax pattern, they are difficult to adjust on a "high" casting and maintain perfect timing of each pod contact. More significantly, the situation becomes impossible if there is any discrepancy in faciolingual or mesiodistal alignment of the casting when inserted in the mouth. Under these circumstances one or more of the pods will be in premature contact, and *one or more of the pods will be out of contact, thus eliminating the "balance" from opposed incline contacts*. The probability that such a discrepancy will occur when the crown is initially fitted is very great. The probability that it will occur within the life span of a good crown is virtually absolute.

In summary, the advantage of the poded centric contact is the ca-pacity that it provides for creating a vertically stable contact in anatomi-cally deep fossae. The disadvantages are that (1) it seldom occurs naturally and (2) it is very difficult to create as a "stable" contact during occlusal adjustment of the natural dentition or of cast restorations. These contacts are usually rendered unstable by the necessity for ad-justment to compensate for error in the initial occlusal relation of

19

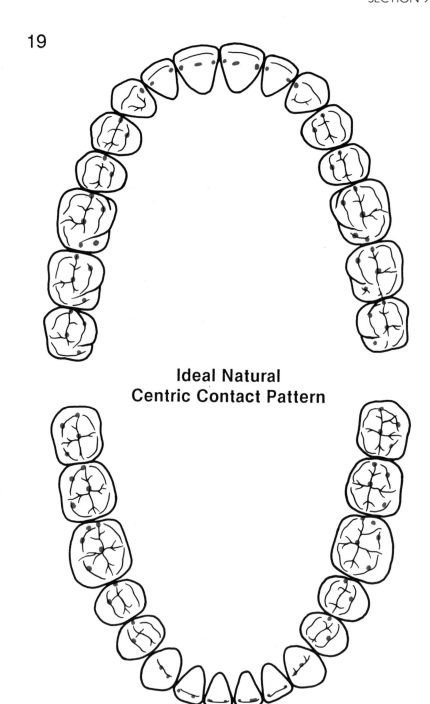

**Ideal Natural
Centric Contact Pattern**

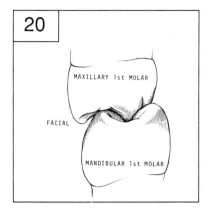

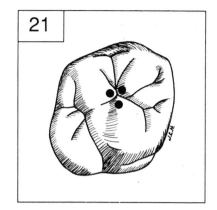

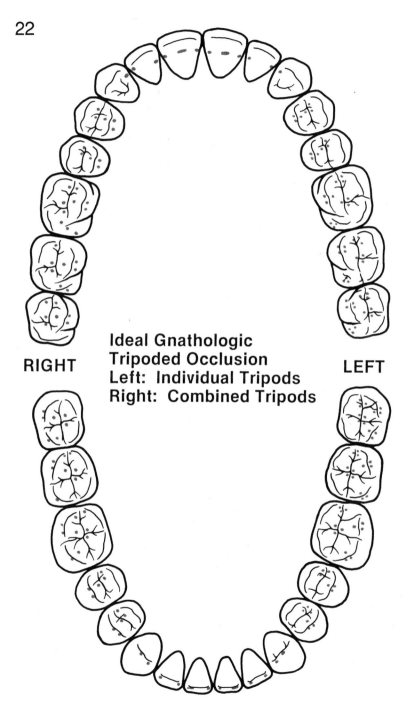

**Ideal Gnathologic
Tripoded Occlusion
Left: Individual Tripods
Right: Combined Tripods**

RIGHT   LEFT

castings and/or subsequent variation due to repositioning of teeth or the lower jaw.

Alternatives to the poded contact include the creation of a horizontal plateau or "saucer" recess in one of the inclines, approximating the base of the central fossa. All other (other than central fossa) posterior contacts can normally be located on proximal marginal ridges.

One group of "occlusionists" (the gnathologists) have until recently advocated (and some of them still do) that all centric holding contacts be cusp-to-fossa poded contacts. To accomplish this, cusps that would naturally contact marginal ridges are warped into the adjacent proximal pit and poded. Obviously such occlusions could only be established when opposed occlusal surfaces were being restored. The current concept of this group is to "scatter" centric contacts on the various inclines and ridges of an occlusal surface with the intent of involving the three faciolingual inclines of the occluding surfaces. If one is able to produce and maintain "equilibrated" contacts in all three ranges in the mouth, vertical stability is achieved.

Figure 22 shows an ideal pattern of individual tripoded centric contacts on the left side of the arches and an ideal pattern of combined tripoded centric contacts on the right side of the arches.

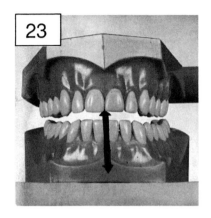 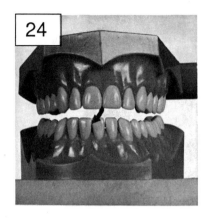 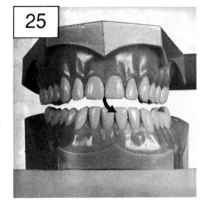 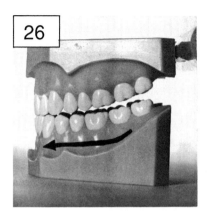

Summary of Requirements for a Successful Centric Occlusion

Regardless of the particular pattern of contact, the important requisites for centric occlusion are:

1. *Distribution*. All posterior opponents should participate in providing a stable centric relationship. Anterior contacts should be passive in relation to posterior contacts.
2. *Location*. Posterior centric contacts should be located such that the forces of vertical closure are resolved along the long axis of opponents.
3. *Timing*. Posterior centric contacts should be timed (equalized) such that they all occur within 10 microns of closure. Anterior contacts should be timed slightly late—that is, should be in passive contact or just out of contact.
4. *Relationship*. Centric contacts should establish a positional relationship of the mandible that places the condyles in a physiologically acceptable position.

ECCENTRIC OCCLUSION (FUNCTION AND NONFUNCTION)

Eccentric means "away from" or "other than" centric. Obviously eccentric occlusion occurs as a result of mandibular movement. Thus an understanding of eccentric occlusion requires knowledge of mandibular motion and the factors that control or determine these pathways of movement. Further, the amount and nature of eccentric contact (articulation) of the teeth depends upon the specific pathways of mandibular movement and the relationship of the occluding surfaces to these pathways.

Mandibular Movement

Although the mandible can make an infinite variety of chewing strokes or motions, there are four basic mandibular functional movements. The most simple chewing stroke is a straight opening and closing motion. The mandible is dropped down by action of the depressor muscles to create space between the maxillary and mandibular teeth. The tongue and cheeks move foodstuff onto the occlusal table of the mandibular teeth. The masticatory muscles then pull the mandible closed against the maxillary teeth with sufficient force to penetrate the particular foodstuff. This is the only chewing cycle used by many people, and it is repeated until the food is sufficiently masticated and ready to be swallowed (**Figure 23**).

More frequently some horizontal movement is associated with the chewing stroke. The other three principle patterns of functional movement all involve such a shift and are identified as *right lateral* (**Figure 24**), *left lateral* (**Figure 25**), and *protrusive* movements (**Figure 26**). During these movements the mandible is lowered and moved to either side or forward by action of the depressor and external pterygoid muscles. During opening, foodstuff is loaded onto the occlusal table of the teeth by action of the tongue and cheeks, and perhaps the lips. Closure is an arc movement that brings the teeth together with a sliding or shearing motion. There may be actual contact of the posterior teeth as

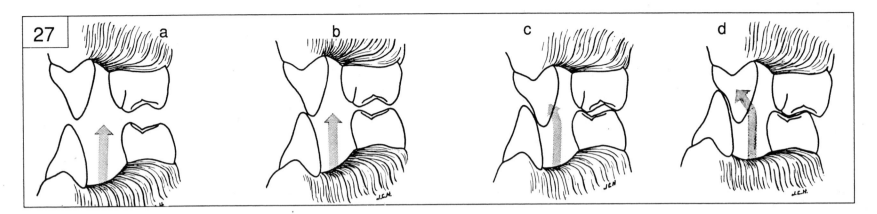

in the segmented-group-function concept, or the teeth may shear by one another with slight clearance between all except the canines as in the canine-guided concept.

Let us consider specifically a left lateral functional movement. The mandible drops by action of the depressor muscles. As it drops, it begins to shift to the left side, primarily by action of the right external pterygoid muscle, which pulls that condyle forward, downward, and inward. During this period the foodstuff is positioned by tongue and cheek. Closure is initiated primarily by the left masseter and temporal muscles. The mandible may shift even further to the left as the lower teeth squeeze the foodstuff against the uppers and begin to penetrate it. At this point the tips of the mandibular facial cusps may be as far or farther to the left than are the tips of the maxillary facial cusps (**Figure 27a**). As penetration continues, the lower canine contacts or approximates the maxillary canine at some point lingual to its incisal edge (**Figure 27b**). This contact deflects and guides the mandible along the inclined surface of the maxillary canine toward centric position in a path that precludes end-to-end clashing of posterior cusps (**Figure 27c**). Once the bracing and guiding influence of the canine contact is established, the forceful shearing closure is effected by all of the closing and retracting muscles of mastication until the closing stroke is terminated by centric occlusion (**Figure 27d**). The importance of the canine relationship in providing the dominant guidance for lateral chewing strokes is a cardinal feature of successful functional occlusion.

The pattern of tooth contact during this closure is often scissor-like. As the mandibular canine continues its slide up the lingual surface of the maxillary canine, the tip of the mandibular first premolar facial cusp contacts just lingual to the occlusofacial cuspal ridge of the maxil-

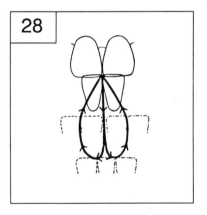

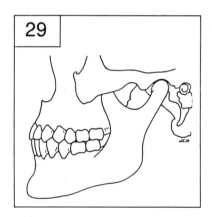

lary first premolar. Next, the second premolars contact as the slide toward centric continues, and then the first molars, and finally the second molars come into shearing contact. The chewing stroke is terminated as the centric contacts are reached. If one were to trace the path of movement of the mandible through bilateral examples of such excursion, it would be found that a teardrop-shaped orbit was described. This orbit starts and stops at centric contact and is termed the *envelope of function* (**Figure 28**).

Because we are concerned here with the specific shape of teeth that governs their contact, we have implied that the teeth actually contact and rub against one another during the full range of their functional relationship. This is not the case during normal mastication. Teeth seldom contact with any significant force or duration when chewing foodstuffs. They are kept separated by the body of the foodstuff and a neuromuscular mechanism that controls the force of closure dependent on the resistance of the foodstuff. For example, when someone chews a tough piece of meat, the jaw closes with the maximum comfortable force. When the force of the closure is equaled by the resistance of the food, the cycle is terminated and repeated until the meat is torn apart sufficiently to permit penetration. At the instant that tooth contact occurs, the force of closure is arrested and the meat remaining between the teeth serves as a cushion to absorb the shock of any further contact. Subsequent chewing strokes are executed at reduced force with the same control until the food is ready to be swallowed. In contrast, soft foodstuffs like mashed potatoes do not have sufficient body to stop or cushion a forceful closure. As a result very little force is applied. In fact, foods this soft are manipulated as much by the tongue as they are by the teeth. In either case the result is the same. Only the force necessary to masticate the particular foodstuff is applied. Consequently the teeth exert pressures against one another, but seldom actually contact. When contact does occur, it is with controlled force of short duration and is cushioned by the foodstuff.

These circumstances in no way minimize the importance of finite occlusal contour and contact patterns. Although the teeth seldom actually contact during chewing, they shear by one another so closely that any discrepancies in interdigitation would very likely result in traumatic conflicts. More important, most tooth contact occurs during habit and tension closure, resulting in nonuseful clenching and "gritting." Discrepancies in occlusal harmony focus and aggravate the trauma imposed by these nonchewing contacts. Accordingly, harmony of centric and functional occlusal contacts is essential to the continued health of the gnathostomatic system.

Function and Nonfunction

At the outset of this section the three basic criteria for a successful occlusion were identified as (1) stable centric occlusion, (2) appropriate functional occlusion, and (3) adequate nonfunctional disclusion. Thus far we have defined and identified the specific contact patterns that might comprise a stable centric occlusion and overviewed the general mechanism of masticatory function. Now we need to identify functional (working) and nonfunctional (nonworking) occlusal relationships, what factors control or determine these relationships, and the specific patterns of potential occlusal contact associated with each.

The logic of the mechanism of occlusion that serves masticatory function can be described rather simply. There are four basic functional movements of the mandible, and four corresponding functional components or segments of the dental arches:

1. Opening/closing arc: entire dental arches
2. Protrusive: anterior segments
3. Right lateral: right half of arches
4. Left lateral: left half of arches

The functional component of the arches is the segment *toward* which the mandible moves. During opening/closing arc (centric) chewing the entire arches are involved in the direction of mandibular movement; thus any or all teeth are intended to be involved in this type of masticatory function. In protrusive function the mandible moves forward, and work is intended in the anterior segment of the arches. In right lateral function the mandible moves to the right, and the teeth in the right half of the arches are intended to accomplish the chewing function; and likewise for left lateral function.

During those excursions involving movement in the horizontal plane (protrusive, right and left lateral) the teeth in the segments *away* from which the mandible moves are *not* intended to function and need to stay out of contact so as not to interfere with contact of the teeth in the functioning segments. This separation of teeth in the nonfunctioning segments is termed *disclusion* (disocclusion) and is just as important to successful function as occlusion.

FACTORS THAT INFLUENCE THE ARTICULATION OF NATURAL TEETH: OCCLUSAL DETERMINANTS

In addition to the action of muscles (as dictated by the proprioceptive/neuromuscular control mechanism), two major groups of factors determine articulation of the teeth. These factors are usually referred to as the *determinants of occlusion*:

A. Primary (controlling) determinants
    Posterior (condylar) guidance
    Anterior (incisal and canine) guidance

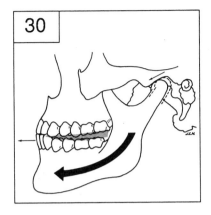

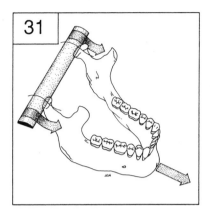

B. Secondary (responsive) determinants
      Arrangement of teeth
      Contour of teeth

Primary Determinants

The primary determinants of occlusion are the factors that determine mandibular position in centric and the pathways of mandibular movement. They are the same factors that adjustable articulators are designed to simulate. Obviously the finite control provided by the neuromuscular mechanism is not available in the articulator. These instruments are thus reduced to approximating the mechanical equivalent of the primary determinants.

Posterior (Condylar) Guidance   There are three significant components to the influence of posterior guidance on articulation: (1) centric relation, (2) contour of the eminentia (horizontal condylar guidance), and (3) Bennett movement.

Centric Relation. Centric relation is the term intended to apply to the position of the mandible in relation to the maxilla and other cranial structures when the condyles are in their anatomically and physiologically correct, fully seated position in the glenoid fossae. This relationship has in the past been variously defined on the basis of how the position was attained—the most posterior, or the most superior position of the condyles in the fossae. More recently efforts have been made to define it as a physiologic positional relationship: the mandible is in centric relation when the condyles are positioned against the postero-superior aspect of the articular slope with the articular disks properly

interposed. This normally results in the condyle being concentrically positioned in the fossa.

Ideally this would be the starting point or home base for occlusion; when the condyles are in centric relation, the teeth should be in centric occlusion. All eccentric excursions would start from and return to centric relation position of the mandible. Unfortunately, in most people maximum intercuspation (centric occlusion) of the teeth forces the condyles out of their centric relationship. This is the basis for what is commonly referred to as a CR/CO skid. The neuromuscular and functional implications of such discrepancies are obviously beyond the scope of this manual. As stated earlier, discussion here is restricted to developing a concept of ideal occlusion—that is, CR = CO.

Contour of the Eminentia (Horizontal Condylar Guidance). The articular eminence is a surface of the temporal bone that slopes downward and forward from the temporomandibular (glenoid) fossa **(Figure 29)**. The inclination of the articular eminence varies from person to person; in rare cases it may be flat. Normally, as the mandible is moved forward, the condyles would be forced to move *downward* along the eminence. Such guidance would obviously cause the mandibular posterior teeth to be separated from the maxillary posterior teeth during any forward movement of a condyle **(Figure 30)**. In the instance of a flat articular eminence, the condyles would move straight forward without causing separation of the posterior teeth.

The forward movement of the condyle along the eminence is termed *translation*. In protrusive movements, both condyles translate along their eminence **(Figure 31)**. In lateral movements the condyle on the nonfunctioning side translates forward along the eminence while the condyle on the functioning side pivots in its fossa **(Figure 32)**. Again, if the articular eminence has significant inclination from horizontal, the translating condyle will be forced downward during its forward movement and thus cause separation of the teeth on the nonfunctioning side. Thus by virtue of its contour and relative inclination to the occlusal plane, the articular eminence provides guidance of mandibular movement that affects the relationship of the teeth in the segments away from which the mandible moves—the nonfunctional segments.

For example, the mandible moves forward (protrusive excursion) in order to function on the anterior teeth. To accomplish this efficiently the posterior teeth need to stay out of contact to prevent interference with the functional contact relationship of the anteriors. In part this disclusion is achieved by horizontal condylar guidance. As the mandi-

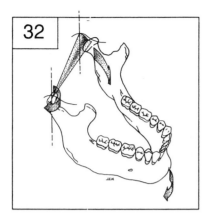
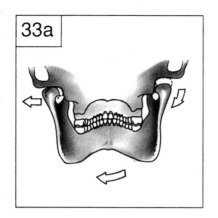
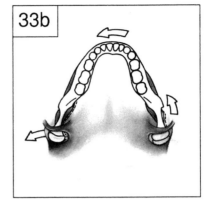
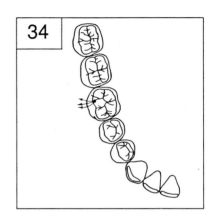

ble moves forward, both condyles translate forward along the posterior slope of their articular eminence (**Figure 31**). The inclination of these slopes causes the condyles to move downward, resulting in the posterior aspect of the mandible moving downward and away from the maxillary arch. Thus this downward motion of both condyles causes the posterior teeth to tend to disengage or disocclude (disclude) bilaterally. In lateral excursion the condyle on the working or functional side (the side toward which the mandible moves) rotates or pivots in its fossa, and the condyle on the balancing or nonfunctional side translates forward, downward, and inward (medially) (**Figure 32**). Again, the downward movement of this condyle causes the mandible to drop down away from the maxilla on the translating or nonfunctional side, resulting in a discluding influence on the posterior teeth on that side.

The simple beauty of this mechanism is now apparent. Translatory movement of condyles causes them to be guided or forced downward by the "inclined planes" of the articular slopes. This downward movement causes separation of the mandibular posterior occlusal table away from the maxillary occlusal table, producing a discluding influence. During protrusive excursion this occurs bilaterally, inducing disclusion of both posterior segments—which is what is needed if contact is to be limited to only the functioning anterior segment. In lateral excursions this occurs unilaterally on the translating side, which is the nonfunctional side and the one that needs to disclude so as to prevent any interference with the functional contact of teeth on the side toward which the mandible has moved. Thus, regardless of direction of excursion, *horizontal condylar guidance influences disclusion of teeth in the nonfunctional segments.*

Bennett Movement. Bennett movement is a bodily side shift of the mandible that occurs during lateral functional excursions (**Figure 33**). The exact anatomic relationships that permit and govern this side shift are debated, but the amount and timing of the shift have a very significant influence on the pattern of tooth contact during lateral excursion. As stated earlier, cusps of the mandibular posterior teeth ideally move between cusps (through the embrasures and grooves) of the maxillary teeth. The direction of travel of the mandibular cusps will be quite different if the lateral movement is a pure arcing movement about a pivoting condyle rather than a combination of arcing movement plus a lateral side shift (**Figure 34**). Timing is as influential as the amount of the shift. If the side shift were to occur progressively throughout the full range of pivoting lateral movement, the effect would simply be to produce an arc of movement of greater radius. But if the shift were to occur all at once during the lateral excursion, the movement might begin as an arc, then have a straight lateral component, and then terminate as an arcing movement. Usually Bennett shift tends to occur in conjunction with initial arc movement.

Intercondylar Distance. Intercondylar distance affects the path of lateral functional excursion of the mandible by virtue of the location of the vertical axis of rotation in relation to the arch. The closer the condyles are to the midsagittal plane, the more acute (posterior) will be the angle of lateral excursion. Conversely, the farther the condyles are from the midsagittal plane, the more obtuse (anterior) will be the angle of lateral excursion. This influence, in conjunction with Bennett shift, controls the actual direction of travel of the mandible in lateral excursions (see **Figure 34**).

Thus inclination of the articular eminence, the amount and timing of Bennett side shift, and intercondylar distance are significant factors

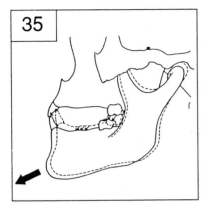
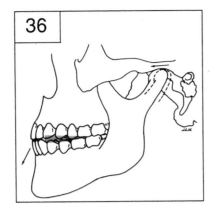
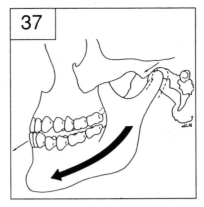
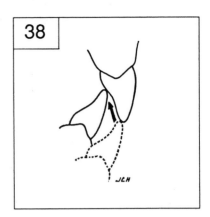

that influence the path of travel of the mandibular cusp tips and hence determine the proper inclination of cusps and the direction and contour of grooves in posterior teeth.

These three components of posterior guidance are known as *fixed factors of articulation*, because they cannot be altered. They are not factors that the dentist or technician can plan to modify in order to improve occlusal relationships. Their significance is that, in conjunction with anterior guidance, they establish the parameters within which the *variable factors of articulation* can be changed.

Anterior Guidance   Anterior guidance is the influence that the canines and incisor teeth have on the direction of mandibular movement. Depending upon their contour and relationship to one another, the upper and lower anterior teeth may permit straight horizontal movement of the mandible or may cause separation of the mandible from the maxilla during protrusive or lateral excursion. Certainly a significant part of this influence is due to the arrangement of these teeth, that is, the amount of horizontal and vertical overlap (see **Figures 27 and 35**). For example, consider the potential of protrusive movement in a situation where there is maximum vertical overlap and minimum horizontal overlap of the incisor teeth—a deep overbite. The mandible cannot move straight forward because the lower anterior teeth contact the lingual surfaces of the maxillary anterior teeth. In such a situation protrusive excursion demands that the mandibular incisors guide downward along the lingual surfaces of the maxillary incisors, thus effecting a separation of the mandible from the maxilla (**Figure 35**). This situation is referred to as *incisal guidance*, and articulation of the posterior teeth is influenced by this guidance. Similarly the maxillary and mandibular canines provide a dominant guiding influence during lateral functional excursions and this phenomenon is called *canine guidance*. The combined effect of incisal guidance and canine guidance is termed *anterior guidance*.

Because teeth can be reshaped and/or replaced, anterior guidance is a determinant that can be controlled by the dentist and is thus recognized as a *variable factor of articulation*. Tooth guidance is the only factor influencing the path of mandibular movement over which the dentist has control.

Summary of Primary Determinants   When a steep condylar guidance is present with a flat incisal guidance, separation of the most posterior teeth will tend to occur during protrusive excursion (see **Figure 30**). When a steep incisal guidance occurs in conjunction with a flat condylar guidance, there will be marked separation of the mandible from the maxilla anteriorly, with very little separation posteriorly (**Figure 36**). When a steep incisal guidance is coupled with steep condylar guidance, the entire mandible is separated markedly from the maxilla during functional excursions (**Figure 37**). Thus in combination these factors determine the steepness of the cuspal inclines which are appropriate to the dentition in question.

Secondary Determinants

Anterior and posterior guidance are recognized as the primary or controlling determinants of occlusion because they determine the pathways of mandibular movement under the control of the neuromuscular mechanism. However, whether teeth contact one another during the given pathways of mandibular movement depends on their shape and arrangement. Thus all factors related to the occlusal contour and positional arrangement of teeth influence whether and how the teeth will occlude during the various mandibular excursions. Occlusal form and arrangement are thus determinants of occlusion, but they are *secondary* or *responsive* to the controlling determinants. They are effective only because of their relation to the paths of mandibular movement.

It is these secondary or responsive determinants that are manipulated to establish occlusion. Occlusal adjustment is a process of reshaping teeth. Occlusion for a denture is accomplished by arranging and shaping the artificial teeth. Occlusion for a crown or fixed bridge is established by positioning and shaping the material that forms the occluding surface. But none of these things can be done correctly unless the occluding surfaces are related to the centric and eccentric positions of the mandible.

Two possibilities exist for relating opponent teeth in centric and eccentric positions. First, obviously, this could be accomplished in the mouth. Secondly, these relationships can also be simulated by casts mounted in an adjustable articulator. *The purpose and significance of articulators is that they can simulate the controlling determinants*: posterior and anterior guidance. It seems inconsistent to say this when anterior guidance is obviously generated by the anterior teeth themselves. However, articulators can be adjusted to duplicate the guidance provided by the anterior teeth on the mounted casts. This is important both because it prevents breakage or wearing away of the anterior teeth on the stone casts and because it permits the anterior teeth to be restored to their original guiding influence in cases where crowns or bridges involving these teeth are required.

Once the controlling determinants are established, development of occlusion in restorations involves proper manipulation of the secondary determinants: the arrangement and shape of the occluding surfaces.

Several factors that influence the articulation of the teeth fall under this category. Included are vertical dimension and the relative vertical position and inclination of the plane of occlusion, horizontal overlap, vertical overlap, arch form (Curve of Spee and Curve of Wilson), and contour of occluding surface.

Vertical Dimension Changes in vertical dimension will alter the relationship of the occlusal plane to the posterior condylar guidance. The effect of this change on cuspal inclination and groove direction is minor. However, increasing vertical dimension is accomplished by

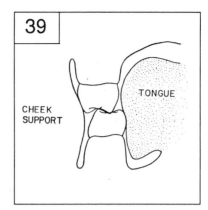
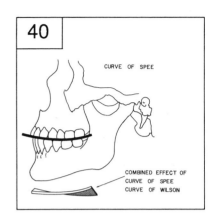

hinge opening of the mandible. Because this is a downward and backward arc movement of the body of the mandible, it results in a more distal relationship of the mandible to the maxilla. Decreasing the vertical dimension creates the opposite effect. Obviously a change in vertical dimension will significantly alter the relationship of the anterior teeth thus changing anterior guidance.

Horizontal Overlap Horizontal overlap (previously termed *overjet*) is the distance that the maxillary teeth overlap the mandibular teeth in a horizontal plane. In some mouths the amount of horizontal overlap is zero: the mandibular facial cusps meet the maxillary facial cusps end to end. In such cases the incisor teeth usually also meet end to end. The term *end-to-end bite* usually refers to this incisor relationship.

Normally the maxillary teeth overlap the mandibular teeth by 2 to 3 millimeters in a horizontal plane. It is this horizontal overlap that provides the potential for useful functional excursion. For example, in the normal protrusive excursion the mandible is moved forward some 2 to 5 millimeters along a combined horizontal and vertical path (an incline) to bring the edges of the incisor teeth into contact. In chewing, a closing stroke along this path permits these teeth to shear by one another throughout this dimension as the mandible closes to centric position. It is this shearing motion that provides incisive function (**Figure 38**). The same is true in lateral functional excursions (see **Figure 27**).

Horizontal overlap is also the basis for preventing tissue impingement during mastication. It serves to prevent cheek and lip biting. The prominent facial surface of the maxillary terminal molar holds the cheek away from the occlusal surface as the mandibular molar closes

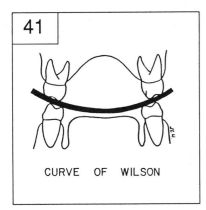

CURVE OF WILSON

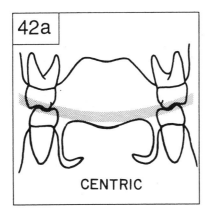

CENTRIC

into the opposing occlusal fossa during the functional orbit. Reciprocally the horizontal extension of the lower posterior teeth lingual to the maxillary teeth prevents impingement of the tongue (**Figure 39**).

In summary, the amount of horizontal overlap determines the dimension of useful range of the functional mandibular excursions and provides protection against impingement of the facial mucosa, lips, and tongue during closure.

Vertical Overlap   Vertical overlap is the amount of overlap of maxillary teeth over the mandibular teeth in a vertical plane. It is vertical overlap, coupled with the amount horizontal overlap, that determines the inclination of incisal or anterior guidance (see **Figures 35 and 38**). The vertical overlap of posterior teeth must be correlated with posterior guidance, anterior guidance, and horizontal overlap if contact along the cuspal inclines is to be provided in function. Obviously no vertical overlap can exist without some horizontal overlap. Clearly the greatest significance of vertical overlap is anterior guidance.

Curve of Spee   The Curve of Spee is the anterioposterior curvature presented by the occlusal surfaces of the posterior teeth as determined by a line beginning at the tip of the canine and extending along the tips of the facial cusps of the lower posterior teeth. Normally the posterior occlusal plane is concave downward in the first molar region (**Figure 40**). (The term *compensating curve* refers to the corresponding curvature of the occlusal plane in artificial dentures.) The upward curvature of the occlusal plane in the terminal (second and third) molar region tends to make this portion of the plane more in line with horizontal condylar guidance (the condylar translatory path), thus negating the discluding influence of horizontal condylar guidance. If this curvature

of the occlusal plane exceeds the combined discluding influence of anterior and posterior guidance, nonfunctional or balancing contact will occur.

The Curve of Spee is a significant factor in causing nonfunctional (balancing) contact in lateral and protrusive excursions. Although this may be desirable for the occlusion of teeth in artificial dentures, such nonfunctional or balancing contacts are undesirable in the natural dentition. To avoid this contact, the influence of posterior and anterior guidance must exceed the influence of the Curve of Spee. Because posterior guidance is fixed and incisal guidance is usually determined prior to development of restorations for posterior teeth, the primary concern in developing an appropriate curvature is to minimize it to the extent that lateral and protrusive balancing contacts are eliminated. Balancing contacts in protrusive are unlikely unless the Curve of Spee is steeper in relation to horizontal than is the condylar guidance. The influence on lateral balancing contact occurs in combination with the Curve of Wilson.

Curve of Wilson   The Curve of Wilson is the cross-arch curvature of the posterior occlusal plane. The lower posterior teeth as positioned in the normal dental arch are usually inclined toward the lingual. As a result, if a line were scribed across the occlusal surface of the mandibular right first molar and extended across the arch through the occlusal surface of the mandibular left first molar, it would form a curve (**Figure 41**). This curve, which is concave upward, is significant in helping to produce the buttressing effect on the teeth as the jaws are closed. The combined effect of the Curve of Spee and Curve of Wilson often produces a notable "twist" in the occlusal plane of a posterior segment (see **Figure 40**).

It should be pointed out that many years ago a Dr. Monson gave recognition to the combined Curve of Spee and Curve of Wilson and identified the shape as a segment of an 8-inch sphere, which was subsequently termed Monson's Curve. In many cases denture teeth have been arranged to conform to this average curvature. Again, it is important to realize that cross-arch curvature (Curve of Wilson) tends to promote nonfunctional or balancing contact. Although desirable in dentures, this curvature is minimized in the restoration of natural teeth, so that posterior and anterior guidance will prevent nonfunctional contact from occurring. **Figure 42a** illustrates a definite Curve of Wilson. **Figure 42b** indicates that nonfunctional contact tends to occur when such a curve is present, because the maxillary lingual cusp is "tipped

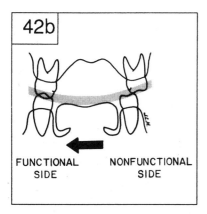

FUNCTIONAL   NONFUNCTIONAL
SIDE   SIDE

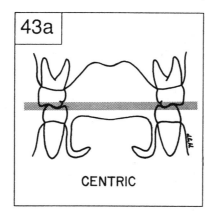

CENTRIC

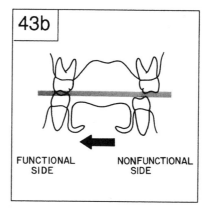

FUNCTIONAL   NONFUNCTIONAL
SIDE   SIDE

down" and the mandibular facial cusp is "tipped up."

In contrast, **Figure 43a** illustrates a relatively flat cross-arch occlusal plane. Because the occlusal plane of the teeth on the nonfunctional side is flatter in relation to the discluding influence of the translating condyle, no nonfunctional contact occurs (**Figure 43b**).

As expected, the arrangement of teeth has many and varied influences on their articulation. These are due primarily to changes in the relative relationship of horizontal and vertical overlap and arch curvatures. The effect of these variables is the rationale for the positioning of denture teeth to provide optimal articulation. These variables are more restricted in fixed restorative procedures, because the position of the natural teeth limits the range of variation.

Contour of the Occluding Surface   Occlusal contact relationships in most fixed restorative procedures are determined primarily by control of the contour of the occlusal surface. Three components of occlusal surface contour are significant in determination of occlusion. Anteriorly these are (1) location of centric contacts, (2) contour of the guiding lingual surface of the maxillary teeth, and (3) incisal length of the maxillary teeth. Posteriorly these components are (1) location of centric contacts, (2) cusp steepness, and (3) groove direction.

Simply stated, anterior guidance depends on the amount of vertical overlap and the inclination or contour of the upper lingual surfaces. Vertical overlap is the distance between centric contact and the incisal edge. This length in conjunction with the contour and inclination of the interposed surface determines the path and amount of anterior guidance. Anterior guidance is essential to a successful functional occlusion in that it is the basis, along with posterior guidance, for disclusion of

the posterior teeth during excursive movements.

The primary requirement of posterior occlusion is to establish and maintain vertical stability of the maxillomandibular relationship. To be physiologically acceptable the vertical holding centric contacts of posterior teeth must be established such that they (1) dissipate the force of closure along the long axis of opponent teeth, with adequate equalization of these contacts between all opponent pairs, (2) permit appropriate occlusion and disclusion during excursions, (3) protect the anterior teeth from the forces of centric closure, and (4) maintain a maxillomandibular relationship in centric that is acceptable to the joints and the musculature. Though simple to list, these requirements may pose the most demanding challenge in restorative dentistry. For example, it is clearly established that some patients can perceive contact discrepancies of dimensions less than 10 microns. Equalizing the multitude of centric contacts between eight and ten opponent pairs of multicusp posterior teeth to less than 10 microns can be an enlightening experience.

Because it is such an important part of establishing an acceptable posterior occlusion, the relationship of cusp steepness and groove direction as determinants of functional occlusion and nonfunctional disclusion deserves further consideration. If lateral functional contact is to be shared by all of the teeth in a posterior segment (group function), their functional cuspal inclines must be exactly in harmony with the guidance provided by the canines. Conversely, if the contact in lateral functional excursion is to be limited to the canines (canine guided function), the steepness of the functional cuspal inclines of the posterior teeth must be less than the steepness of the canine guide path. Because nonfunctional or balancing contact is not desirable in the

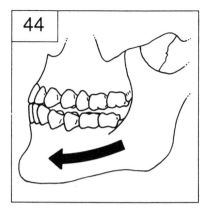

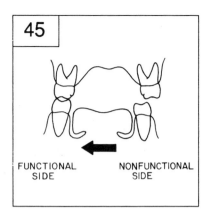

FUNCTIONAL　　　　　NONFUNCTIONAL
SIDE　　　　　　　　　　SIDE

natural dentition, nonfunctional cuspal inclines must be less steep than the combined influence of posterior and anterior guidance.

Grooves are basically *escapeways*. Along with the occlusal embrasures they help foodstuffs escape from the occlusal interface during mastication and serve as pathways for the cusps to move through, thus preventing occlusal interferences. As such they constitute selected or precisely located zones of reduced cusp steepness that permit steepest cuspal elevations (cusp tips) to articulate without interference. This interrelationship is rather precise and serves to increase masticatory efficiency both by allowing cusps to be steeper and by the shearing action of cusps passing at close tolerance through the grooveways.

Summary of Occlusal Determinants

Because of the number of occlusal determinants and their complex interrelationships, only experience can teach one to recognize the significance of each in establishing proper occlusion in fixed restorations. However, it should be recognized at this point that there are two distinct possibilities.

First, it is a relatively simple matter to establish appropriate occlusion for single restorations or small bridges when all of the determinants of occlusion are present. As an example, consider the development of a crown for a mandibular first molar. Posterior guidance is fixed and unalterable: horizontal condylar guidance (inclination of the eminentia) and Bennett shift are established. Assuming there is a full complement of teeth, anterior guidance is established. Likewise vertical dimension, horizontal and vertical overlap, and curvature and form of the arches are also known quantities. The only unknown quantities

that must be established are the pattern of contact and the contour of the individual occlusal surface in question. These variables are easily determined by virtue of the adjacent and opposing teeth. Usually rather simple approaches may be taken to indicate the opposing occlusion for such a restoration at the laboratory bench. These are discussed in Section 10, which deals with relating opposing tooth surfaces to the working cast.

Secondly, as a contrasting possibility, consider a large maxillary bridge that restores and/or replaces all of the teeth in the maxillary arch. Again posterior guidance, being a fixed factor, is provided. However, all other determinants—anterior guidance, vertical dimension, horizontal and vertical overlap, and to some extent arch curvature and arch form—must be established by the bridge. (Admittedly the latter two determinants will largely be indicated by the existing lower arch.) Certainly the best means of establishing occlusion for such a bridge is to use an adjustable articulator that has been set to simulate or reproduce the one known determinant—posterior guidance. Though important for the development of such complex restorations, the technique and use of fully adjustable articulators is beyond the scope of this manual. We must concentrate here on the more simple challenge of registering the influence of established primary determinants and providing by management of secondary determinants the appropriate pattern of occlusion.

ECCENTRIC CONTACT

Functional (Working) and Nonfunctional (Balancing) Occlusion

As mentioned above in discussion of mandibular movement, there are three basic pathways of movement of the lower jaw: (1) forward (protrusive), (2) to the right (right lateral function or right-working), and (3) to the left (left lateral function or left-working). Similarly, and most appropriately, there are three functional segments of the dental arches: (1) anterior (protrusive functional segment), (2) right posterior (right lateral functional segment), and (3) left posterior (left lateral functional segment). Basically the division of these functional segments occurs at the canines—hence in part the basis for their being termed the "cornerstones" of the dental arch. The canines function both as part of the anterior segment and as a component of the posterior segments, a dual role that justifies their being referred to as the "functionally most important teeth in the dental arches."

The correlation of anatomy and function is readily evident in the three anatomic/functional segments of the arches. In an ideal occlusion the anatomic arrangement is such that when the mandible is protruded for incisive function, only the anterior teeth do the work. The posterior teeth "stay out of the way" (**Figure 44**). Similarly, when the mandible is swung to the right, only the teeth in the right posterior segment do the work. The other teeth stay out of the way. And likewise for the left lateral functional excursion (**Figure 45**). *Thus functional occlusion occurs in the segment toward which the mandible moves.* To prevent interference with functional occlusion, *teeth in the nonfunctioning segments must disocclude (nonfunctional disclusion).*

Two more fundamental concepts must be reviewed before considering the specifics of eccentric occlusal contacts. First, in normal function people do not rub their teeth together as they chew. The teeth penetrate the food mass and shear by one another quite closely to the position of "almost" or "very lightly" touching in centric occlusion, at which point the jaw either immediately opens and negotiates another chewing stroke, or the teeth come into contact to brace the jaw in centric position for swallowing. Thus in the normal individual chewing normal foodstuffs, the teeth seldom if ever touch except when swallowing. Most people do, however, exhibit some degree of nervous or habit contact—either *clenching* (nonuseful tension between the arches of teeth in centric occlusion), or *bruxing* (nonuseful rubbing or "gritting" together of the teeth). There are many other types of occlusal habits—biting fingernails, chewing on pencils, pipestems, and other objects, biting threads, holding implements with the teeth, and the like. Categorically all such habits produce *parafunctional occlusal contacts.* It is these parafunctional contacts that bring about the major portion of wear on teeth.

Secondly, movement contacts of the teeth occur in two ways. In *functional movement* the jaw is opened, moved to the position that will be useful for the masticatory stroke (straight open, protrusive, or lateral), and then closed through the foodstuff back toward centric. In *parafunctional movement* (bruxing) the jaw is moved with the teeth held together, thus creating rubbing or grinding contact. Because it is convenient and affords greater control, the dentist examines occlusal contact relations by having the patient rub the teeth out to the excursive relation to be observed. This is called a *test excursion* and duplicates in reverse the functional path movement of the mandible. Thus essentially all comments and discussion relative to functional occlusion are predicated on test-excursion paths of movement (from centric toward eccentric), rather than natural functional excursion (from eccentric toward centric).

In summary, functional or working contacts are eccentric contacts that occur between teeth in the segment toward which the mandible moves. There are three functional segments of the dental arches, and hence three specific categories of functional occlusion: (1) right lateral function, (2) left lateral function, and (3) protrusive function.

Nonfunctional or balancing contacts are eccentric contacts that occur between teeth in the segment(s) away from which the mandible moves or, stated more practically, any contacts between teeth other than those in the functional segment.

Concepts of Eccentric Occlusion

Three major concepts or patterns of eccentric tooth contact have been recognized: fully balanced occlusion, canine guided occlusion, and group function occlusion.

Fully Balanced Occlusion   One of the earlier concepts of eccentric occlusion, referred to as fully balanced occlusion, provided for simultaneous contact of all teeth on both the functional side and the nonfunctional side during lateral mandibular excursion, as well as simultaneous contact of both anterior and posterior teeth in protrusive excursion. This concept was promoted by the original gnathologists but was soon abandoned as far as the natural dentition was concerned. However, balanced occlusion is desirable in full denture occlusion to help prevent tipping of the dentures during eccentric occlusion.

Canine Guided Occlusion   Modern gnathologists have termed the functional relationship between anterior and posterior teeth *mutually protective occlusion*. Posterior teeth provide stability of vertical dimension by virtue of their positive centric contacts and thus protect the anterior teeth, which are poorly positioned to resist the forces of vertical closure. Correspondingly—hence the term *mutually protective*—the anterior teeth protect the posterior teeth from torque forces during lateral and protrusive excursions by virtue of the guiding contact of maxillary and mandibular incisors and canines. A cardinal feature of the gnathologic concept of occlusion is dominant guidance by the canines in lateral excursions. This is termed *canine guidance* and is a characteristic of most normal, unworn dentitions.

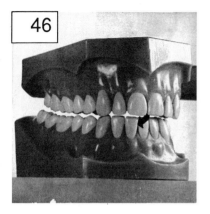
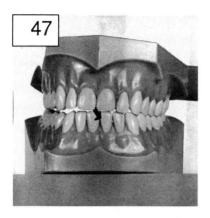
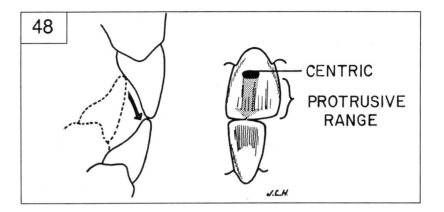

Figure 46 According to the gnathological concept, canine guidance should provide for immediate and total disarticulation of all posterior teeth at the moment lateral mandibular excursion is initiated. This means that in this occlusal arrangement there is no eccentric contact of posterior teeth on either the functioning or nonfunctioning side. The timing and inclination of the canine lift is such that the posterior cuspal ridges pass just by one another, providing a shearing action without actual contact. At termination of the chewing stroke closure, the centric holding cusps penetrate and mash the food against their opposing marginal ridges or fossae, thus stopping the vertical closure.

Group Function Occlusion In this arrangement (Figure 47) all posterior teeth on the functional (working) side contact as a group during the lateral excursion. The anterior teeth (incisors and canines) contact as a group during the protrusive excursion. In short, the group of teeth that makes up the functioning segment share the occlusal contact.

Once again it is interesting to note the dual capacity of the canines. They function with the posterior teeth during the lateral or working excursion, and function with the anterior teeth during the protrusive excursion. This, of course, is due to their unique position at the corners of the dental arches.

Patterns of Eccentric Contact: Functional Contacts

Protrusive Functional Contacts In test excursions, protrusive function begins as the lower incisal edge leaves centric and tracks forward and downward along the lingual surface of its maxillary opponent. This range of contact terminates as the incisal edges meet end to end (Figure 48).

Ideally all six mandibular anterior teeth will track in harmony along the lingual incline of their opponents throughout the full range of the excursion. Marking would thus leave a stripe on the maxillary linguals from each centric forward onto the incisal edge (Figure 48). Ideal contact marking on the lower teeth would be at the facioincisal angle. In actuality this contact may vary—from moving down the facial surface (deep vertical overlap), to moving incisally across the edge (less vertical overlap, more horizontal overlap). Obviously the rubbing, protrusive contact will cross the area of centric contact on the lower occlusal, thus causing wear of the centric contact. This phenomenon is one of the significant reasons that approximately half of our population do not have actual contact in centric on their incisors. However, the incisors will erupt to compensate for wear to the extent permitted by either centric or functional contact.

Although shared protrusive contact among the six maxillary and six mandibular anterior teeth is the classic ideal pattern for functional contact in the anterior segment, a significant variation frequently occurs naturally or is purposely created in restorations. As mentioned earlier, centric contact of the mandibular first premolar facial cusp occurs ideally on the mesial marginal ridge of the maxillary first premolar. Frequently, however, it is slightly more mesially positioned and contacts the distal marginal ridge area of the maxillary canine. In either case, during protrusive excursion the mesial arm of the lower first premolar facial cusp may track anteriorly across the lingual surface of the canine (Figure 49). Such contact may be very important in occlusions with an "open bite" incisor relationship or when a six-unit (ca-

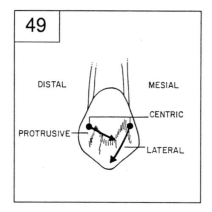

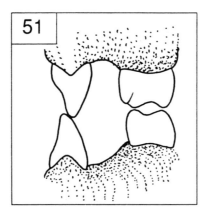

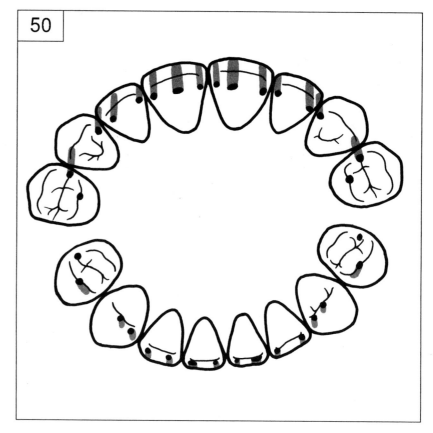

nine-to-canine) anterior bridge is being made. With this variation in mind, it may thus be said that *ideal distribution of protrusive functional contacts will involve the six maxillary anterior teeth and the eight most anterior mandibular teeth* (**Figure 50**).

Another concept relating to functional excursion needs to be introduced here: the *range of contact*. As already explained, functional and nonfunctional occlusion occurs in the form of dynamic paths of contact. As such, these contacts have a linear dimension, or range, that varies depending upon the location of centric contact on anterior teeth and the length of cuspal inclines on posterior teeth. Because harmony of contact is the desired occlusion when a group of teeth are in function together, it is important to be able to compare contacts on all involved teeth throughout the full range of potential contact. This is commonly done by mentally dividing the potential contact range into three components—early, middle, and late. As usual, this is done in relation to test excursion. Accordingly, early range is adjacent to centric, and late range is the terminal one-third approximating the end-to-end position.

Lateral Functional Contacts   Lateral functional contacts occur on the side toward which the mandible is moved. This is basically an arc movement, the center of rotation being in the functional or working side condyle. All teeth in the half arches on the functional side have the potential for lateral functional contact.

Anterior teeth are important participants in the lateral functional excursion, even though they are not the teeth that are intended to do the work. They provide the *guidance* which in conjunction with condylar guidance produces disclusion of the teeth on the opposite (nonfunctional) side. Thus *anterior guidance* is one of the most important

aspects of functional occlusion.

There are two basic concepts regarding the pattern of lateral functional contact and other naturally occurring variations.

Canine Guided Lateral Function. A common occurrence in the young or unworn dentition is that canines on the functional side are the only posterior teeth that contact in lateral function (**Figure 51**). The adjacent lateral and central incisors may passively share contact throughout the functional range, but the other posterior teeth in the functional segment are discluded throughout the range of movement by the guiding "lift" of the canines. The result is that only one to three teeth (the canine and adjacent incisors) in each arch make contact in the lateral excursion. In an ideal occlusion the functional contact path of the cusp tip of the lower canine extends obliquely from the point of centric contact on the mesial aspect of the lingual surface of the upper canine laterally and posteriorly toward the cusp tip (**Figure 52**). These contact

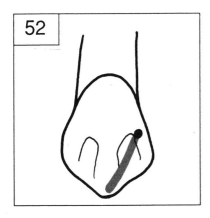
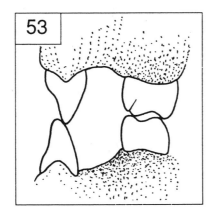

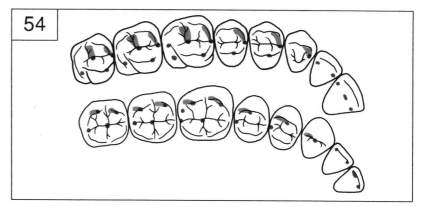

paths usually have a more posterior (distal) orientation than the path of lateral mandibular movement. This is because of the contour of the lingual surface of the maxillary canine. Depending upon the amount of vertical and horizontal overlap, the contact area may extend down onto the facial surface of the lower canine and/or across its incisal edge. In addition it normally migrates from the point of centric contact along the distal arm of the lower cusp.

Lateral Segment Group Function. Usually referred to as segmental group function or just group function, this concept of lateral functional contact involves a sharing of contact by all teeth in the functional segment throughout the functional range. (This has already been described as the ideal arrangement for protrusive function.) Classic group lateral function contact provides dominant guidance by the canines, with contact being shared by all other teeth in the functional segment (**Figure 53**). There are two ranges of such contact on the multicusp posterior teeth—a *facial range* and a *lingual range*—just as there were two ranges of centric contact on these teeth (**Figure 53, molars**).

The facial range of lateral functional contact involves tracking of the lower facial cusps obliquely, laterally, and posteriorly across the lingual inclines of the upper facial cusps. Thus this is a facial-cusp-to-facial-cusp relationship. Just as with the canines, the functional contact path is more posteriorly oriented than the path of mandibular excursion, because the contact area migrates distally along the distal arm of the lower facial cusp. The contour of the lingual incline of the upper facial cusp promotes this migration because of the rise of the triangular ridge. The functional path or track of each lower facial cusp can thus be traced from the point of centric contact facially and distally across the mesiolingual incline of each upper facial cusp (**Figure 54**). If such tracks are

carefully observed in an ideal occlusion, it is evident that they become progressively shorter on the more posterior teeth in the segment. This is to be expected, as they are closer to the center of rotation. Thus just as the anterior teeth separate on hinge opening at a ratio of about 3 millimeters to 1 millimeter of separation for the second molars because they are farther from the center of rotation, they also usually have a lateral contact path that is longer than that of the second molars. The anatomy of the teeth reflects this functional geometry, as the length of the facial cusp inclines usually becomes shorter in the most posterior teeth.

The lingual range of lateral functional contact involves tracking of the upper lingual cusps from their point of centric contact up the facial inclines of the lower lingual cusps. This contact area migrates from the upper lingual cusp tip lingually and usually somewhat mesially (**Figure 54**). Ideally *these contacts will not occur in the natural dentition group function occlusion.* Although they may be desirable in denture occlusion, the anatomic form and functional efficiency of the natural dentition do not warrant actual contact in lingual range lateral function. Instead the lingual cusps of the upper premolars would ideally pass through the opposing lingual occlusal embrasures without contact. The mesiolingual cusps of the upper molars would pass through the occlusolingual groove of the lower molars. And the distolingual cusps of the upper molars would pass through the lingual aspect of the occlusal embrasure of the opposing lower molars (**Figure 54**). Thus lingual range lateral functional contacts are very much like nonfunctional contacts. They can and do occur, but are undesirable in the normal natural occlusion. However, the potential for these contacts must be recognized so that they may be identified and eliminated in occlusal adjustment or avoided in developing restorations for the natural dentition.

Summary. In summarizing the two basic concepts of lateral functional contact, several comparisons and contrasts are important. First, in both occlusal arrangements the canines should provide the dominant guiding influence. In both arrangements the length of the contact range on the canines should exceed that of all other teeth. In canine guided occlusion the "lift" or steepness of the canine guidance is greater than that of the posterior teeth, thus effecting their immediate disclusion. In both arrangements the lift of the canines should be sufficient to disclude the posterior teeth in terminal range, that is, before they reach the end-on (cusp-tip to cusp-tip) relation (see **Figures 27, 51 and 53**).

In grouped lateral occlusion contact the steepness of facial range functional inclines of the posterior teeth should be in harmony with the canines out to the terminal functional relationships. However, the range of contact should be shorter than the canines', so that cusp tip collisions are positively prevented in the chewing stroke. As noted previously, to accomplish this the functional range must become shorter as it moves posteriorly in the arch. In addition the "pressure" of functional contact should diminish posteriorly. In fact, many dentists purposely eliminate actual test-excursion contact on the second molars and perhaps even the distal aspect of the first molars. Under heavy functional loading these teeth, because of their proximity to the joints and musculature, will be brought into contact by torquing of the mandible.

Figure 55 is summary example of functional contacts. It identifies the full range of potential protrusive functional contacts in the anterior segments. The full range (both facial and lingual) of potential lateral functional contacts is illustrated in the left posterior segments. The right posterior segments identify desired patterns of lateral group function contacts.

Nonfunctional Contacts

Nonfunctional or balancing contacts are undesirable in the natural dentition. Conversely, they are purposely developed in full denture occlusions to help prevent tipping of the dentures off their respective ridges. Harmonized nonfunctional contacts may be desirable in bizarre natural occlusions (severe Class II or III occlusions) when they are the only means of providing adequate tooth guidance for mandibular excursions or when the teeth cannot be discluded by available anterior guidance.

Although normally undesirable because they impose useless torque

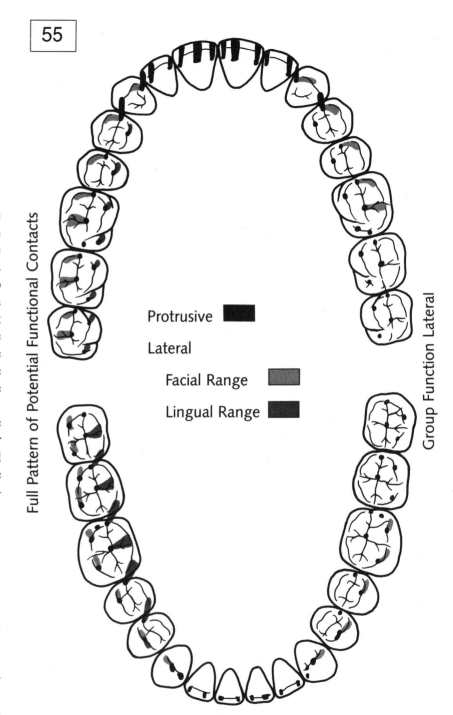

55

Protrusive

Lateral

    Facial Range

    Lingual Range

Full Pattern of Potential Functional Contacts

Group Function Lateral

stress on teeth, periodontium, musculature, and joints, nonfunctional contacts can and do occur in the natural dentition. One must know the location for these "potential" contacts, so that they may be readily recognized during evaluation or adjustment of occlusion and development of restorations. Knowing where to look for nonfunctional contacts is quite simple. *Nonfunctional contacts cannot occur on normally aligned anterior teeth*. They can occur in either or both posterior segments except when they are in centric or functional relationship.

Protrusive Nonfunctional Contacts Nonfunctional contact during protrusive excursion may occur in either or both posterior segments. Such contacts occur on the arms of centric holding cusps. As a result there are two ranges of protrusive nonfunctional contact potential—facial and lingual—just as there are two ranges of centric and lateral function.

Facial Range Protrusive Nonfunctional Contacts. As the mandible moves forward for functional contact in the anterior segment, the mesial arm of the lower facial cusps (the facial range centric holding cusps) may run into the distal slope of the triangular ridge of the maxillary facial cusps. These contacts serve no useful purpose, as the intended function is occurring in the anterior segment. Thus they are termed nonfunctional and may in fact interfere with the functional contact relationship of the anterior teeth. Because these nonfunctional contacts are made by the lower facial cusps as they move forward, markings will extend from the point of centric contact on the upper tooth anteriorly across the distal slope of the triangular ridge of the upper facial cusps. And because the arches are somewhat triangular in shape, converging anteriorly, a straight anterior movement of a lower facial cusp will take it obliquely toward the facial of the maxillary opponent (**Figure 56**), not through the central groove zone.

Lingual Range Protrusive Nonfunctional Contacts. The lingual range of protrusive nonfunctional contacts is created by the distal arm of the upper lingual cusps (the lingual range centric holding cusps) rubbing against the mesial slope of the triangular ridge of the lower lingual cusps as the lower teeth move forward in the protrusive excursion. Markings will extend distally from the point of centric obliquely lingually and distally on the mesial slope of the triangular ridge of the lower lingual cusps (**Figure 56**).

Lateral Nonfunctional Contacts Lateral nonfunctional contacts are unique. Thus far all posterior occlusal contacts discussed have had two ranges, involving the facial and lingual range centric holding cusps.

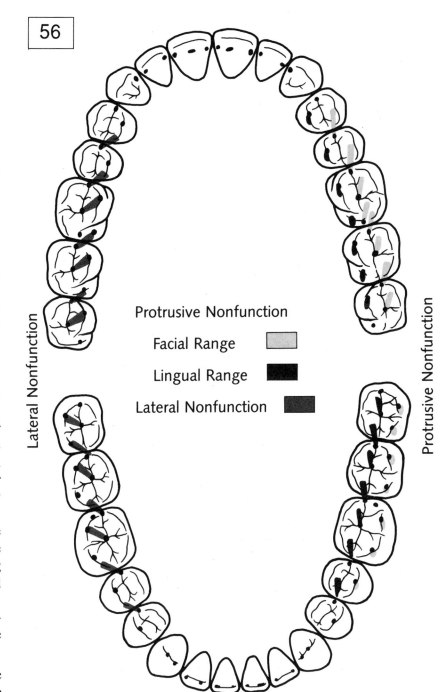

56

Lateral Nonfunction

Protrusive Nonfunction

Protrusive Nonfunction
Facial Range
Lingual Range
Lateral Nonfunction

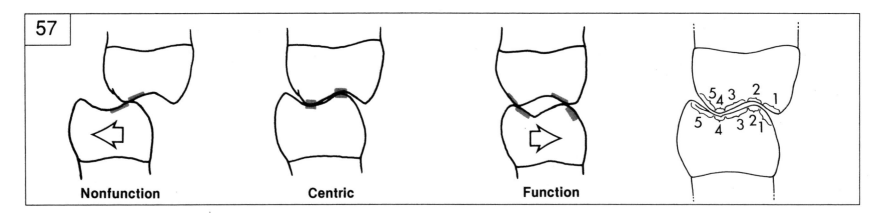

Nonfunction   **Centric**   **Function**

There are two ranges of centric, two ranges of lateral function (protrusive function has only one range but involves anterior teeth), and two ranges of protrusive nonfunction. Lateral nonfunction, by contrast, involves both the facial and lingual range centric holding cusps but *has only one range*. This is because lateral nonfunctional contacts involve the opposed inclines that lie between the two zones of centric contact. These are referred to as the *included inclines* (because they are included between the two zones of centric) and specifically are the lingual incline of the lower facial cusps and the facial incline of the upper lingual cusps. Thus there is one range on the lower teeth and an opposing single range on the upper teeth.

When the mandible moves into lateral function, the lower facial cusps may contact the lingual incline of the upper facial cusps and the upper lingual cusps may contact the facial incline of the lower lingual cusps on the functional side. On the nonfunctional side the lower facial cusp moves lingually toward the upper lingual cusp. Thus the lower facial cusp may create a contact marking that runs obliquely mesially and lingually across the facial incline of the upper lingual cusp. Reciprocally the upper lingual cusp may create a contact marking that runs obliquely facially and distally along the lingual incline of the lower facial cusp. This rubbing contact of the opposed included inclines may terminate with direct contact between the opposed centric holding cusps (see **Figure 56**).

Review of Posterior Contacts

A rather simple means is available to organize understanding of posterior occlusal contact potential. The various types of contact can be related to the area or zone of the occlusal surface on which they occur (**Figure 57**):

Zone 1: Facial incline of lower facial cusps against lingual incline of upper facial cusps: facial range function.
Zone 2: Lower facial cusp tip against upper central groove zone: facial range centric.
Zone 3: Lingual incline of lower facial cusp against facial incline of upper lingual cusp: lateral nonfunction.
Zone 4: Upper lingual cusp tip against lower central groove zone: lingual range centric.
Zone 5: Lingual incline of upper lingual cusp against facial incline of lower lingual cusp: lingual range function.

A simple cross-sectional diagram of any opponent pair of posterior teeth can be used to identify all contact zones except protrusive nonfunction. One should learn to name the zones of the occlusal surfaces of both upper and lower teeth and the specific type of contact that occurs or has the potential to occur on each. One should also learn to identify these zones and potential contact points on diagrams and models.

Thus there are two ranges (facial and lingual) of centric and lateral function, but only one range of lateral nonfunction. Of course there are also two ranges of protrusive nonfunction (facial and lingual) that are not represented by a cross-sectional diagram (see **Figure 56**).

The types and location of potential contacts can also be represented by outline.

A. Centric
   1. Facial range: lower incisal edges against upper incisor lingual

surfaces, and lower facial cusps against upper central groove zone (marginal ridges and fossae).

2. Lingual range: upper lingual cusps against lower central groove zone (marginal ridges and fossae).

B. Protrusive
1. Function: lower incisal edges and mesial arms of lower first premolars against upper incisor linguals (only one range).
2. Nonfunction:
   a. Facial range: lower facial cusps (mesial arm) against upper facial cusps (distal slope of triangular ridge)
   b. Lingual ridge: upper lingual cusps (distal arm) against lower lingual cusps (mesial slope of triangular ridge)

C. Lateral
1. Function:
   a. Facial range: lower facial cusps (distal arm) against upper facial cusps (mesial slope of triangular ridge and mesial arm)
   b. Lingual range: upper lingual cusps (mesial arm) against lower cusps (facial inclines)
2. Nonfunction: lingual inclines of lower facial cusps against facial inclines of upper lingual cusps (only one range).

Recognition of these zones of contact will greatly facilitate development of patterns and correction of castings to produce the desired pattern of contact. For example, assuming a normal arrangement of the teeth, such knowledge should immediately indicate that when carving a mandibular molar, a check for centric contact should produce markings only on the tips of the facial cusps and in the central groove region. One should recognize immediately that a registration of eccentric contact on the lingual incline of the facial cusp of this lower molar pattern is undesirable lateral nonfunctional contact and must be eliminated. Thus recognition of the normal pattern or zone of contact is an indispensable aid in the buildup and/or correction of the pattern for a restoration. The composite of centric, lateral function, protrusive function, and potential nonfunctional contacts for all teeth is shown in **Figure 58**. The classic pattern of centric is identified by black dots. Eccentric contact pathways are outlined. It may be helpful to color code these so that protrusive and lateral functional and nonfunctional contacts can be readily distinguished.

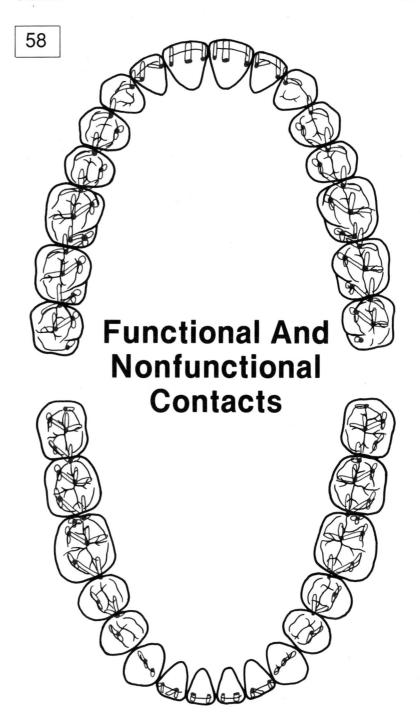

58

Functional And Nonfunctional Contacts

REVIEW QUESTIONS

1. Define occlusion as related by Ramfjord and Ash.
2. What constitutes ideal occlusion? What are the results of these ideal relationships?
3. What are the two aspects of the term *functional occlusion*?
4. List the three basic criteria for a successful functional occlusion.
5. Name the four things an ideal centric occlusion provides.
6. Describe the three basic functional movements of the mandible and the functional segments or components of the dental arches for each movement.
7. Enumerate the "determinants of occlusion," primary and secondary.
8. Name the major concepts or patterns of eccentric tooth contact.

SECTION 10

Establishing Occlusal Relationships with the Working Cast

Of all chairside dental procedures, the techniques used by dentists to register occlusal relationships for fixed restorations are among the most variable. Although specific techniques are too numerous and extensive to identify here, general categories can be described and examples given. It is the responsibility of the dentist and the dental laboratory technician to recognize the potential of any given occlusal registration and utilize it to maximum advantage in developing the restoration at hand.

Familiarity with the clinical procedures for producing the various occlusal registrations is necessary before one can expect to make use of them knowledgeably in the laboratory. Unfortunately the terminology used to describe various occlusal registrations is often confusing because of contradiction and variation from one section of the country to another. An attempt should be made to standardize terminology for ease of communication. A case in point is the term *wax bite*. This undesirable, but routinely used, term can have many meanings depending on the procedure involved. It may relate to the interocclusal records used to mount edentulous or dentulous casts, or to any one of several types of occlusal registrations used to identify the occlusion in patterns for fixed restorations.

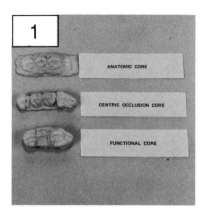
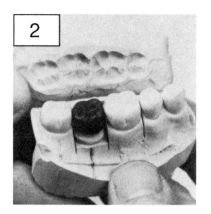
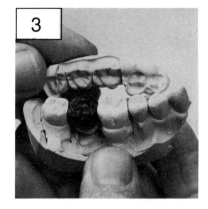
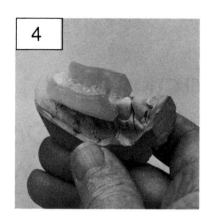

DEVELOPMENT OF OCCLUSION AS RELATED TO THE THREE BASIC TECHNIQUES FOR PATTERN DEVELOPMENT

Direct Technique

A term common to occlusal registrations for fixed restorations is *wax chew-in*. Originally the wax chew-in was simply a step in the development of a direct pattern for an onlay. Wax was placed in the prepared tooth, and the patient was requested to chew into the wax until all interferences were removed. The pattern was then completed directly on the tooth, sprued, removed, and cast without the necessity of a die. At the time that this technique was popular most dentists using it completed the casting themselves. The transition to greater utilization of dental laboratory technicians for fixed restorative procedures began with their involvement in casting direct patterns.

Indirect Technique

Such wax chew-ins have subsequently become known as *wax occlusal registrations* and have been adapted for use in the *indirect technique* for making cast restorations. The wax chew-in (wax occlusal registration), made with inlay wax in the mouth, is often positioned on the die in a working cast. The occlusal surface of the wax occlusal registration is appropriately refined, and axial contours are carved in relation to the die and the adjacent teeth. As an example of the *direct-indirect* approach, this procedure requires that *only* occlusal relationships be established directly in the mouth. A working cast is available to permit development of all other aspects of the pattern in the laboratory.

The incorporation of the wax occlusal registration in the pattern has many disadvantages. It is often difficult to remove the chew-in from the tooth and position it on the die without distortion. Internal adaptation is frequently poor. This is especially true with registrations for a full crown, because they lack stability on the tooth during the "chewing in." The primary disadvantages become apparent when completing the pattern on the working cast in the laboratory. It may be difficult to determine exactly what modification of the wax occlusal registration (chew-in) is necessary to maintain correct centric and functional occlusal contacts. There are no guides for correcting errors made in carving the occlusal surface. In addition there is no way to evaluate or correct the casting and, should a miscast occur, there is no possibility to remake the casting without having the patient make another visit to the dentist (unless a duplicate chew-in was made initially).

Because of these disadvantages and the need to delegate development of castings, the wax chew-in technique has been made even more indirect. Today dentists are using procedures for recording occlusal relationships that are more suitable for the completely indirect approach, and most castings are made by dental technicians. Accordingly, the focus here is on examples of indirect procedures.

OCCLUSAL CORES

Many of the disadvantages of converting the wax occlusal registration into the restoration pattern can be overcome by making a stone index of the registration.

These stone indexes are made by placing quick-setting stone over the

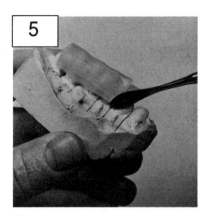
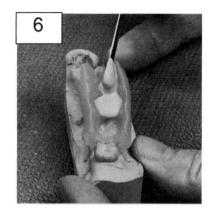
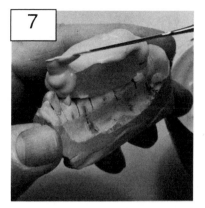
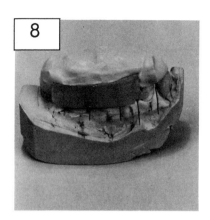

wax occlusal registration, either *directly* in the mouth (by the dentist) or *indirectly* after the chew-in has been transferred to the working cast (by the technician). The stone index makes an excellent permanent record of the wax registration. Its use permits a pattern to be completely developed on the die thus improving the internal adaptation and allowing repeated checks and corrections of the occlusal carving. Sites of sprue attachments and other errors in the occlusal surface of the casting can be checked and corrected, and should it be necessary, repeated patterns can be developed until an adequate casting is obtained.

These stone indexes have been termed *cores*. The wax chew-ins (wax occlusal registrations) from which they are developed have come to be called *functionally generated path registrations*.

The concept of creating a stone occlusal counterdie from a wax registration of the full range of occlusion on a given tooth or segment of teeth has been employed to create counterdies of other types of occlusal registrations as well. Specifically, three types of cores can be identified (**Figure 1**). In selected instances an index may be made of a tooth before it is prepared, so that the original occlusal contours may be reproduced. This is termed an *anatomic core*. A *centric occlusion core* is made from a registration of the teeth in centric occlusion. The occlusal core developed from the functionally generated path registration is termed a *functional occlusal core*.

Anatomic Core

The anatomic core (**Figure 2**) is simply a negative stone duplication of the occlusal surfaces of the involved and adjacent teeth prior to preparation (a preoperative stone impression). Often a practical proce-

dure for onlays, the anatomic core is seldom adequate for the full crown restoration, because few teeth requiring the full crown as a restoration present an occlusal surface deserving of duplication. However, when appropriate, the anatomic core is easily established by conveying quick-setting stone over the occlusal surfaces of the tooth or teeth that are to be prepared and at least one adjacent tooth on either side. The resulting stone index can be precisely related to an accurate working cast and can thus be used to form the occlusal portion of the wax pattern. If contours and occlusion are optimal prior to preparation, the anatomic core is an excellent, simple means of establishing occlusal contours, provided the index can be made and used with precision. Thus the anatomic core provides a means of duplicating the original form of the occlusal surface of the tooth being restored.

Centric Occlusion Core

A centric occlusion core (**Figure 3**) is developed from nothing more than a centric occlusion wax, zinc oxide–eugenol paste, or impression material record like that used to relate anatomic casts. However, rather than making a separate impression of the opposing arch and relating the resulting cast via the bite record, the centric occlusion core is developed by positioning the registration on the working cast (**Figure 4**), stabilizing it (**Figure 5**), and pouring stone into the depressions representing the opposing teeth (**Figures 6 and 7**). The result is an anatomic model of the opposing teeth related to the working cast in centric occlusion. This relationship can be maintained by mounting the casts, still related and unseparated (**Figure 8**), on a suitable articulator.

A different technique is to trim the bite record at either end to expose

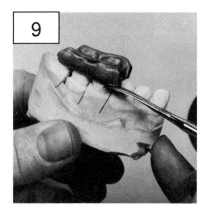
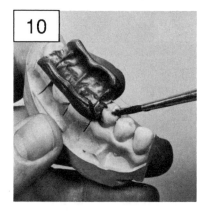
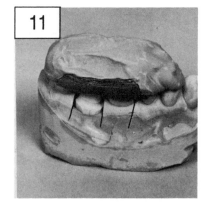
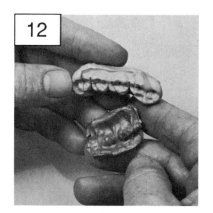

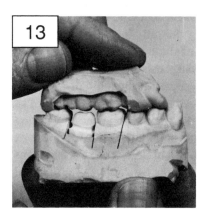
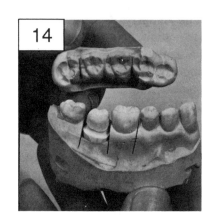
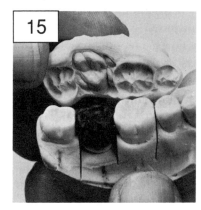
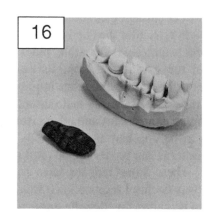

a definite "stop" on the occlusal surface or land area of the working cast adjacent to the prepared teeth (**Figure 9**) and apply a suitable separating medium before pouring the stone core (**Figure 10**). The core is poured in stone (**Figure 11**), allowed to set, and then separated from the bite registration (**Figure 12**). By this latter approach the core is indexed to the working cast with precision and can be hand articulated (**Figures 13 and 14**). If the occlusal demands of the restoration involved are simple enough to permit fabrication based on adjacent anatomy and centric occlusion, the centric occlusion core is a simple means of providing occlusal relations. It does, however, require adjustment of the casting in the mouth to accommodate functional relationships.

Functional Occlusal Core

Without doubt, the true objective of the concept of occlusal coring is the functional occlusal core (**Figure 15**). Developed from a wax chew-

in (functionally generated path registration), the functional core is a *static record of the full range of centric and eccentric occlusal contact*. Before proceeding, it must be pointed out that the functional core indicates the *maximum amount of occlusal contact that can occur between teeth without causing interference with mandibular movement or centric position*. Modifications must be made to provide ideal anatomic form: occlusal pits and grooves must be established or defined by carving away some of the wax, and the position of maxillary facial and mandibular lingual cusps must be determined by adjacent teeth or an opposing anatomic model, as the functional core affords no indication of the position and contour of axial surfaces.

A very serious problem is often associated with use of a core from functionally generated path registrations. In many clinical situations conflict exists between properly located centric contacts and functional or nonfunctional interferences. In these cases the eccentric interfer-

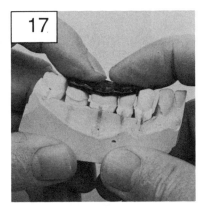
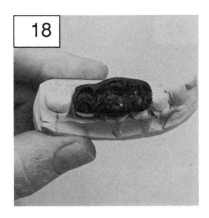
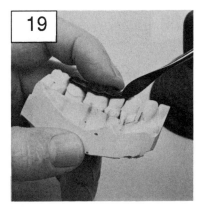
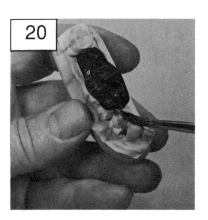

ences will rub away the centric holding portions (cusp tips) of the wax registration. The resulting core will dictate a wax pattern with deficient centric holding contacts. The answer to this problem is knowledgeable assessment of the occlusion by the dentist prior to deciding to use a functionally generated path occlusal registration. Such problems cannot be readily recognized by the laboratory technician.

Most importantly, it must be understood that although the functional core (or any other core or mounted cast for that matter) is a static record, the contacts thus represented are, when in the mouth, potential dynamic forces. Said differently, these are not just points or areas of intermittent touch contact, but moving points of contact involving moving varying forces, which often present a complex multiplicity of components.

Webster's Dictionary defines *dynamics* as a "branch of mechanics that deals with forces and their relation primarily to the motion but sometimes also to the equilibrium of bodies of matter." Thus we are dealing with a subject that is well termed *occlusal dynamics*. To use the functional core, one must have some appreciation of how the dynamics of occlusion are accommodated by such a registration.

The accuracy of a functional core is directly dependent upon the accuracy and completeness of the functionally generated path registration. The greatest problem in establishing an accurate registration is stabilization of the wax. Usually difficult enough in the single crown situation, this problem is particularly apparent in the bridge situation, where wax must be supported across an edentulous space if a functional occlusal recording is to be obtained. Dentists use several methods to stabilize wax for functional registrations, with varying degrees of success. Although these procedures may at times involve the service of a

technician to make one of the many types of bite platforms, they are primarily clinical and thus are not covered in this manual. Once the registration is established, the dentist may make the functional core by carrying quick-setting stone into place over the wax and adjacent teeth *directly* in the mouth.

Figures 16 and 17   The functional core may also be developed *indirectly* (in the laboratory) by seating the wax registration carefully on the working cast.

Figure 18   If necessary, the ends of the wax registration are trimmed to leave sufficient exposure of adjacent teeth or land area of the cast to provide a positive index.

Figure 19   Stability of the wax may be ensured by luting it to adjacent teeth.

Figure 20   Stone separating medium is applied to the areas that will form the index.

Figure 21   The stone core is carefully poured. It is important that the stone mix be firm, so that it does not slump and flow down over the wax registration onto the dies. For the same reason, the use of vibration must be carefully controlled.

Figures 22 and 23   When set, the core and wax registration are separated and the core is repositioned on the working cast. This core, properly related to its working cast, can be used to establish the maxi-

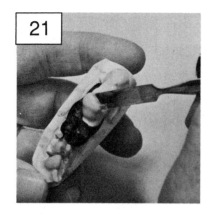
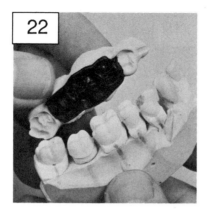
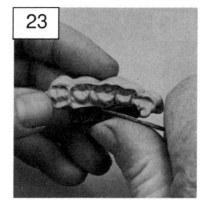
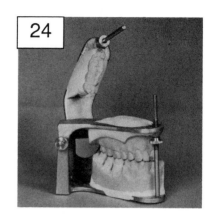

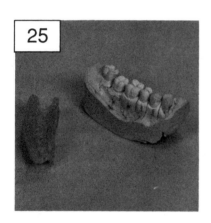
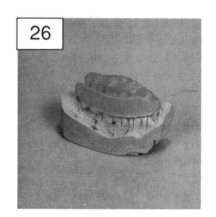
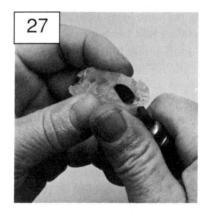
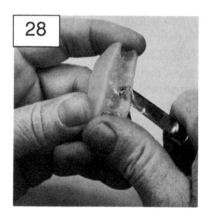

mum dimension of occlusal contours that will not interfere with mandibular excursion or centric position.

Use of Occlusal Cores

As suggested, developing the core provides some definite advantages over the direct-indirect approach of transferring a partially complete pattern from mouth to cast. First, the core is permanent. If the wax pattern is lost, broken, inadvertently overcarved, or miscast, the core is still available to permit correction and/or recarving of the pattern. Secondly, the core permits checks and correction of the casting to eliminate errors due to expansion, sprue placement and removal, and other factors. If this can be done accurately in the laboratory, time-consuming intraoral corrections can be virtually eliminated. It is the dentist's responsibility to deliver an accurate functionally generated path registration and the technician's responsibility to use it correctly.

Because an occlusal core is a stone counterdie that is indexed against the working cast, its inherent design normally permits it to be hand-articulated. For single restorations, this is accomplished by indexing the occlusal surfaces of adjacent teeth. In multiple-unit or small bridge situations where no unprepared tooth remains distal to the prepared teeth, the occlusal core can be indexed against the land area of the working cast.

Cores may also be related to the working cast with a simple hinge articulator. In fact, because of the need for an anatomical opposing cast in conjunction with the functional core, one hinge device has been made to receive a quadrant arch working cast with dual opposing hinges for an anatomic cast and a functional core (**Figure 24**). This articulator permits relating both a functional core *and* an anatomic opposing cast to a working cast.

Because anatomic cores are made directly in the mouth and are

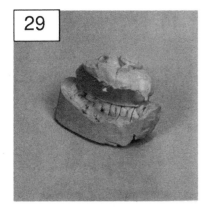

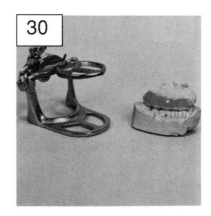

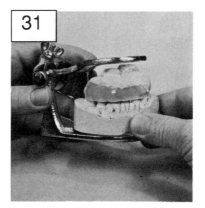

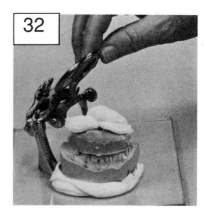

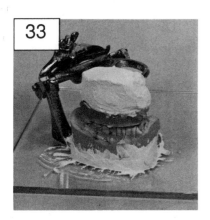

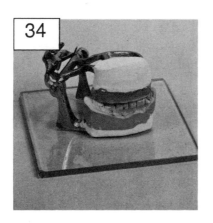

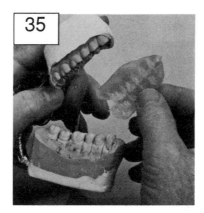

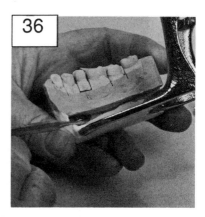

normally used in the laboratory by seating them directly on the working cast, no preparation by the technician is required. However, they can be used mounted in a simple hinge articulator. If this is desired, they must be prepared and mounted as described for the centric occlusion core.

Figures 25 and 26   When it is desirable to mount the working cast and a centric occlusion core on a simple hinge articulator, the wax registration is carefully seated on the working cast to insure accurate position.

Figures 27 and 28   If necessary, the record is trimmed with a sharp knife to eliminate or minimize any conflicts that might occur. *Occlusal records should never be allowed to contact soft-tissue areas of the cast.*

Figure 29   When correct position of the registration is assured, the

centric occlusion core is poured without extending it to contact exposed areas of the working cast. It is allowed to set.

Figures 30 through 34   With the working cast and core still related, the assembly is mounted on an appropriate hinge articulator.

Figure 35   When mounting is complete, the wax registration is removed.

Figure 36   Access to the ends of the dowel pins should not be blocked by the articulator framework. Access through the mounting plaster can easily be maintained by positioning a rope of utility wax over the dowel ends before mounting. The dowels can then be easily reached by removing the utility wax. In this illustration access was established through the lingual surface of the mounting.

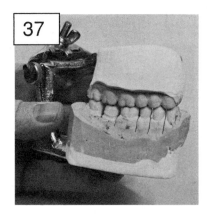
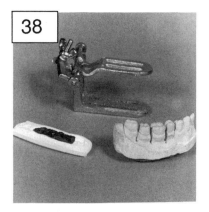
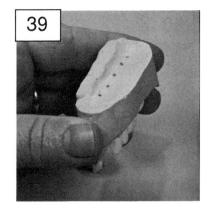
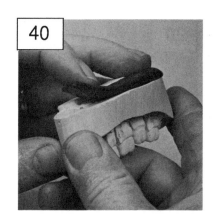

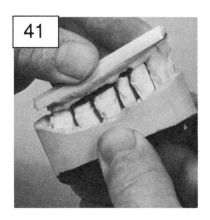
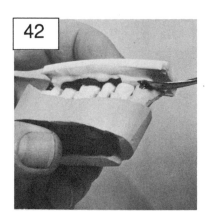
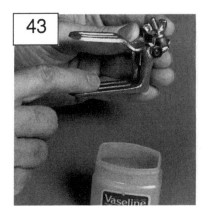
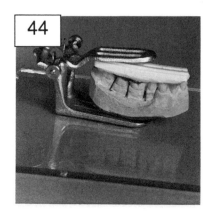

Figure 37   The working cast and opposing anatomic cast, related in centric occlusion, are now mounted.

Figure 38   Note the quadrant working cast with inlay preparations in the mandibular second premolar and the first molar, and a full crown preparation on the second molar. Note also the functional core with the wax chew-in still in position. The functional core was made *directly* in the mouth, using quick-setting stone carried into place in a tray designed for the purpose.

Figure 39   The working cast has been developed so that access to the end of the dowel for each removable die can be obtained from the facial aspect of the cast.

Figure 40   Strips of utility wax are placed to permit access to the dowel ends after mounting is completed.

Figure 41   The core is carefully related to the working cast. Normally the wax registration is removed from a "direct" core before it is related to the working cast. However, with exceeding care, the wax registration can often be left in position to enhance stability of the core on the working cast. When the core is developed indirectly (that is, on the working cast), it can simply be left unseparated in position on the cast until mounting is completed.

Figure 42   Once correctly positioned, the core is firmly luted to the working cast.

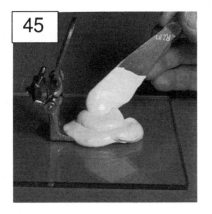

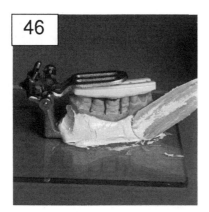

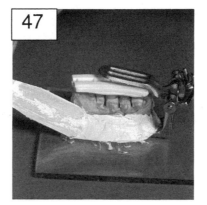

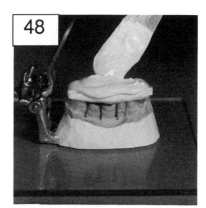

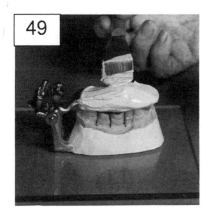

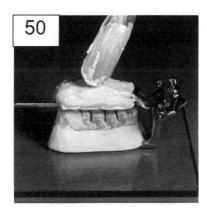

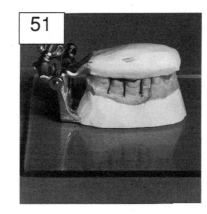

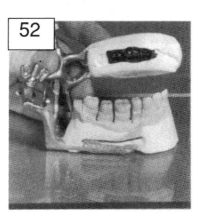

Figure 43　The mounting arms of the simple hinge articulator are lubricated for their protection and to facilitate subsequent removal of the casts.

Figure 44　The joined cast and core are trial-positioned in the assembled articulator. The utility wax used to maintain access to the dowels facilitates this positioning.

Figures 45 and 46　The joined core and cast are then mounted on the lower member of the articulator with quick-set plaster. Excess plaster is removed.

Additional working time for mounting procedures can be gained by mixing regular and quick-set plaster.

Figure 47　The mounting plaster is extended and smoothed to provide a clean mounting with sufficient retention of the working cast.

Figure 48　The mounting plaster is added to the core prior to the attachment to the upper member of the articulator.

Figures 49 and 50　The upper member of the articulator is closed and plaster is extended to cover the member and the core on both the facial (**Figure 49**) and lingual (**Figure 50**). The plaster is smoothed and the articulator stabilized in position until the plaster is set.

Figure 51　The mounting procedure is completed.

Figure 52　The upper and lower members of the articulator are separated and checked for accuracy of mounting.

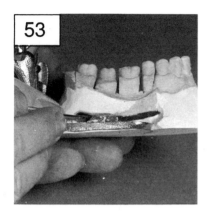
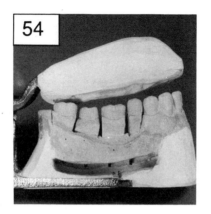
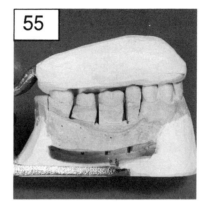
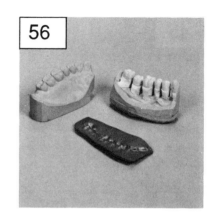

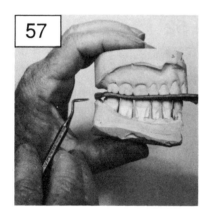
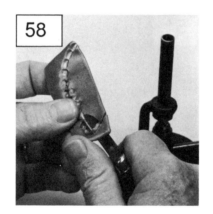
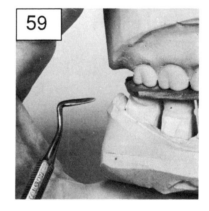
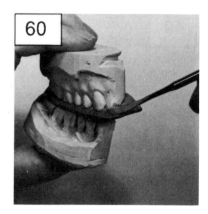

Figure 53   The utility wax is removed to provide access to the dowel pins.

Figures 54 and 55   If not previously accomplished, the wax registration is removed from the core and the instrument reassembled (**Figure 54**). When the articulator is closed, the core should be perfectly indexed against the working cast.

ANATOMIC OPPOSING CASTS

Instead of the simple wax chew-in or some type of occlusal core, a full or partial arch opposing cast (or an impression for same) may be provided. In addition, unless both the working cast and the opposing cast are full arch and the complement and interdigitation of teeth are sufficient to index hand articulation, some type of interocclusal registration must also be provided.

Partial Arch Casts

Figure 56   In the single onlay, crown, or small bridge situation involving partial arch casts an interocclusal registration will often be in the form of a centric occlusion wax bite. Pictured here are a half arch working cast, an opposing cast, and a wax registration.

When mounting is to be accomplished on a simple hinge (nonadjustable) type of articulator, this wax bite must provide centric occlusion—the position of maximum occlusal interdigitation. The probability for

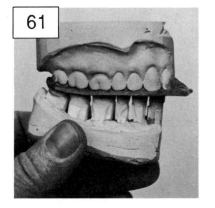

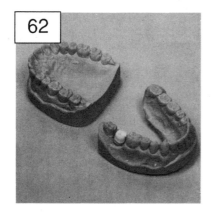

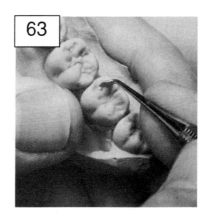

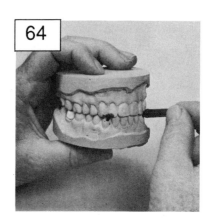

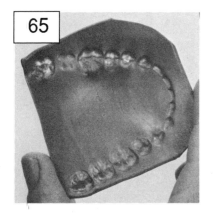

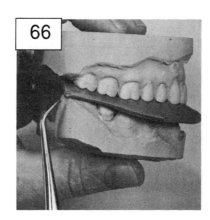

interocclusal registration are the retromolar pad area in the mandibular arch and the tuberosity and incisive papilla area in the maxillary arch.

Figures 58 and 59 To eliminate soft tissue conflict, trim the wax so that it contacts *only* the teeth.

Figures 60 and 61 Once the casts are accurately related in the registration, they are firmly luted together by melting appropriate areas of the registration wax or by the addition of sticky wax. When the relationship of the casts is stabilized, they are ready to be mounted on the instrument of choice.

Full Arch Casts

Figure 62 Full arch casts with sufficient complement and interdigitation of teeth may at times be hand articulated for mounting if a centric occlusion relationship is desired.

Figure 63 All blebs should be detected and removed before any articulation is attempted.

Figure 64 Once in correct relationship, the casts are firmly luted together to facilitate mounting.

Figure 65 If an interocclusal record is provided, it should be carefully studied for indications of any soft tissue contact. In this record there is evidence of such contact distal to the terminal molar at the upper left-hand corner of the record.

some error in mounting with such a wax registration is quite high, due to errors in making the registration (such as the patient's closing in an eccentric position, condylar displacement, distortion of the record during removal) as well as in using it to relate the casts (such as mispositioning the casts in the registration). Ideally the casts should be related by the dentist, as only the dentist is familiar with the occlusion presented by the patient. However, if this procedure is left to the laboratory technician, only good judgment and very careful observation can effect a complete and accurate seating of the casts.

Figure 57 Note in particular and remove any blebs (positive errors) on the cast (see also **Figure 63**). Areas where the wax contacts the soft tissue portion of the cast must also be noted, as the wax may have compressed this tissue in the mouth but of course cannot compress the stone cast. The most common areas for such soft tissue contact with an

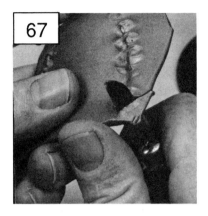
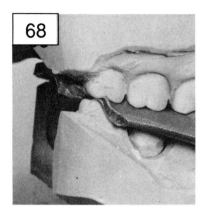
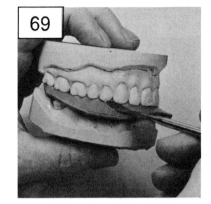
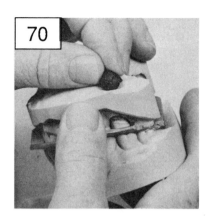

Figure 66 These areas of soft tissue contact may be verified by observation of the record on the cast.

Figures 67 and 68 *All areas of a registration that contact soft tissue must be trimmed away.*

Figure 69 When correctly related in the record, casts are luted together to facilitate mounting.

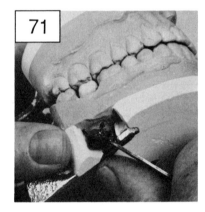
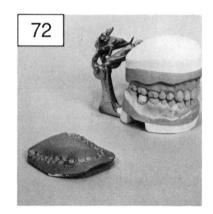

Figures 70 and 71 Consideration is always given to maintaining access to the dowel pins of all removable dies. This is readily done by the appropriate positioning of utility wax, which is removed once mounting is completed.

Figure 72 The mounted casts should be carefully inspected to verify the accuracy of their relationship. If sufficient teeth are present, uniform distribution of tooth contact should indicate accuracy of relationship.

Mounting Casts on Adjustable Articulators

Full arch casts are often mounted on an adjustable articulator when multiple individual restorations or a bridge restoration is being made. Use of such an instrument is indicated whenever eccentric occlusal relationships need to be evaluated or established during development of the restoration pattern.

Adjustable articulators fall into two categories: semiadjustable and fully adjustable. Description of all the available instruments and the techniques for their adjustment and use is far beyond the scope of this

manual. As a cursory example, the mounting of casts on the Hanau H-2 articulator is described here.

For an adjustable articulator to offer any advantage, the maxillary cast must be mounted via a face-bow transfer. The mandibular cast is then mounted by means of hand articulation or an interocclusal record. Although a centric occlusion record is common to the mounting of casts on simple hinge articulators, one of the primary advantages in use of an adjustable articulator is a centric relation (centric jaw position) mounting of the casts. Adjustment of the instrument depends on which instrument and technique are being used and the records provided.

Figure 73 Pictured here are the Hanau H-2 articulator and records and armamentarium necessary for mounting full arch casts. In addition to the casts there is a face-bow transfer record and a protrusive checkbite record.

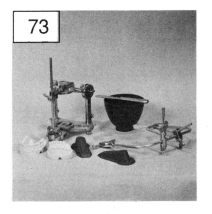
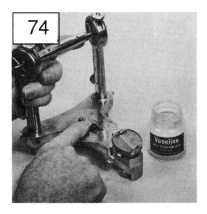
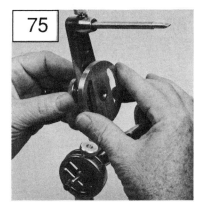
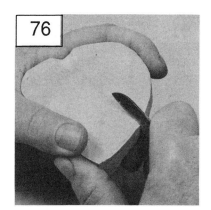

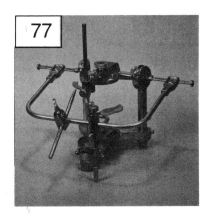
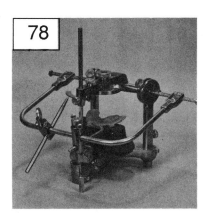
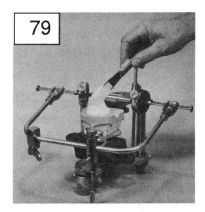
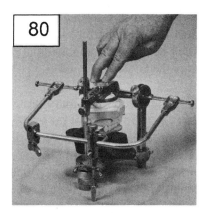

Figures 74 and 75   The articulator is lightly lubricated and mounting rings *securely* positioned before initiating the mounting procedure.

Figure 76   Unless the casts have been poured on some type of slab or template that provides an indexing contour to their base surfaces, they are notched on either side and posteriorly to facilitate indexing should it become necessary to remove and reposition the casts on their mounting.

Figure 77   The face-bow transfer record is assembled on the instrument. The condylar rods are positioned to center the face-bow on the instrument. This is done by adjusting the position of the face-bow to provide the same reading on each calibrated condylar rod. The vertical position of the face-bow record is determined by the orbital pointer. This position is adjusted until the pointer is even with the orbital plane guide.

Figure 78   Once the face-bow is properly adjusted, the position of the bite plane record should be supported to resist the weight and pressure of mounting the maxillary cast. This can be accomplished conveniently by use of two small wedge-shaped rubber doorstops as shown. The maxillary cast is carefully positioned in the transfer record.

Figure 79   Fast-setting plaster is quickly mixed to a creamy consistency and placed on the surface of the cast in a quantity sufficient to engage the mounting ring.

Additional working time for such mounting procedures can be gained by mixing regular and quick-set plaster.

Figures 80 and 81   The upper member of the articulator is quickly hinged closed such that the incisal guide pin is firmly seated on the incisal table. It is imperative that the plaster mix be loose enough that it

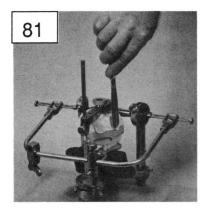
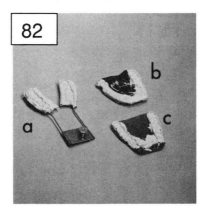
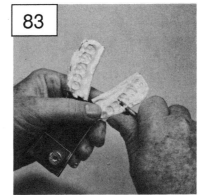
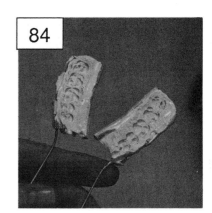

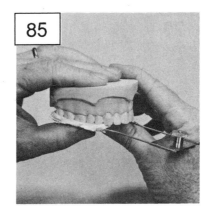
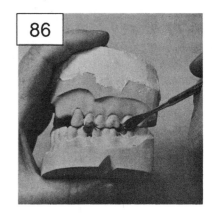

will not cause movement or displacement of the cast. The retentive slots in the mounting ring should be checked to make sure they are filled with plaster, and then the surface of the mounting may be gently smoothed.

As soon as the maxillary cast mounting is completed, the mandibular cast can be related to it for mounting. If the lower cast is to be mounted in centric occlusion and a sufficient complement of teeth are present to provide a stable interdigitation, the cast can be positioned by hand articulation. Because most patients present some discrepancy between centric relation and centric occlusion position, a CR interocclusal record may be provided to permit a centric relation mounting. Depending upon the nature and amount of the CR/CO discrepancy, centric relation records may of necessity be relatively thick. In such cases the thickness of the record anteriorly is estimated and the incisal pin is usually lowered so as to open the articulator by that approximate amount (normally 4 to 5 millimeters). After mounting, closure to contact of the casts will return the incisal pin approximately to its normal position—that is, the upper member of the instrument will be approximately parallel to the lower member.

As mentioned earlier, interocclusal records are most frequently made with some type of wax. However, dentists are rapidly switching to the use of various impression materials due to their greater accuracy. These materials are usually carried into place on a gauze or paper mesh (something quite thin to permit uninhibited tooth contact) suspended in an appropriate frame when *centric occlusion* is to be recorded (**Figure 82a**). These materials are usually conveyed on a wax, metal, or impres-

sion compound wafer when *centric relation* is being recorded (**Figure 82b**).

Zinc oxide–eugenol paste records offer the advantages of more accurate detail and resistance to distortion by virtue of their being rigid when set. However, this enhanced detail and rigidity demand comparable accuracy of the cast if indexing is to be correct. Even more than with wax registrations, it is important that points of interference be carefully noted and relieved until both casts can be fully seated in such indices (**Figures 83, 84 and 85**). In fact it is usually best to trim zinc oxide registrations so that only the tips of the cusps are contacted by the record.

Figure 86 The casts being mounted in this example are full arch dentoform casts that demonstrate no discrepancy between centric rela-

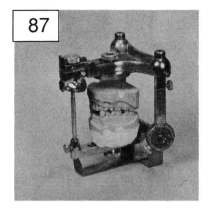

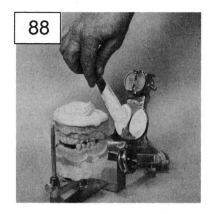

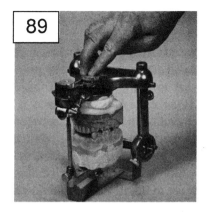

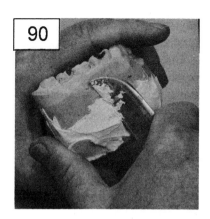

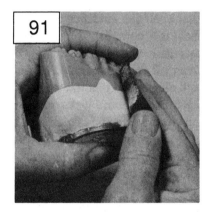

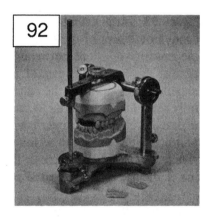

tion and centric occlusion. Hence they have positive interdigitation and they are being hand articulated.

The cast should be indexed and moistened by the application of a wet paper towel to the base or immersion of the base of the cast in a shallow level of water. Once the lower cast has been properly related to the maxillary cast, this position is fixed with sticky wax to facilitate mounting.

Figure 87 The articulator is inverted to facilitate mounting the lower cast. For the Hanau instrument a jig is available to provide additional stability for this inverted position as shown. The upper cast is repositioned on the instrument, making sure that the mounting ring is firmly tightened. *It is important that articulators be adjusted in centric position before mounting a lower cast*. If appropriate, *lock the instrument in*

this position. The articulator should only open and close with no lateral shift or wobble.

The incisal guide table should be set at zero (flat), and the incisal guide pin set at zero or at an increased vertical dimension appropriate to accommodate an interocclusal record if used. When these adjustments are made, the instrument should be trial-closed to be sure that the incisal guide table will clear the lower cast. The lower mounting ring should again be checked to ensure that it is firmly secured.

Figure 88 An appropriate quantity of a thin creamy mix of fast-setting plaster is applied to the mounting ring and cast as shown. Plaster must be pushed into the spaces in the mounting ring.

Figure 89 The instrument is promptly closed while the plaster is still loose, so that no displacement of the mandibular cast occurs. *Be sure that the lower cast does not move in the registration during the mounting procedure*. Additional plaster is added and smoothed as indicated to complete the mounting.

Figure 90 Excess plaster may be removed with a knife. This is most easily accomplished while the plaster is still "green" (after setting but before drying).

Figure 91 Final smoothing can be readily accomplished with wet sandpaper.

Once mounting is completed, the instrument can be adjusted. Semiadjustable articulators are usually adjusted by the use of eccentric interocclusal records termed *checkbites*.

Checkbites are static interocclusal records (like centric occlusion or centric relation records) that record isolated eccentric mandibular positions. Adjustable articulators can be set to duplicate these isolated positions of the mandible, but there is no record of, and hence no possibility of duplicating, the path of travel of the mandible between these positions. For example, a lateral checkbite records the relative position of the mandibular teeth in relation to the maxillary teeth at the given point of lateral mandibular excursion at which the registration was made. The instrument can then be set to duplicate this intertooth positional relationship.

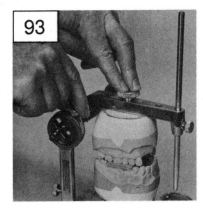 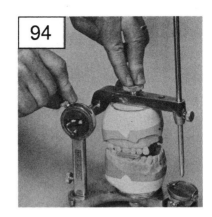

Figure 92   Because the Hanau H-2 is a semiadjustable instrument, it is set with checkbites. It is pictured here with casts mounted and a two-piece wax protrusive checkbite, which is commonly the only checkbite used in setting this instrument. (**Figure 82c** shows a one-piece protrusive record made of wax and zinc oxide paste.)

The protrusive checkbite is used to set the horizontal condylar guidance of the instrument. The Hanau is a so-called straight-line tracking instrument. That is, the condylar element of the instrument travels in a straight track, rather than along a curved path as is found naturally in the articular eminence, the curved bony contour along which the condyles glide during lateral or protrusive mandibular excursions. The correct position for the starting point of the condylar path has already been determined by virtue of the centric mounting. The protrusive checkbite indicates the location of the condyles at some protruded mandibular position by using the teeth to index the positional relationship of the mandible to the maxilla.

Said another way, the protrusive record indicates the position of the condyles at a given point of protrusion by indexing the relationship of the teeth at this protruded position. Thus two points of condylar position are identified: the point of origin (centric position) and a protruded point. Two points determine a straight line, and if this line is oriented to a plane (in this case the Frankfort Plane) an angle is determined. Thus the inclination of a straight-line path of condylar travel during protrusive excursion in relation to the maxillary occlusal plane is determined by the protrusive checkbite. In the Hanau technique this inclination is referred to as *horizontal condylar guidance*.

Figure 93   Adjustment of the horizontal condylar guidance for each condylar element of the Hanau instrument is accomplished by placing the protrusive record between the casts and, with pressure applied against the upper member of the instrument over the center of the maxillary cast, rotating the condylar path element so that the teeth are fully seated in the record. To accomplish this the centric locks must be released such that the upper bow of the instrument can be carried into a protruded relationship to permit the teeth to be positioned in the protrusive record. The thumbscrews that lock the horizontal condylar tracking elements are then released so that these may be rotated.

Figure 94   While pressure is applied over the center of the maxillary cast to facilitate finding the seated position of the maxillary teeth in the index, the condylar tracking element is rotated backward and forward by the thumbscrew.

Figure 95   The rotation of the tracking element produces an anterioposterior rocking of the maxillary cast. This rocking is continued until the most stable position of the maxillary cast in the checkbite can be obtained. Usually a "neutral zone" with a range of about 5° is felt at the point of correct positional relationship of the maxillary cast. This is a result of "slack" or "play" in the instrument and record. When such is the case, set the horizontal condylar guidance at the lowest reading in the slack zone. When the condylar element on one side has been adjusted and the thumbscrew tightened, this procedure is repeated for the other. After adjustment of the second element, the first should always be rechecked.

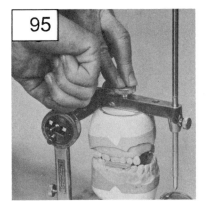

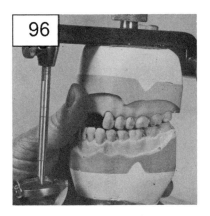

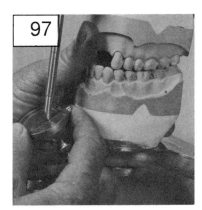

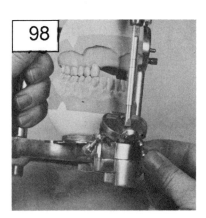

A discrepancy in the reading between the right and left elements often results. This may be real, but it may also result from having recorded a protrusolateral mandibular position rather than a straight protrusive position. In such situations one condyle will have traveled farther down its articular eminence than the other, thus resulting in a greater indicated angulation. This possibility can be easily verified by checking the dental midline with the casts in centric position and then replacing the protrusive checkbite and again observing the dental midline relationship. If the mandible had deviated significantly to one side when the protrusive record was taken, the discrepancy will be evident. In such cases a greater angulation could be expected on the side opposite that toward which the mandible has deviated (the non-functional or balancing side). The safest procedure in such situations is to get another record. If this cannot be done, an alternative is to reduce the greater angulation to equal the lesser, or split the difference if the discrepancy is very large.

Figure 96 When the inclination of horizontal condylar guidance is determined, the incisal or anterior guidance for protrusive excursion can be set. This is accomplished by carrying the instrument into a protruded relationship as pictured. There are no incisor teeth on this maxillary working cast, but the distal arm of the maxillary canine is related to the mesial arm of the mandibular first premolar facial cusp. This protruded relationship will normally cause the incisal guide pin to be elevated from the incisal guidance table.

Figure 97 The incisal guidance table is rotated into contact with the incisal guide pin in the protruded position. Obviously, the teeth are

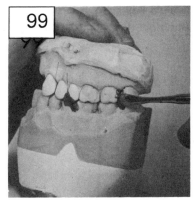

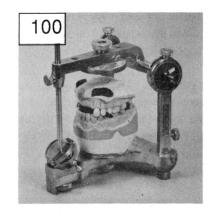

providing the incisal guidance. The table is being set for two reasons: (1) to protect the teeth on the cast against abrasion during manipulation of the instrument, and (2) because the canines, which are providing the anterior guidance at this point, will subsequently be prepared. By setting the instrument with these study casts, it will be properly set when the working cast, which has no incisal guidance (due to absence of the incisors and preparation of the canines), is substituted.

Figure 98 After the protrusive inclination of the incisal table is set, lateral guidance is adjusted by carrying the instrument into an end-to-end lateral relationship and setting the wings of the incisal guidance table to contact the pin. This adjustment is, of course, made for both sides. The rationale and purpose of the lateral adjustments are the same as for the protrusive adjustment.

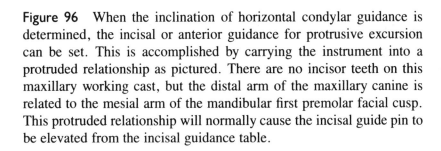

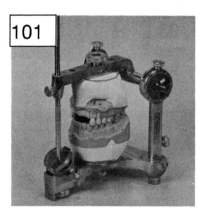

Figures 99 and 100   Once the instrument is adjusted, it is a simple matter to substitute a working cast for either the maxillary or the mandibular study cast.

Figure 101   The working cast is now mounted in an instrument that has been adjusted to simulate posterior and anterior guidance, even though the teeth that would normally establish anterior guidance are missing and/or prepared.

REVIEW QUESTIONS

1. List three types of occlusal cores.
2. Describe an anatomic core.
3. Functionally generated path registration provides contacts that are undesirable in the natural dentition. What are these contacts called, and how are they corrected?
4. Name two types of errors that can occur when mounting full arch casts using a centric occlusion wax-bite interocclusal record.
5. In using the semiadjustable Hanau H-2 articulator, what type of interocclusal records are used to set the horizontal condylar guidance?

SECTION 11

Contour

In general statement, *contour* is the aspect of a tooth or restoration that relates it to its environment. Considered in full perspective, contour includes the anatomic or morphologic relationship of the tooth or restoration, its functional relationship, and its esthetic quality.

General consideration was given to all of these factors in your study of dental anatomy. Occlusal functional relationship has received further specific attention in the preceding sections of this manual. The general features of esthetic contour are common to all of us as a result of observation of our own dentition and that of others (**Figure 1**). Practical experience in applied knowledge of the anatomic arrangement of teeth occurs in removable prosthodontics. However, the challenge to generate anatomic form of individual teeth to provide function and esthetics is much greater in a fixed restorative prosthesis.

ANATOMIC CONTOUR

Occlusal Contours

The primary consideration in establishing occlusal contour for a restoration is to provide a pattern of contact that is functionally consis-

tent with the other occlusal components. To a great extent functional consistency dictates anatomic consistency. For example, a restoration carved with steep cuspal inclines cannot provide proper centric contact and functional relationships with adjacent and opposing teeth that present flat occlusal surfaces (**Figure 2**). Conversely, a restoration developed with a flat occlusal configuration cannot function in harmony with adjacent and opposing teeth that have steep cuspal inclines (**Figure 3**). Thus, occlusally speaking, to be functionally consistent with its environment, a restoration must be anatomically consistent. Adhering to this concept offers little challenge when normal occlusal anatomy is present, but because we are conditioned to think in terms of ideal or normal anatomy, a malposed or flat occlusal surface often seems difficult to accommodate.

Experience with flat or monoplane denture teeth shows that even a flat occlusal surface can be made more functionally efficient by placing pits and grooves in it (**Figure 4**). It is difficult to describe fully the significance of the primary pit-and-groove pattern of the posterior occlusal surface in the efficient mastication of foodstuff. It is even more difficult to describe the importance of secondary occlusal anatomy. However, it is often the secondary groove or depression that permits a cusp tip properly located for centric contact to pass along an

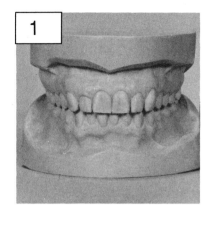
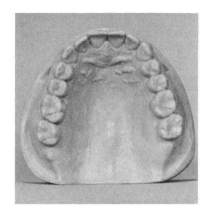
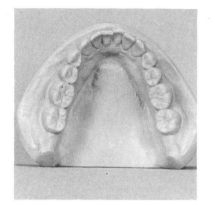
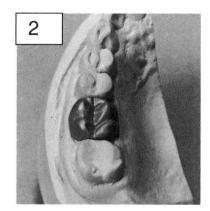

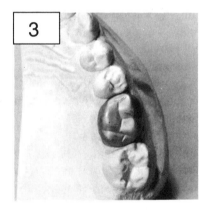
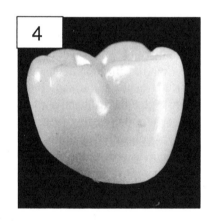
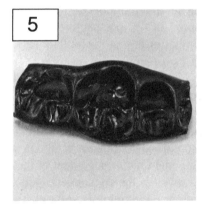
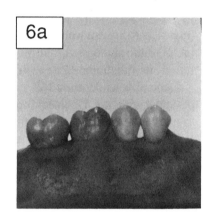

opposing cuspal incline without conflict during mandibular excursion. One needs only to observe the detail and frequency of such secondary pathways in functionally generated path registrations (functional chew-ins) or cores to begin to understand the importance of these contours in occlusal function. It is often amazing to see how completely and accurately the properly positioned opposing tooth can carve an occlusal surface in a functional wax chew-in (**Figure 5**). Familiarity with the ideal or normal occlusal anatomy, together with the ability to modify and locate these contours to be functionally compatible with the opposing dentition, is the secret to proper development of occlusal contour.

Axial Contours

Once the occlusal surface of the pattern has been related to the opposing teeth, it becomes relatively easy to establish axial contours. The axial surface connects occlusal contour with the gingival margin of the preparation. Lack of attention to appropriate contour of the axial surfaces of restorations can significantly impair the normal function of the tooth.

Proximal Contour and Contact Area   A positive landmark to be established in axial contour is the proximal contact relationship with adjacent teeth. The normal proximal contact between adjacent teeth is formed by two curved surfaces touching each other (**Figure 6**). These are known as the *proximal surfaces*, and the area where they touch each other is the *proximal contact point* (or *area*). In older people proximal

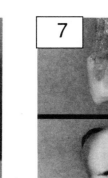

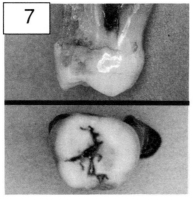

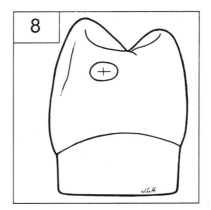

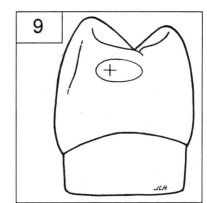

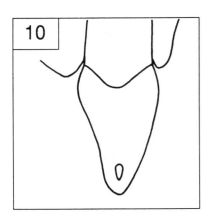

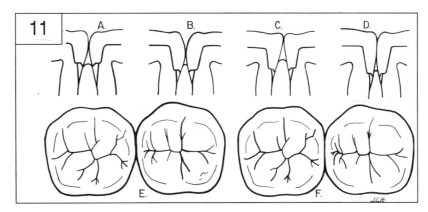

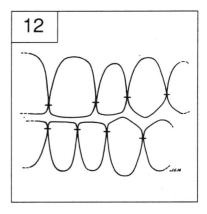

contacts become areas rather than points, as a result of wear produced as adjacent teeth rub against one another (**Figure 7**).

In general, posterior contact areas have a dimension of 1 to 2 millimeters occlusogingivally and are oval in outline. The long axis of the oval contact area is oriented faciolingually and is normally located at the junction of the facial and middle third of the proximal surface (**Figure 8**). Variations toward a more midline position are common, especially as wear expands the area of contact (**Figure 9**). In anterior teeth, proximal contact is usually smaller and may be round in outline or have an incisogingivally oriented oval outline (**Figure 10**).

Contacts must not only be of proper form but also must be placed in the correct position. The location and size of the contact area are important to correct function. The contact areas between the posterior teeth are normally located on the facial half of the proximal surface.

Thus the lingual embrasure is normally about twice as long faciolingually as the facial embrasure (**Figure 11e**).

Occlusogingivally posterior proximal contact areas are normally located at or about the junction of the occlusal and middle thirds of the proximal surface (**Figure 11a**). The incisogingival location of anterior proximal contacts is much more variable due to variations in contour and position of the teeth. As a rule of thumb, the contacts on maxillary teeth are in the incisal one-third mesially, and on the distal surface are closer to the junction of the incisal and middle thirds (**Figure 12**). The contacts between mandibular incisors are in the incisal one-third, often extending to the incisal edge due to wear of the incisal surfaces.

Interproximal Embrasures   There are four recognized interproximal embrasure spaces: occlusal, facial, lingual, and gingival. Because they

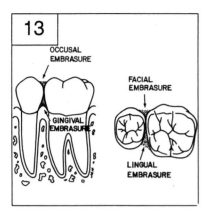

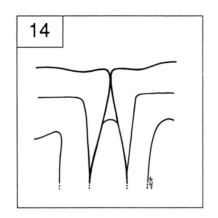

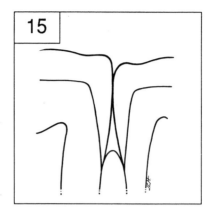

are created by apposition of convex surfaces, these embrasures are pointed V-shaped spaces (**Figure 13**).

Occlusal embrasure. The occlusal embrasure is formed by the contour of adjacent marginal ridges and the location of the occlusal margin of the interproximal contact area. When the adjacent marginal ridges are left as square or sharp angles, they restrict the normal dimension of the occlusal embrasure (**Figure 14**). Such contour is usually associated with a flat occlusal surface area in the region of the adjacent proximal pit. The resulting occlusal embrasure is essentially a crack in a flat surface rather than a curved V-shaped crevice between two rounded marginal ridges. A poorly contoured sharp-angle marginal ridge is almost always accompanied by a wide (faciolingually) proximal contact area (**Figure 11f**). As already suggested, such contour restricts the normal spillage of foodstuff into the adjacent embrasures. The net effect of this altered function is the impaction of food material (especially stringy foods) through the contact area into the interproximal space. Impaction of food debris is a serious problem, as it produces irritation of the interproximal tissue, with resultant pocket formation that may eventually cause loss of the teeth.

Another cause of interproximal food impaction is the uneven marginal ridge relationship (**Figure 15**). When one of two adjacent marginal ridges is higher than the other, foodstuff becomes packed into the angle thus formed and tends to be forced through the proximal contact into the interproximal space. Because of the severe consequences of this impaction, marginal ridges, if possible, should always be developed to be even in their occlusal height, thus eliminating the "backboard" against which food may become impacted and forced through the proximal contact. Accordingly, *marginal ridge compatibility takes pre-*

cedence over occlusal contact.

Centric contacts are often properly located on proximal marginal ridges. However, if establishing such a contact dictates elevation of the marginal ridge in question above that of its neighbor, the occlusal contact should be forfeited and the marginal ridge developed even with the adjacent marginal ridge. Conversely, if the opposing cusps dictate that a marginal ridge should be carved lower than its neighbor, (1) the opposing cusp must be reduced to permit carving of the marginal ridge at a compatible level (**Figure 16a**), or (2) the adjacent marginal ridge must be reduced so that it is compatible with the involved marginal ridge when it is carved to proper relationship with the opposing occlusion (**Figure 16b**).

The decision as to which one or both of these procedures should be effected must be based on an evaluation of the position and occlusion of the adjacent teeth. Such decisions should be made by the dentist. However, it is often difficult to anticipate such problems, and when repeated communication with the dentist is not feasible, the technician may have to resolve the question independently. Under these circumstances, the best choice would probably be to relieve the opposing tooth, develop the marginal ridge in question to a height compatible with that of the adjacent marginal ridge and advise the dentist of what has been done. This approach leaves the dentist with the ultimate choice: either to accept the restoration as developed and reduce the opposing tooth, or to reduce the marginal ridges of the restoration and adjacent tooth. This sort of "play it safe" thinking and planning can resolve many of the minor questions that the laboratory technician faces.

Facial and lingual embrasures. The form of the facial and lingual

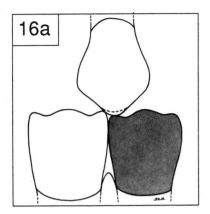
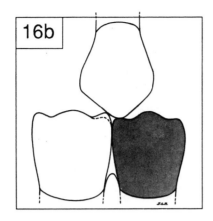
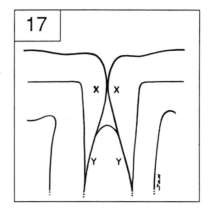
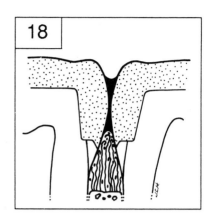

embrasures must, for practical purposes, be considered concurrently, because their determinants and functional implications are essentially the same. The form and relative size of the facial and lingual embrasures are determined by three factors: (1) the convexity of the adjacent proximal surfaces, (2) the prominence or sharpness of the proximal line angles of these surfaces, and (3) the size and location of the proximal contact area.

Because the posterior interproximal contact is located on the facial half of the proximal surface, the lingual embrasure is larger than the facial embrasure. Hence the primary excursion of foodstuff occurs through the lingual embrasure toward the tongue. The tongue can easily return the food onto the occlusal table in preparation for the next masticatory stroke. If the facial embrasures were larger than the lingual and the pattern of horizontal overlap of the upper and lower teeth were reversed, the greater portion of foodstuff would be directed into the facial vestibule, where the return of foodstuff to the occlusal table by the cheeks is less efficient. Broad faciolingual contacts reduce the dimension of the embrasures and thus restrict the excursion of foodstuffs from the occlusal tables and inhibit adequate stimulation of interproximal tissues (**Figure 11f**).

Gingival embrasure. The largest of the interproximal embrasures is the gingival embrasure. Grossly triangular in shape, the vertex of this embrasure is again the result of apposition of convex proximal surfaces as they meet at the proximal contact area (**Figure 17x**). However, the sides of the lower portion of the gingival embrasure are formed by opposed, diverging, concave tooth surfaces. It is this concave outline of the proximal surface of a tooth just at and above the cervical line that accounts for the greater dimension of the gingival embrasure space

(**Figure 17y**). This space is important because it determines the configuration and size of the interproximal papilla. Normally this space is completely filled by the interdental papilla. Reduction of the gingival embrasure space by overcontouring the proximal surfaces of restorations or by locating the gingival extent of the proximal contact area too far apically may crowd the interproximal papilla, resulting in inflammation and subsequent periodontal breakdown (**Figures 11b and d**). Thus it is vitally important that the normal bell shape or pear shape of the proximal surface of a tooth be faithfully reproduced in any restoration.

The problem of crowding of the interdental papilla by excessive occlusogingival dimension of the proximal contact area is particularly evident in the soldered or cast connection of adjacent restorations. It is often difficult to provide adequate strength in such connectors by virtue of their dimension without crowding the gingival embrasure space (**Figure 18**). Every effort should be made to keep these connectors as high as possible, because *occlusal* embrasure form is not significant when there is rigid union between adjacent restorations (**Figure 19**).

Even under ideal conditions, the gingival embrasure is the most difficult area in the mouth to clean. This problem is compounded by the rigid union of adjacent restorations, which precludes the conventional approach of introducing dental floss through the proximal contact area. In these circumstances access to the interdental area beneath contact must be gained from the facial or lingual. Such access is essentially impossible when the gingival embrasure space has been significantly restricted by an overcontoured connector. If in doubt as to proper contour when establishing the proximal surfaces of a posterior restoration, one should remember that it would be quite difficult, if not impossible, to have too much embrasure space if any semblance of

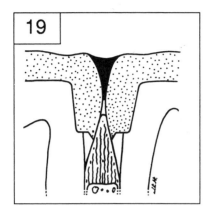

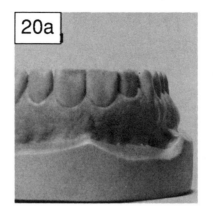

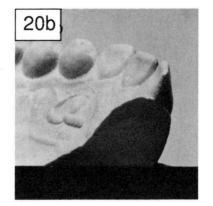

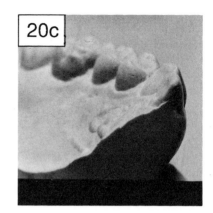

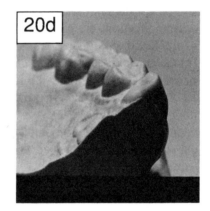

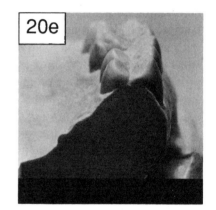

normal proximal contour is maintained. In other words, *too much gingival embrasure space is much healthier than not enough.* This general rule may not be applicable to anterior restorations because of esthetics and phonetics.

Facial and Lingual Surfaces   On the laboratory bench only two guides exist to dictate the proper form of facial and lingual surfaces: the contour of adjacent teeth, and a thorough knowledge of dental anatomy. Normal soft tissue contour cannot be duplicated on the die of a preparation that has a subgingivally positioned margin. Hopefully, contour of the adjacent soft tissue and teeth will have been faithfully reproduced in the working cast so that it can serve as a guide to appropriate contour for the restoration at hand.

Recorded, unprepared tooth structure apical to the margin may also indicate appropriate contour for the gingival portion of a pattern (see **Section 7, Figure 20**). Even so, the exact location and amount of height of contour of the facial and lingual surfaces necessary to protect the subjacent gingival tissues will remain in question. Because it is much easier to correct slightly excessive contour of a restoration by reduction than to correct deficient contour by addition, the safest procedure for the technician is to be sure that adequate heights of contour do exist on the facial and lingual surfaces of the restoration. It is interesting to note, however, how little contour is required to "protect" the investing gingival tissues properly. It is practically impossible to identify all combinations of tooth/tissue contour.

Figures 20 and 21 show serial sections of the rather "ideal" casts pictured in **Figure 1**. Note the amount and location of facial and lingual contours and variation in axial (long axis) orientation as the sections progress about the arches (**Figure 20a–h**, maxillary right central through second molar; **Figure 21a–h**, mandibular right central through second molar). These examples are especially interesting because the casts from which they were made are not (as one might expect) those of a teenager, but rather those of a forty-six-year-old woman.

CONTOURING FOR ESTHETICS

Although functional contour and esthetic contour are closely related, it is quite probable that a restoration that has been developed with very adequate functional contour may not satisfy requirements for esthetic

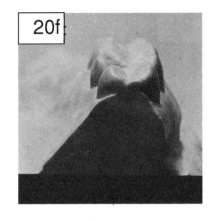

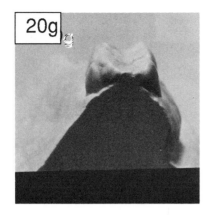

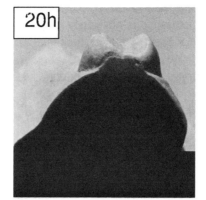

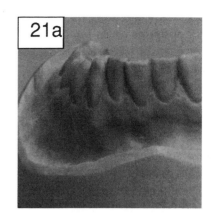

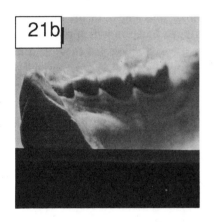

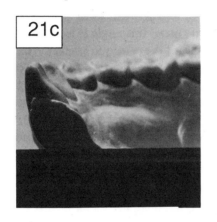

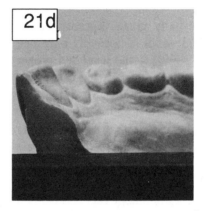

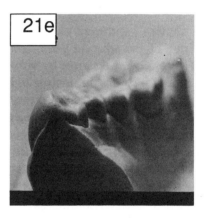

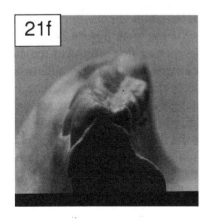

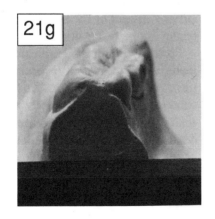

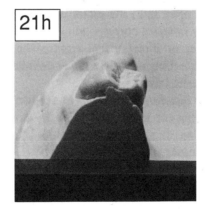

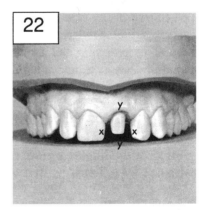

contour. Contouring for function may well be considered more critical for posterior teeth, but contouring for esthetics is obviously essential for anterior teeth. Hence discussion here focuses on the fundamental factors of contour that influence the esthetic character of anterior teeth. These same principles of course also apply with lesser significance to posterior tooth contour.

Contouring for esthetics is an art and very dependent upon an individual's artistic ability. Nevertheless several specific fundamentals that are significant in obtaining desired contour can be readily identified and evaluated. There is also a logical sequence to the consideration and development of these contours.

General Contours

Certain perimeters of contour are usually given. Specifically, by virtue of the adjacent teeth, mesiodistal width is normally indicated (**Figure 22x**). Likewise, by virtue of gingival tissue level and proper occlusal relationship, incisogingival length is normally indicated (**Figure 22y**). These contour dimensions are primarily functional, but they do contribute to the esthetic dimensions of the restoration and should be considered first, as they are known dimensions that can be readily established. Of course, there are situations when these dimensions are not definitely indicated. For example, when diastemas are present the mesiodistal width of the restoration may have to be arbitrarily established by observation unless an exact measurement can be obtained from a corresponding tooth in the arch. Likewise, when no occlusion is present (as in the case of an anterior open bite) the establishment of incisogingival length may be arbitrary unless a corresponding tooth is present to permit actual measurement or direct visual comparison. Normally, however, indications for these dimensions are rather definite and accordingly they should be established first.

In effect, we have just described the *absolute dimensions* of a crown: mesiodistal width as indicated by adjacent teeth, and gross incisogingival length as indicated by occlusion. In addition, the contour of a portion of the lingual surface of an upper incisor can usually be determined by function as well as the facioincisal aspect of the lower incisors.

More important esthetically are the *apparent dimensions* of the restoration. One of the most important dimensions of esthetic contour is apparent mesiodistal width. Whereas actual width of the tooth is determined by proximal contact location, apparent width is determined by

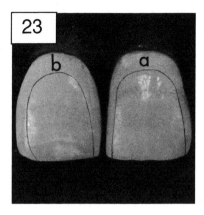
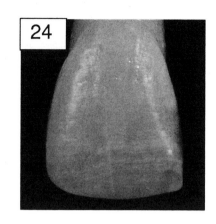

the location and form of the facioproximal line angles of the tooth. If the facial line angle is left as a right angle, its location will approximate that of the proximal contact. This makes the tooth look just as wide as it actually is (**Figure 23a**). If, however, the line angles are markedly rounded, thus moving their height of contour in toward the center of the facial surface of the tooth, the apparent width of the tooth can be markedly reduced (**Figure 23b**). Close observation of an incisor tooth (or any tooth for that matter) soon reveals that the contour of the facial line angles varies from the incisal to the gingival. The actual width of a tooth in the incisal or occlusal area is greater; moreover, it *appears* wider because the line angles are sharper or more acute. Conversely, even though the actual width of the tooth is less at the gingival level, its apparent width is even narrower because of the marked rounding and curving inward of the line angles. This variation in contour of the line angles is one factor that gives character to the tooth (**Figure 24**).

Probably the most significant single contour that influences the esthetic value of a tooth (especially an anterior tooth) is the silhouette form of the incisal edge. This is true because the incisal outline or silhouette is the most readily and discretely observable contour presented by the tooth. The reason for this is quite simple: the marked contrast of the color of a tooth against the dark background of the oral cavity permits immediate appreciation of contour or silhouette form by even casual observation. To appreciate this, look at the incisal edge contour of your teeth in a mirror. Note how discretely these edges are outlined against the oral cavity. Now close sufficiently to permit the maxillary incisors to overlap the mandibular incisors, or simply place a finger tip behind the incisal edges of the maxillary teeth. Observe how the definition of the incisal edges is diminished by virtue of reduction of

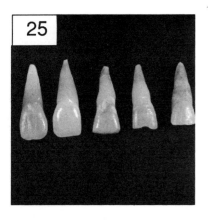
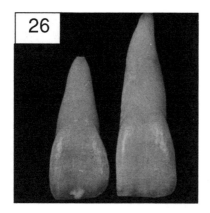
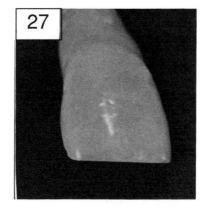
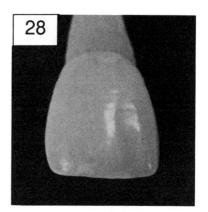

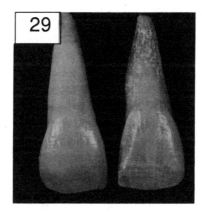
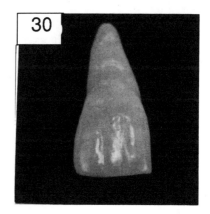

contrast. Obviously, even the most minute changes in incisal edge contour are readily observable; hence they strongly influence the esthetic value of the tooth. Contour of the edge, whether it is straight or curved, smooth or irregular, has a distinct influence on the character of the tooth (**Figure 25**).

The incisal corners are particularly significant esthetically. They contribute to the contour of both the proximal outline and the incisal edge. It is specifically the contour of the incisal corners that creates the form of the incisal embrasures. These embrasure outlines are important esthetically because they are one of the unique features of the overall incisal silhouette pattern. Exact contour of incisal corners may be difficult to create because of a greater, third-dimensional influence. Being a part of the proximofacial line angle, which is the determinant of apparent width of the tooth, sharp or right-angled corners yield a significant increase in apparent width, while rounding of the corners is effective in apparent reduction of width (**Figure 26**).

The incisal area of the tooth has one other third-dimensional influence: the apparent thickness of an anterior tooth is primarily a product of the contour of the incisal edge. This is readily observable on the lower incisors, where the contour and dimension of the incisal edge is directly visible and is thus an absolute value. The incisal edge of the maxillary incisor, however, is not directly visible and as such has an apparent value. If the facioincisal angle or edge is sharp and distinctly longer than the linguoincisal angle, the incisal edge will appear sharp and hence the tooth will appear thin (**Figure 27**). Conversely, if the incisal edge is bluntly rounded or flat, so that even though not directly visible there is obviously some tooth structure apparent lingual to the facioincisal angle, the incisal edge (and hence the tooth) will appear

thick (**Figure 28**). Again we are dealing with an apparent value, as the effect is more the result of contour rather than actual dimension.

Once the actual and apparent contour and dimension of the proximal and incisal surfaces have been established, one can begin to consider the contour of the facial surface proper. Although much of the character of a tooth is determined by the perimeters discussed above, the relative convexity or flatness of the facial surface per se is also a prominent factor in creating the impression of tooth form. The range of tooth forms available for dentures—square, tapering, ovoid, and their modifications—offers only a basic overview of the possibilities.

In general, the more round or convex the facial surface, the softer or more feminine and narrow will the tooth appear to be. Conversely, the flatter the facial surface, the more bold, masculine, and wide the tooth will seem (**Figure 29**).

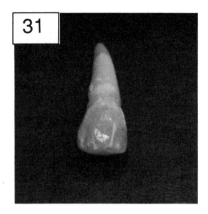 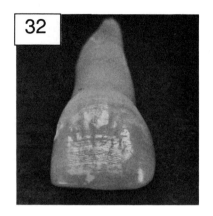 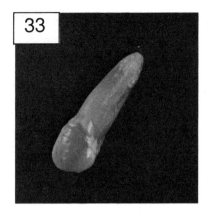 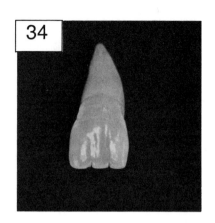

Discrete Contours

In addition to the influence of general contour on apparent tooth form, discrete contours or markings on the facial surface can strongly influence the character of tooth appearance. Notable among these are the subtle, usually somewhat linear, depressions that suggest the division of developmental lobes—generally termed *developmental grooves*. The presence of such concavities lends to the bold or masculine appearance of the tooth (**Figure 30**). Smaller, flat or concave *facets* on the facial surface contribute little to general form but are significant in that they change the pattern of reflection and/or refraction of light and hence contribute to surface character (**Figure 31**).

Surface character is often also strongly influenced by the presence of *perikymata*. These appear as very fine, wavy, parallel ridges running transversely across the facial surface and result from the incremental deposition of enamel. Although these minute ridges have no specific bearing on general form, they are significant in creating the appearance of a textured surface (**Figure 32**).

The grooves between these minute ridges are known as *incremental lines* (Lines of Retzius) and at times are exaggerated in size giving rise to another recognized facial marking. This group of larger transverse grooves are identified as *imbrication lines*. These are very shallow rounded linear depressions, usually less than six or eight in number, that traverse the height of contour usually in the gingival half of the facial surface. Though sometimes in evidence, they are not nearly so prevalent or obvious as it seems they have been reputed to be (**Figure 33**).

To be complete in listing facial markings, it is probably appropriate to identify the developmental grooves and lobes that constitute the mamelons on the incisal edges of young anterior teeth. Although they are a very positive marking when present, mamelons are normally worn away during the early years of life and are thus not present at those ages when restorations are usually made, unless an abnormal occlusal relationship exists (**Figure 34**). Mamelons are rarely reproduced on restorations.

Facial markings added to restorations should duplicate the appearance of adjacent or corresponding teeth. When no such teeth are present for comparison, the skilled and knowledgeable technician may selectively apply appropriate facial markings to provide a desired effect.

Gingival Contour

Only one perimeter of the esthetically significant surface of the tooth has not yet been considered: the gingival contour and outline. Seldom is any true consideration given to gingival outline, either actual or apparent, as neither can be controlled at the time the restoration is being made. Actual outline of the gingival contour of a crown is of course determined by the contour of the prepared margin. Because the margin is normally located subgingival, the apparent outline is created by the gingival tissue rather than by the crown itself. Although many factors may ultimately influence the contour of the gingiva, certainly not the least of which is the contour of the crown, seldom is any procedure actually executed for the specific purpose of changing the gingival outline. Where necessary or desirable this can be done, however, either by purposely altering the gingival height of contour on the crown, or more positively by surgically recontouring the gingival tissues.

REVIEW QUESTIONS

1. What are the three elements that contour includes?
2. Discuss occlusal contour as it concerns the relationship between functional consistency and anatomic consistency.
3. Discuss proximal contour as related to the proximal contact area.
4. Name the four embrasure spaces.
5. Discuss the concept of marginal ridge compatibility, including its relation to occlusal centric contacts.
6. Discuss the contour and width of the facial and lingual embrasures as related to the excursion of food.

SECTION 12

Wax Patterns

The technical procedures considered thus far have all been directed toward the development of dies and working casts sufficient to permit creating a pattern of the restoration. The ultimate objective is a casting that restores form and function, and maintains the integrity of the breached tooth. These features must be established in the pattern, as it will form the mold for the casting. The accuracy of the casting is wholly dependent on the accuracy of the pattern from which it is developed. The accuracy of the pattern, in turn, is dependent on the accuracy of the die and working cast and the skill and artistic ability of the technician.

In times past, patterns for cast restorations were created by the dentist directly on the tooth in the patient's mouth. During the early years of dentistry this was the only appropriate means for pattern development, as technicians and suitable impression materials were not available. Very few patterns are made via the direct technique today.

We are concerned here with the indirect technique for pattern development. Since the advent of elastic impression materials, the advantages of this technique have been routinely recognized and enjoyed. The more significant advantages are:

1. The saving of chair time.
2. The capacity to develop more complicated patterns, that is, full crown, bridge, and multiple adjacent patterns.
3. Improved axial contours and accuracy of gingival margins, due to better accessibilty.
4. The capacity to check, correct, and, if necessary, remake castings before returning to the patient.
5. The opportunity to assemble complicated prostheses and place

veneering materials without having to return to the patient for repeated relationship impressions and similar adjustments.

PREPARATION OF THE DIE

Identification of the Margin

For it to be possible to develop an accurate indirect pattern for a cast restoration, the die must present a definite duplication of the preparation margins. In addition to being identifiable, the margin must present a cavosurface angle sufficient to facilitate carving the wax to termination exactly coincident with the marginal angle. If such an angle is not present by virtue of the prepared form and/or the natural contour of the tooth, it should be created by trimming the die (see Section 7).

Figures 1 and 2   To further identify the margin, a good-quality colored pencil may be used to outline the marginal angle. The pencil should be used by letting the *side* of the point find the height of the cavosurface angle. An indelible or regular lead pencil should not be used because of the tendency to smear and not leave a clearly defined line. Margins that are not clearly defined may usually be identified by reading the bur marks or diamond striations on the die. Any portion of the die that duplicates a portion of the tooth that draws and has been surfaced should be included as part of the preparation. The very best light and highest magnification available should be used in making such identifications.

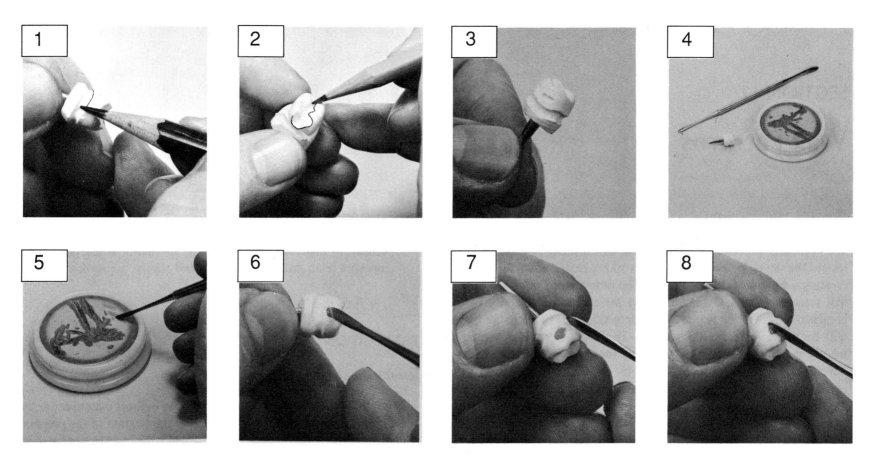

Elimination of Undercuts

Many dies contain undercuts because of carious involvement or previous restorations in the tooth. These undercuts must be eliminated by blocking them out with suitable material in order to permit removal of the wax pattern. These definite undercuts should not be confused with boxed or grooved forms that will draw and can be used to enhance the retention of the preparation.

Figure 3   The undercut on this die is the result of cervical decay that penetrated the tooth beyond the level of the preparation. It must be blocked out to prevent extension of the pattern into the recess. This should be done before the die is lubricated.

Figure 4   Undercuts are most easily relieved by using an "undercut wax." Many of these materials contain clay and, although they do not flow readily, they are thermoplastic and can be built up and carved to contour. However, the undercut wax must not become part of the completed wax pattern, because some types do not completely volatilize and will therefore contaminate the casting.

Other so-called undercut or block-out waxes are thermoplastic resinous materials. Although they are more completely volatile and thus not likely to contaminate the casting, they too should not be incorporated in the pattern.

Figures 5 and 6   A warmed wax spatula is used to pick up a small portion of undercut wax and place it in the depression on the die.

Figure 7   The material is placed in excess to facilitate subsequent carving.

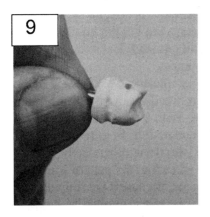
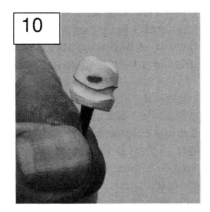
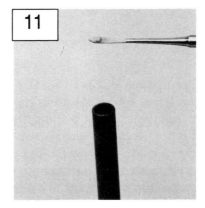
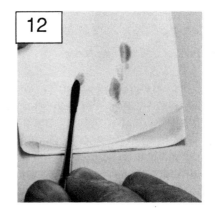

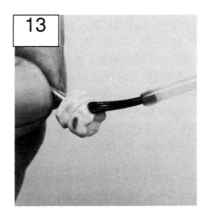
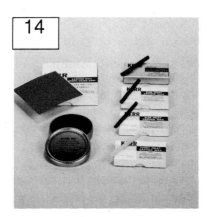

Figure 8   Excess undercut wax is carved to form with a warm spatula.

Figure 9   The undercut has been contoured so that its surface draws with the remainder of the die.

Figure 10   The margin has been clearly identified, and the die is ready to be lubricated in preparation for development of the pattern.

Figures 11 and 12   These illustrations of undercut wax that has been held in a Bunsen flame for an extended period show that the wax does not volatilize completely but leaves a sandy residue that would contaminate a casting.

Casting Relief: Die Spacer

The purpose of the die spacer is to provide space for the cementing medium between the casting and the tooth when the restoration is permanently placed. There are several commercial die spacers available. The die spacer is a material that is similar to varnish, to which coloring agents such as silver and gold have been added so that the material is easily identifiable. The die spacer should be about 0.2 millimeter in thickness, which is about two thin coats of material. The die spacer should *not* be placed any closer to the gingival margin than 1 to 2 millimeters, because this can adversely affect the marginal adaptation of the restoration to the tooth.

Application of Die Lubricant

The purpose of a die lubricant is to keep the wax from sticking to the die, so that the pattern can be removed. These lubricants not only permit separation of the wax pattern from the die but also reduce surface tension, which permits wax to flow freely on the die. A heavy-bodied lubricant is not desirable, as it prevents close adaptation of wax to the die. Die lubricant should be used by following the manufacturer's directions.

Figure 13   The die lubricant is applied in excess and allowed to soak into the die surface for a few minutes. The excess lubricant is then removed from the die by using a brush from which the lubricant has been expressed, or by a gentle air blast.

If the initial application of lubricant soaks completely into the die, another light coat is applied before waxing is begun. Excess lubricant, however, must be removed before waxing, to permit close adaptation of the wax pattern to the die.

WAXING

Properties of Inlay Wax

The American Dental Association Specification Number 4 for Dental Inlay Casting Wax is divided into three types: Type A, a hard or low-flow wax that is used in some indirect techniques; Type B (formerly Type I), used for direct techniques; and Type C (formerly Type II), used for indirect techniques in the production of inlays and crowns. These different physical properties are required because of the different ways in which the waxes are used and the variations in temperature to which they are subjected. Many waxes do not fit any exact classification but fall somewhere between in their physical properties.

Casting wax, usually referred to as inlay wax, is available in the sticks, cones, or bulk containers, as well as in sheets of various thicknesses. Several varieties of inlay wax are illustrated in **Figure 14**. These waxes are available in a variety of colors, but blue and green are most common. Generally, green waxes are softer. Ivory inlay wax contains no pigment and is used primarily to construct patterns for acrylic jacket crowns and acrylic facings, because the absence of pigment ensures that no colored residue remains to discolor the resin material during its processing.

Flow, expansion, thermal conductivity, plasticity, ductility, and warpage are among the properties to consider when selecting an inlay wax. These properties determine the behavior of the pattern during and after its formation.

Because wax has a low thermal conductivity, both the heating and the cooling cycles of wax occur slowly. Sufficient time must thus be allowed to heat the wax to proper working consistency and then to cool it so that flow and plasticity are at a minimum when the pattern is removed.

When wax cools, it contracts or shrinks. This contraction may be controlled (directed toward the die) by pressure on the wax during its solidification. However, the resultant compressive stresses tend to be released over a period of time and may cause distortion unless they are carefully controlled.

Inlay waxes may be permanently deformed without breaking. This ductility increases with an increase in temperature. In good waxing procedures the pressure on the wax and the temperature of the wax should be kept as uniform as possible throughout the entire technique. When wax is being carved, the carving instrument should be warm enough that thin areas of the pattern, particularly margins, are softened sufficiently to be carved easily to contour, but not hot enough to melt the wax. A warm carving instrument will introduce less stress and strain into the pattern than an unheated instrument.

Wax has one of the highest thermal coefficients of expansion of any commonly used dental material. Thus small changes in temperature will cause large changes in dimension. With a direct wax pattern, the thermal contraction from mouth temperature (99° F) to room temperature (77° F) is important because wax shrinks approximately 0.4 percent. Contraction is less of a problem when the wax pattern is made at room temperature in the indirect technique, because it is manipulated at only one temperature. In any event such shrinkage must be compensated in the investing and casting technique.

Warpage of wax results from uneven stresses that occur during the manipulation of any wax. These stresses result from the natural tendencies of wax to shrink upon cooling from the shape of the wax during the molding of the pattern, or from any manipulative procedure (such as heating, application, carving, remelting, or removal of the wax pattern from a tooth or die). Any procedure may result in residual stresses being introduced into the pattern; there will always be a tendency for these stresses to be relieved with consequent warpage. All techniques for applying wax to make a pattern are designed to minimize these unwanted stresses and thus prevent distortion.

Another important property of any material used as a pattern for a casting is that it must volatilize and leave no residue other than carbon at temperatures normally used for wax elimination. A nonvolatile residue of no more that 0.1 percent should remain after a sufficient period of burnout at a temperature of 932° F. Excess residue in the investment mold will cause a defective casting, usually occurring at the margin.

Manipulation of Inlay Wax

Inlay wax should always be softened with *dry heat*. It must not be softened in a water bath, as some of the constituents may be leached from the wax, causing changes in its properties that may result in crumbling and flaking.

Wax may be applied to a die for formation of the pattern in several ways. It may be heated in bulk form by rotating a stick of wax above the tip of the Bunsen flame until it is softened throughout. The softened wax is then pressed into the die and held under pressure until it hardens. This procedure is identical to the method used by the dentist to make a direct wax pattern in the patient's mouth.

Another method of application is to use a heated spatula to melt the wax and flow it onto the die.

Still another method is to dip the die into molten wax. This procedure is appropriate for full crowns or copings but is not appropriate when making onlay patterns.

In any procedure, the amount of heat applied to the wax must be such that no ingredients of the wax are volatilized. The temperature is too high if the wax smokes or boils. Conversely, the wax must be sufficiently heated to be uniformly soft throughout, to avoid building up unwanted stresses. This is particularly significant in the press-on technique.

To minimize introduction of internal stresses, wax should be manipulated at the highest acceptable temperature consistent with the chosen waxing procedure. In the direct technique the dentist must heat the inlay wax so that it reaches a working temperature (of about 125° F) and has the proper amount of flow. In the mouth the temperature must be kept low to avoid injury to the tooth and soft tissue. In the indirect technique wax may be heated to a liquid state, placed on the die and then held under pressure. This procedure results in a *relatively* stress-free pattern.

When a metal die is used, the temperature of the die is critical if a flow-on waxing technique is used. Unless the die is warm, the wax tends to cool rapidly and shrink away from the die, with resultant poor adaptation. The temperature of stone or resin dies is not as critical, as these materials are poor thermal conductors.

Other Pattern Materials

Acrylic resin material, such as Duralay, may be used to construct various parts of the pattern. Such resin materials are applied by a brush-on technique. They harden quickly into a pattern that does not distort easily under subsequent manipulation. The resin is used primarily for the core portion of the pattern, and wax is added to form the occlusal surface, contact areas, and particularly the margins of the pattern. Resin materials will burn out cleanly, but a high-heat investment and burnout technique is desirable to eliminate the resin completely and to provide the correct amount of mold expansion.

Prefabricated occlusal forms are available that can save time in developing a cusp-capping onlay, three-quarter crown, and full crown pattern. These forms are made of a dead soft plastic or wax. The die is lubricated and covered with a thin coating of inlay wax. The desired occlusal form is selected and adapted to the wax-coated die with light finger pressure. The die is placed into its cast, and the opposing cast or core is closed into occlusal relationship. Pressure is used to adapt the occlusal form to the correct occlusion. Any excess portions of the form are trimmed away, and wax is used to complete and refine the pattern.

SEQUENCE OF WAXING

Most technicians develop a systematic approach to the production of wax patterns. First the wax is usually flowed onto the prepared area of the die to create a *coping* with a thickness of approximately 0.5 millimeter or a *thimble* 0.5 millimeter thick on a full crown preparation. Then the wax is allowed to cool under pressure of the fingers and thumb. Occlusal contours are established next, using opposing casts or cores. Finally, the axial contours with proximal contacts are developed. The pattern is brought to final contour and then the margins are refined. The last step is to smooth and finish the pattern. The sequence of steps in producing a pattern is not important as long as the desired final product is obtained. However, the sequence described above is the most logical approach.

Occlusal Contours

Wax may be formed into a given shape in one of two ways, either by starting with an excess amount and reducing it to proper size (*negative waxing*), or by building the wax to the desired shape by the addition of small increments (*positive waxing*). These terms are particularly significant when related to waxing occlusal contours.

In negative waxing, as usually accomplished, excess wax is placed on the occlusal surface and uniformly softened. The opposing cast or core is then closed against the wax to displace excess and mold gross form. The softening and molding may have to be repeated several times until the occlusal surface is established at the correct vertical dimension.

Stresses are almost certain to be introduced into the pattern by this procedure. The best means to avoid any significant effect from these stresses is to use a softer wax for the occlusal portion of the pattern. If soft wax is not used, the gross pattern should be completely solidified. The occlusal surface should then be thoroughly softened before it is occluded with an opposing cast or core.

Positive waxing is usually initiated by building up the centric holding cusp tips until their correct position and height has been established. Cusp slopes and marginal ridge contours and the noncentric cusps are carefully added to complete the occlusal form. Softer wax is commonly used with this occlusal buildup technique to reduce thermal and mechanical stresses.

In positive waxing the small increments of wax are carefully placed with an explorer or small waxing instrument. The placement of each increment is checked immediately with the opposing cast or core, thus ensuring that any displacement of the occlusal form will be effected against only a small amount of softened wax. This helps to eliminate the incorporation of stresses into the pattern.

The positive wax technique is the better approach for establishing full occlusal patterns, provided that the articulation of the opposing cast or core is accurate enough to warrant the additional effort. This technique was introduced by Dr. Everitt Payne and is described at length later in this section.

Axial Contours

Once the occlusal table of the pattern has been completed, axial contours are developed. The first step in developing these contours is to remove most of the excess wax at the margins of the preparations. With the marginal and occlusal outlines thus established, the axial contours and proximal contacts can be established in keeping with the requirements identified in Section 11.

Axial contours may be established by negative or positive waxing. Some technicians add an excess of wax and carve their contours while others build their contours with smooth increments of wax.

Margins

The margin of the pattern (via the resultant casting) seals the breach in the tooth created by its preparation. Inadequacy of this seal results in the failure of restorations even though they have been perfectly executed in terms of occlusal relationships and axial contours. To date there is no dental cement that is impervious to oral fluids. Consequently, only near-perfect adaptation of the margins of cast restorations prevents dissolution of the cement, which may result in failure of the restoration and potential loss of the tooth.

Extreme care is mandatory for waxing the margins. First the wax pattern is removed, and the marginal area of the die is *lightly* relubricated. The pattern is then firmly replaced on the die and very carefully checked to ensure that it is fully reseated.

There must be a continuous adaptation of wax to the margins, with no voids, folds, or faults. To ensure this, the marginal wax should be pooled to a distance about 2 millimeters above the margin and held under progressively firmer pressure until it solidifies. If this is done to one surface at a time with sufficient overlap between surfaces, a continuous accurate adaptation of the wax about the entire marginal circumference of the die may be obtained. If necessary, more wax should be added during the remelting procedure to ensure a slight excess of contour and extension beyond the margin.

Wax along the margins is then carved with a warm wax spatula that does not have sharp edges. A warm spatula permits carving of the marginal wax with light pressure so that the die margins are not damaged. The technician will soon learn just how much to heat the spatula for smooth and effective carving of the wax to margin.

The unprepared trimmed die surface just beneath the cavosurface margin is used to guide the carving instrument. The attitude or angulation of the carving instrument should relate it to this die surface just beneath the prepared portions of the tooth, and not to the marginal angle itself. Carving directly against the cavosurface angle of the margin will likely result in abrasion of this most critical area of the die. Where possible, the blade of the carving instrument should be guided by the unprepared tooth surface recorded beyond the margin of the die.

After the external surface of the margin has been completed, the internal surface should be checked for smoothness. Voids and irregularities of the internal surface close to the margin must be corrected before the pattern is invested. Care should be taken that no portion of the thin wax margin cracks or breaks away during removal and reseating of the pattern.

Smoothing the Pattern

Proximal contacts must be adequate in the finished casting. Many dentists request that a slight excess be placed on the proximal contact area. Approximately 0.2 millimeter of excess wax provides an adequate bulk for polishing and fitting. However, for this thickness to be advantageous, it must be carefully added. Usually there are slight depressions evident at the contact areas. A light film of wax at just the right temperature should be wiped across the surface so that it just fills this concavity and blends to a smooth, convex form. Application of a discrete drop of wax is of no advantage, as it would likely be completely removed in attempting to blend its contour and eliminate the junction line between it and the rest of the casting surface.

The time required to finish the casting is significantly reduced if the pattern is smooth before investing. This is particularly true in the gingival margin areas, because irregularities and roughness may be difficult to remove in the casting without jeopardizing the integrity of the margins. Some people flame the wax lightly to smooth it. This produces a smooth pattern surface but may alter the occlusal and proximal relationships. Even more critical is the distortion that will occur at the marginal areas. This invariably occurs due to the thin cross-sectional dimension of this portion of the pattern.

A safer method of smoothing a pattern is by rubbing. Many technicians use the end of the finger with a few rubbing motions to achieve a satisfactory smoothness on the accessible surface of the wax pattern. A cotton applicator or a small piece of damp cotton may also be used. Sometimes the occlusal surface contour may be smoothed by using a small piece of warm, damp cotton wrapped around the end of a toothpick. Probably the most commonly employed material is a piece of nylon or silk stocking wrapped over the fingertip. This has a slightly abrasive effect on the wax and produces a smooth surface. *It must be used sparingly, however, as it can also easily abrade the sharp marginal angle of the die.*

Whatever the technique used, a few moments spent smoothing the wax pattern will save many minutes of finishing time after the casting is produced and probably will result in a more accurate final contour.

WAXING TECHNIQUES FOR PATTERN CONSTRUCTION

There are many ways in which a wax pattern may be constructed. Several are illustrated in the succeeding portions of this section. Variations from these techniques are common, but the principle of constructing a wax pattern to be a precise model of the desired casting must be followed.

No matter what technique is used, *cleanliness* is important. A clean work surface, clean instruments, a dust-free atmosphere, and clean wax are essential to success.

Wax Chew-in Technique

The *wax chew-in technique* is shown in the following illustrations by demonstrating the construction of a MOD wax pattern on the mandibular right second premolar. When this technique is followed, the technician will have received an impression or working cast and a wax chew-in from the dentist. An opposing cast may or may not be provided. When available, it may be in the form of an anatomic opposing cast with interocclusal record, or an anatomic, functional, or centric occlusion core, or the registration for same. Whichever is provided, when the wax chew-in technique is used the purpose of the opposing model is to verify the occlusion of the pattern developed from the wax chew-in before it is invested and to facilitate correction of the casting.

When two or more adjacent teeth are prepared, the wax chew-in is made in one piece and must be separated into individual tooth segments. Separation is accomplished by removing the wax that extends into the gingival interproximal areas. The wax is then grooved around the occlusal, facial, gingival, and lingual areas of the proposed segments. The deepest groove is placed on the gingival side, and when the groove is almost through the wax, the segments are broken apart with light finger pressure. Care should be taken to avoid distortion of the wax during this procedure.

The use of a functional wax chew-in as part of a wax pattern is not a desirable procedure because unknown and uncontrolled stresses are present in the wax chew-in. Additionally, tooth dust and debris may have been incorporated in the wax, and the properties of the wax may have been changed if the dentist inadvertently overheated the wax. Nevertheless, because of the simplicity of obtaining such an occlusal registration, the wax chew-in is often employed, especially for inlays that have limited occlusal coverage. Better procedure would be to develop a functional core from the wax chew-in, so that the wax pattern could be generated completely on the die.

Figure 15   The cast with removable dies and opposing centric occlusion core, prior to making the wax pattern. (As described in Section 9, a centric occlusion core is an opposing anatomic cast that has been indexed against the working cast.)

As will be seen more clearly later, this working cast contains dies of three prepared teeth. The second premolar presents an MOD inlay preparation, the first molar has a DO inlay preparation, and the second molar has been prepared for a full crown. This combination permits illustration of some of the considerations that are necessary when multiple adjacent patterns are being developed.

Figure 16   The wax chew-in for the MOD pattern on the second premolar, positioned on the lubricated die. Its stability and accurate seating on the occlusal portion of the die must be verified.

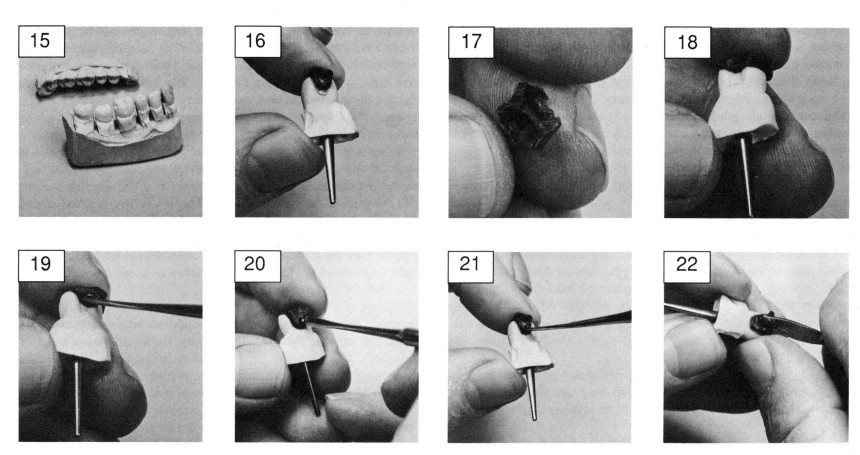

Figure 17 If the chew-in fits correctly, it is removed to check the internal adaptation of the pattern to the cavity preparation.

Figure 18 If the internal angles and surface of the chew-in are not correctly adapted to the cavity surface, the chew-in is reseated on the die and the wax in the proximal box portion removed. The contact areas of the proximal surfaces are maintained.

Figure 19 Without disturbing the occlusal portion, a hot instrument such as a number 23 explorer or a small waxing spatula is used to readapt the wax to the prepared form. The hot instrument should penetrate the wax to its internal depth, with the tip resting gently against the die surface.

Figure 20 Wax is added to fill the voids and discrepancies between the

pattern and die. The same procedure is used to adapt a wax chew-in for any type of restoration—inlay, onlay, partial crown, or full crown.

Figure 21 After adapting the chew-in to the die, a hot waxing instrument (number 7 spatula or number 3 Hollenbeck carver) is used to readapt the wax around the margin of the die. Additional wax is placed where the chew-in is shy of contour or margin. The wax is added in increments to permit the use of finger pressure on the wax immediately after the surface solidifies.

Figure 22 Gross excess wax may be removed with a carving knife.

Figure 23 Final excess wax is removed from the proximal margins with a warm instrument.

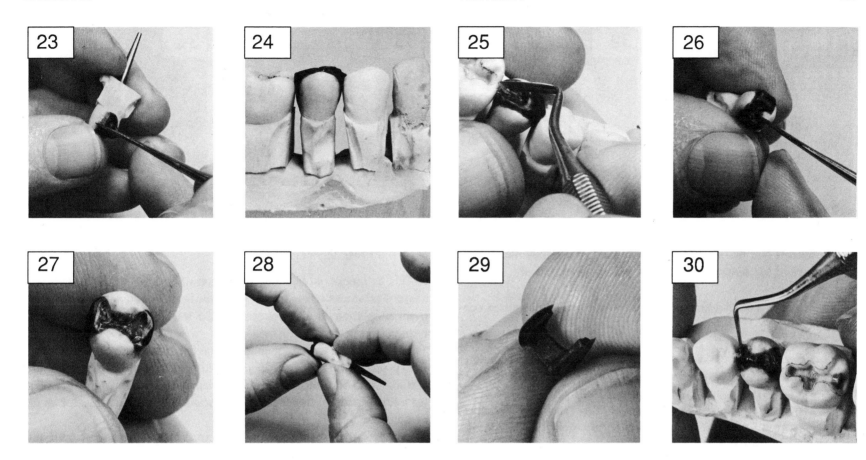

Figure 24 The die is replaced in the cast to verify proximal contact and marginal ridge relationships.

Figure 25 Any occlusal excess is removed and the height of each marginal ridge is established, using the height of the adjacent marginal ridges as a guide. Consideration must be given to maintenance of centric occlusion contacts.

Figure 26 The wax is then carved back to the occlusal margin with a warm instrument.

Figure 27 Excess wax has been removed and the pattern has been carved to margin.

Figure 28 The die is removed from the pattern using the thumb and forefinger, with the other fingers (middle, ring, and little) braced against each other. The wax pattern is held passively with one hand and the die is held tightly in the other hand. The die is removed from under the pattern, *not* the pattern from the die, because the pattern tends to break if it is removed forcefully from the die.

Figure 29 The internal portion of the pattern is examined for adaptation. Any discrepancies must be corrected by remelting the area and applying pressure to bring about adaptation. Retention, especially in small, short-walled inlay preparations, is critically dependent on adaptation of the casting.

Figure 30 The pattern is replaced on the die and the occlusal surface anatomy is defined, using the functional or anatomic core as a guide to the maintenance of occlusal contact—especially centric. The axial con-

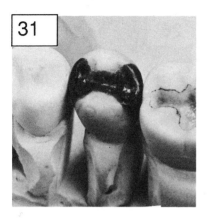 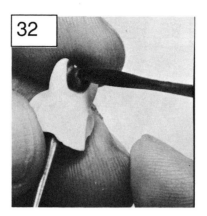 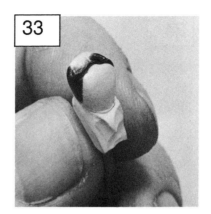 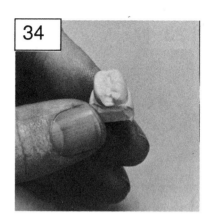

tour is refined and the margins are completed in a sequential manner and rechecked for adaptation. The wax pattern is smoothed.

Figure 31   The completed wax pattern with correct anatomical contour.

Figure 32   A slight excess of wax may be added to the contact areas to insure proper contour and proper contact of the casting. It is much easier to remove part of this contour during insertion than to add solder in the event the contact is shy. However, the careful, experienced technician can establish proper contacts if provided an accurate tray impression or working cast.

Figure 33   The MOD wax pattern is completed.

NEGATIVE WAXING

The following series of illustrations demonstrates negative waxing, or the wax-reduction technique. In negative waxing wax is added until contours are overdeveloped and then carved back to the correct form and contour. Whether to use negative or positive waxing depends upon individual preference and the extent of the restoration being made. Negative waxing is best suited for small restorations; positive waxing is best used for crowns and large onlays. (The previously described procedure for using a wax chew-in is essentially a negative waxing technique, the only difference being that a portion of the pattern was molded directly in the mouth.)

Flow and Press Technique

This technique is a preferred method of making a wax pattern because it produces fewer internal stresses in the wax and permits maximum adaptation. It also assures that the wax pattern is clean and will burn out properly.

The technique varies depending upon the size of the cavity. A small cavity preparation is overfilled quickly with liquid wax. After the surface wax solidifies (which may be hastened by blowing gently on it for a few seconds), finger pressure is applied and maintained for about one minute.

In larger cavity preparations wax increments are added until the pattern is overcontoured. In this technique the wax increment being flowed onto the previously applied wax must be hot enough and placed rapidly enough to blend the increments together. Otherwise voids and wrinkles on the internal cavity surface and lamination of the wax will result. As soon as the cavity is filled, finger pressure is exerted until the wax completely solidifies. On multiple-surface patterns, this may have to be done on one surface at a time.

When flowing wax onto a die with a spatula, consideration must be given to maintaining an even temperature. Routine technique is to warm the spatula tip and place it against the inlay wax until a large molten drop can be picked up and carried to the die. Often by the time this molten drop is conveyed to the die, the instrument and wax have cooled to the extent that the wax does not readily flow onto the die surface. In this event the instrument with wax should be gently flamed on the way to the die such that the wax is quite molten, flows easily on the die surface, and blends smoothly with the wax already placed. Adequate heating is important for good wax manipulation, but over-

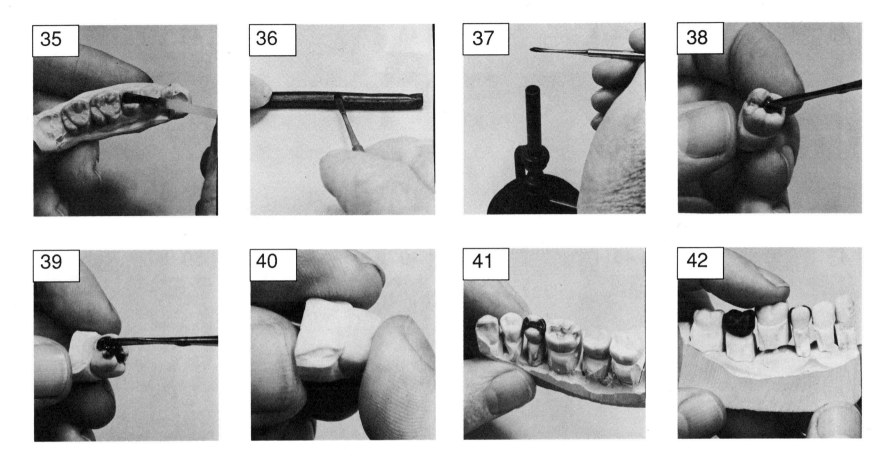

heating must be avoided. Never heat the spatula to a temperature that causes the wax to smoke and never flame wax to ignition.

The flow and press technique of negative waxing is illustrated in the development of the DO pattern capping the distal cusp of the first molar.

Figure 34   The die containing the DO preparation is removed from the cast and inspected. Margins of the preparation are marked and undercuts filled as necessary.

Figure 35   The die, adjacent teeth, and the opposing casts are coated with die lubricant.

Figure 36   A heated spatula is used to pick up a drop of inlay wax.

Figure 37   If necessary, the wax is reheated in the flame on the way to the die. Avoid overheating.

Figure 38   The wax is flowed into the preparation.

Figure 39   Wax is added immediately in successive increments until the cavity is overfilled.

Figure 40   As soon as the surface solidifies, progressive pressure is applied to the pattern. Fingers are placed on both the proximal and occlusal surfaces during this procedure. Note that the middle finger of the right hand is on the occlusal surface and the middle finger of the left hand is on the proximal surface.

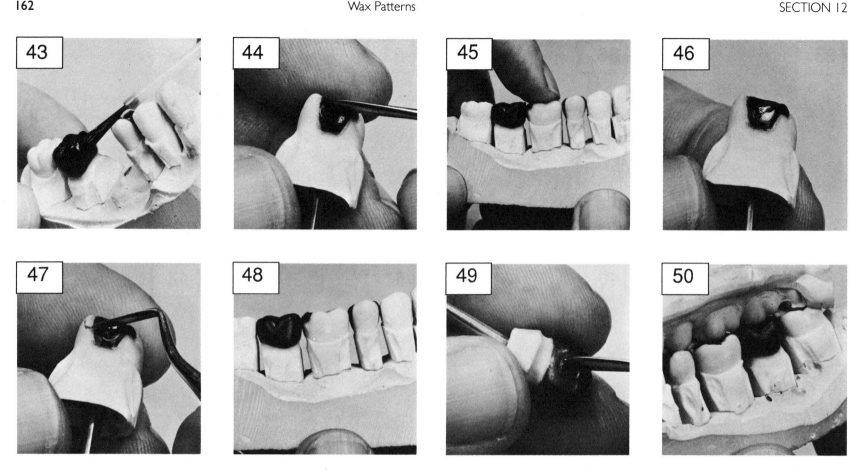

Figure 41   This brings us to consideration of development of adjacent patterns. When adjacent proximal surfaces are involved, as they are here, both proximal surfaces must be created before either can be presumed completed. Assurance of proper form of embrasures and location of proximal contact requires that either surface be subject to change after comparision with the other. To demonstrate this, a pattern for the full crown preparation has been developed and placed on the adjacent second molar. (The procedure for developing a full crown pattern is covered in the final portion of this section.)

Figure 42   The mesial surface of the crown has been carved to what has been judged to be correct contour. However, excess contour between the two molar patterns prevents seating of the first molar die. This is *not* caused by the second premolar pattern, as that has already been completed, including a check of its proximal contact relationship

with the first molar. If in doubt in such situations, other adjacent patterns and dies may be removed, leaving only the contact to be established in question. A decision must be made as to which pattern is most properly contoured and whether one or both patterns must be changed to correct the excessive contact. The contour of the established pattern is changed if indicated.

Figure 43   When contour of the established proximal surface is verified, a film of wax lubricant is applied.

Figure 44   The contact area of the proximal surface to be established is softened with a heated spatula.

Figure 45   The die with pattern is seated in the cast. Note the incorrect proximal contour between the molar patterns.

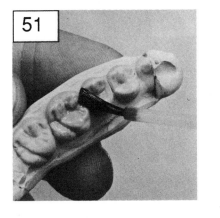

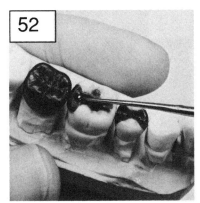

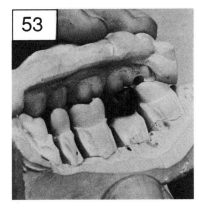

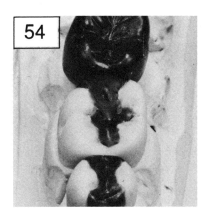

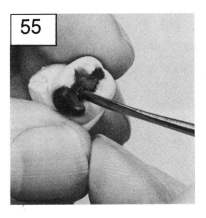

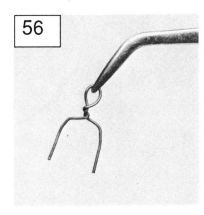

Figure 46 The incorrect concave contact area is further illustrated in this photograph.

Figure 47 The excess wax is trimmed so that the proximal surface will assume its correct convex form. A warm instrument is used to carve the margins.

Figure 48 The die and pattern are reseated in the cast. Note the correct surface contour in the distal contact area. The capped distal cusp is also evident in this photograph.

Figure 49 If it is determined at this point that one proximal surface is overcontoured in relation to the other, it can be reduced and the contact-forming procedure repeated by adding wax to the other pattern.

Figure 50 The opposing core is placed to check the occlusion. Note that it does not occlude correctly because of excess wax on the occlusal surface of the first molar.

Figure 51 If necessary, the occlusal surface of the core is relubricated.

Figure 52 The conflicting area of the occlusal surface of the wax pattern is reheated with a warm spatula.

Figure 53 The lubricated opposing core is seated in the correct occlusal relationship.

Figure 54 The occlusal surface shows an indentation made from the anatomic core. Care must be exercised during such registrations to ensure that the opposing core is correctly positioned on the working cast.

Figure 55 Excess wax is carved from the occlusal margin with a warm instrument. The opposing core is used to check and refine the occlusal surface until it is correctly carved. White zinc stearate powder can be dusted carefully onto the occlusal surface with a brush to reveal occlusal areas that need correction, using the core to identify the clear premature areas that are wiped clean by the closure of the core onto the surface of the wax.

Figure 56 Some patterns may be grasped and separated from their dies by the fingertips as shown in **Figure 28**; others may be removed by

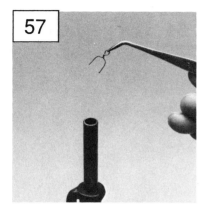
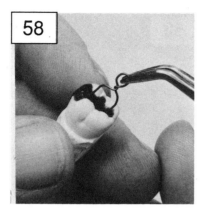
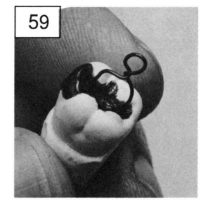
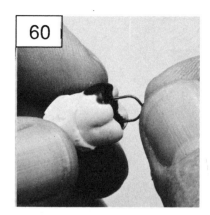

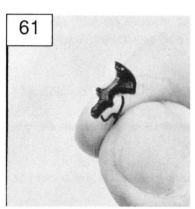
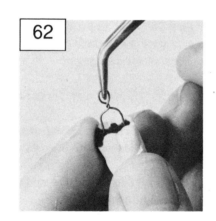
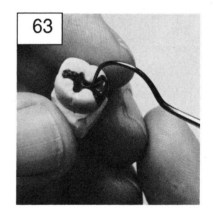
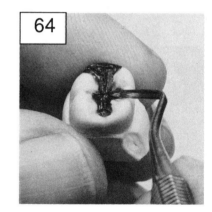

using the sprue as a handle. However, these techniques are not always suitable. The use of a *U-wire* is often necessary when removing a one- or two-surface inlay pattern if distortion is to be avoided. A U-wire is simply a handle with which a pattern can be removed from tooth or die. When used with direct patterns, the wire is usually left incorporated in the pattern and subsequently has its ends incorporated in the casting. This, of course, demands a noble wire; 21-gauge gold alloy wire (Zephyr wire) is conventionally used. U-wires used with the indirect technique can be recovered from the pattern before investing (**Figure 62**); thus copper wire of about 24 gauge is ordinarily used for these. A piece of the appropriate wire 1 to 1½ inches in length is bent to the form shown in this illustration. The legs of the U should approximate the distance between the mesial and distal pits, so that the U-wire can be attached to the pattern to provide a direct pull that will withdraw the pattern without distortion or fracture. The U-wire not only aids in

withdrawal but serves as a handle for holding the wax pattern while the internal surface is inspected.

Figure 57   The legs of the U-wire are heated slightly.

Figure 58   The heated U-wire is placed in the mesial and distal pits of the occlusal portion of the pattern and held until the wax begins to solidify.

Figure 59   Once properly placed, the wire is left undisturbed until completely cooled.

Figure 60   The U-wire is grasped by the thumb and forefinger and tension applied so that the pattern is removed in a straight occlusal direction.

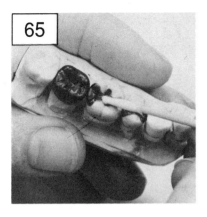
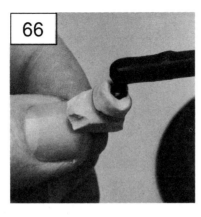
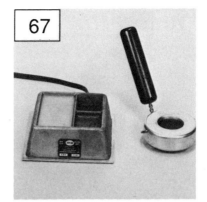
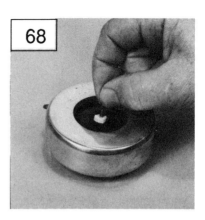

Figure 61   The pattern is examined for proper internal adaptation.

Figure 62   The pattern is returned to the die and fully seated. To remove the U-wire, tweezers are first heated and then used to grasp the U-wire. The heat will be transferred to the U-wire, and after a few moments a very light pull will easily remove it from the pattern.

Figure 63   The holes remaining in the pattern are filled with wax by using the tine of an explorer that has been properly heated.

Figure 64   If necessary, the occlusal anatomy is redefined.

Figure 65   The occlusal surface is smoothed with wet cotton applied to a toothpick. The entire wax pattern is then smoothed using wet cotton or a fine-textured cloth. The pattern is now ready to be sprued.

Full-coverage Patterns

In addition to the flow and press technique, wax may be added for copings and full crown patterns by dripping it on the die, or by dipping the die in molten wax.

Wax Dripping Technique   Dripping is accomplished simply by flaming the end of a stick of inlay wax until it just becomes molten. The liquid wax thus formed is spread on the appropriate surface of the lubricated die (**Figure 66**). With practice, subsequent additions can be brought into place rapidly until the die is adequately covered with about 0.5 to 1.0 millimeter thickness of wax. Pressure may be applied after application to each surface, or after the entire die is covered.

This approach is obviously very similar to the flow-on technique using a spatula. Elimination of the spatula can speed up application. However, the wax-dripping technique is only appropriate to the waxing of exposed flat surfaces. Recesses such as grooves and boxes must first be filled by discrete placement of wax with a spatula to insure good adaptation.

Dipping-the-die Technique   This technique is specifically appropriate only to full crown preparation dies. It is accomplished by melting clean inlay wax in a suitable vessel and repeatedly dipping the lubricated die into the molten wax. The wax must be melted slowly and evenly to avoid overheating as evidenced by smoking or boiling.

Figure 67   Wax may be melted in an electric heater or a metal vessel over a flame. Melting with a flame should be accomplished in a metal vessel that has sufficient bulk to retain heat for a prolonged period.

Figure 68   The lubricated die is immersed in the molten wax to the desired level. Most technicians using this technique prefer to let the wax engage the ditch or natural undercut beneath margin. This permits the wax to lock beyond the margin and helps focus contraction toward the die.

Figure 69   The die is removed to allow the adherent wax to chill slightly; then it is quickly dipped again to pick up another layer of wax. The first dipping of the die should be somewhat slow, to allow thorough coverage. Subsequent dips should occur only after the applied wax has chilled, and the immersions must be rapid enough to prevent excessive solution of previously applied wax.

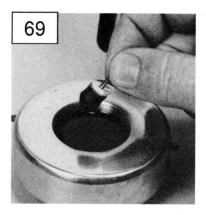 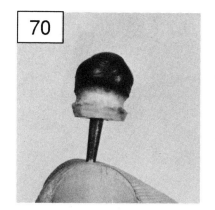 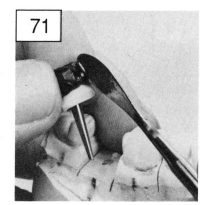 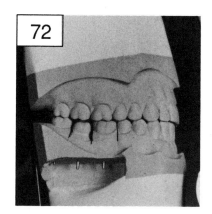

Figure 70 Dipping is continued until a sufficient bulk of wax (about 0.5 to 1.0 millimeter) is established.

Figure 71 Gross form of the buildup may need to be completed by controlled additions with a wax spatula.

POSITIVE WAXING

The controlled addition of wax to build a pattern progressively to an exact form is a most effective technique for developing full occlusal coverage restorations. Consequently this approach is advocated for the development of patterns for cusp-capping onlays, three-quarter crowns, and full crowns except when the functional core (functionally generated path) technique is employed.

The primary advantage of the wax-added or positive waxing approach is that it affords the opportunity knowledgeably to generate and test each component of the occlusion for any given restoration. Some examples of this should be evident in the following sequence, which involves the development of a full crown pattern on a lower molar.

Figure 72 Working and opposing casts have been mounted on a semi-adjustable articulator. Such a mounting is the only means by which the full potential of the wax-added technique can be realized. Mounting on a simple hinge articulator would permit only an accurate identification of centric occlusion. Functionally generated path registrations provide

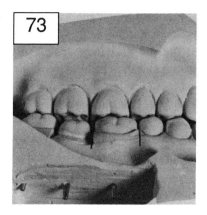 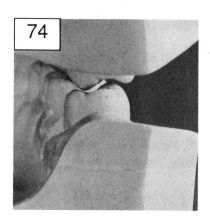

for maximum excursive contact but do not necessarily permit control in locating centric contacts and eliminating nonfunctional contacts. Mountings on semi- or fully adjustable articulators permit control of centric and eccentric contact in direct relation to the accuracy of the mounting and guidance of the instrument. If such mounting and guidance provide an accurate duplication of the patient's occlusion, the technician has complete control over the occlusal relationships of the restoration being developed. This circumstance is seldom actually achieved but often approximated.

Figure 73 The dies of the prepared second molar and the adjacent teeth have been made removable. Evaluation of the mounted relationship reveals a normal mesiodistal interdigitation. However, the amount of horizontal overlap seems minimal, and the lower facial cusps do not appear to directly oppose the upper fossae.

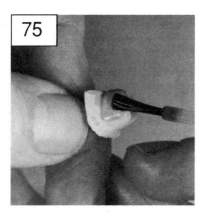 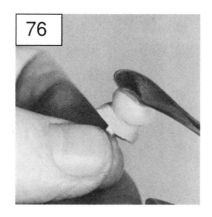 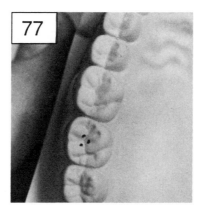 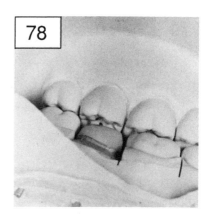

Figure 74 The articulator has been slightly opened to facilitate a lingual and posterior view of the faciolingual interdigitation. Note that the facial cusps of the terminal lower molar are facial to the central groove region of the opposing upper molar. Correspondingly, the upper lingual cusp is lingual to the central groove region of the lower molar. This pattern of insufficient horizontal overlap prevails for the entire posterior segment. However (referring back to **Figure 73**), the second molar has been reduced sufficiently to permit locating the facial cusps in the opposing central groove. An ideal centric contact pattern should thus be possible.

Forming the Pattern Base

Regardless of whether the positive or negative waxing technique will be employed to develop occlusal relationships, the base portion (coping, thimble) of the pattern, consisting of a layer of wax 0.5 to 1.0 millimeter thick, must be established on the die with good internal adaptation. Whether this is accomplished via the flow and press, dripping, or dipping-the-die technique depends on the type of preparation and preference of the technician.

Figures 75 and 76 By whatever technique desired, the base portion of the pattern is developed on a properly lubricated die. In this case it is being constructed with ivory wax to facilitate photography in subsequent steps.

Forming the Centric Contacts

The prime thrust of the wax-added technique is the development of exact, planned occlusal relationships. Hence each component of the occlusal relationship is identified and individually executed.

The first occlusal component to be established for posterior restorations should always be the centric holding cusps. Molars have two centric holding cusps, one of which ideally opposes a central fossa and the other a marginal ridge area. Normally the holding cusp opposing the central fossa is the most significant for several reasons: (1) it is more centrally located and therefore more important to the transmission of axially oriented forces; (2) it is the cusp that must escape through an occlusal embrasure; (3) it is the cusp that most frequently contacts when nonfunctional conflicts occur; and (4) it often has a more complicated pattern of centric contact because of the steeply inclined walls of the opposing fossa. Because of these unique relationships the fossa-related cusp is best established first. For the lower molars the fossa-related centric holding cusps are the distofacial cusps. For the maxillary molars they are the mesiolingual cusps.

Figure 77 Because the cusps must be formed to produce a specific pattern of contact, the desired location of the contact on the opposing tooth must be discretely identified. In this example, the distofacial cusp of the lower second molar must contact the central fossa of the upper second molar. Because of the depth of this particular fossa, it is inappropriate to plan for a single mortar-and-pestle type of contact. As a result a three-point contact, taking advantage of the three primary inclines of the tooth surrounding the central pit, has been identified.

Figure 78 The relationship between the desired contact location on the opposing tooth and the pattern base is observed to permit good judgment in placing the cusp cone.

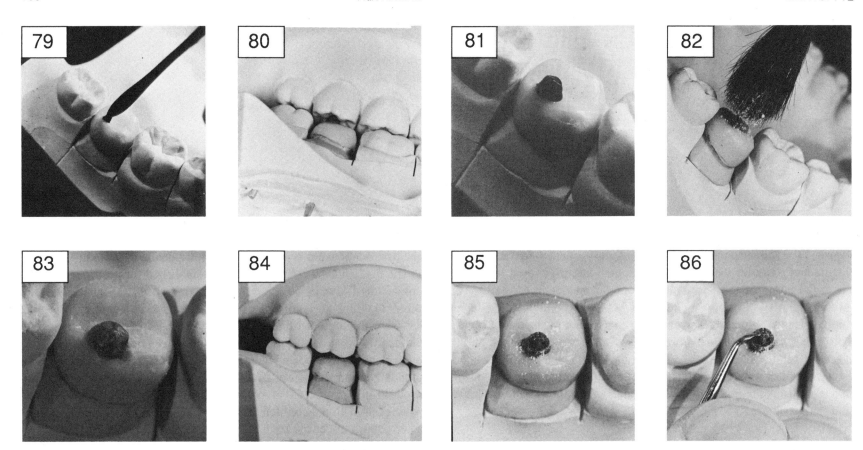

Figure 79 A cusp cone is created by obtaining an appropriate quantity of wax at the right temperature on the spatula tip and gently placing it like a droplet at the correct location on the pattern base. The tip of the spatula is *not* removed from the wax, however. As the wax cools, the dimension of the base of the cone can be enlarged by gently moving the spatula tip in a circular fashion to enlarge the area of contact between the cone and the base. Finally, when the wax has cooled almost to the point of solidification, the spatula tip is slowly lifted to draw the wax into a cone. Blowing gently on the wax can help synchronize solidification with removal of the spatula tip.

Figure 80 The articulator is closed while the wax is still soft, to form the cone for proper contact.

Figure 81 If the cone is deficient in size or improperly located, addi-

tions are made as indicated and the articulator is again closed; this procedure is repeated until adequate contact is established.

Figure 82 The pattern of occlusal contact can be precisely checked by dusting the pattern with talc or zinc stearate powder. The latter is preferred as it will readily decompose during burnout, thus eliminating any possibility of contaminating the casting.

Figure 83 Dusting leaves the cone covered with a thin layer of white powder.

Figure 84 A test closure is made by gently tapping together the articulated casts.

Figure 85 Points of contact are readily identifiable as clear spots on the dusted surface.

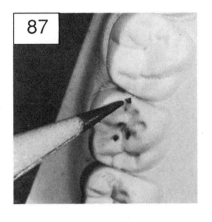
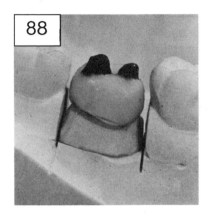
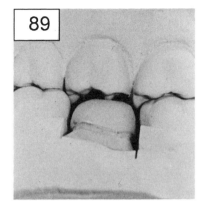
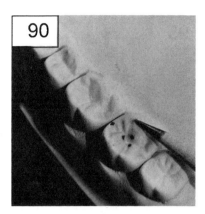

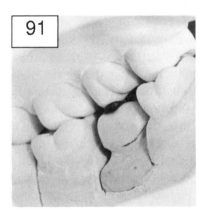
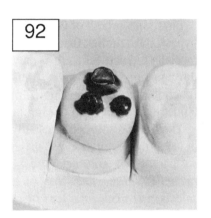
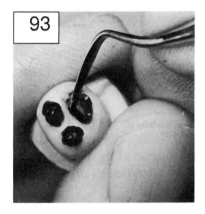
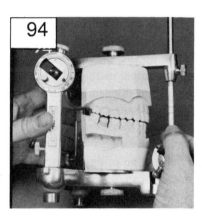

Figure 86 Excess is carved away with care to leave the contacts precisely located.

Figure 87 The proper location of the contact of the second centric holding cusp—the mesiofacial cusp—is the mesial marginal ridge of the upper second molar. The exact position desired should be identified and, if need be, marked. An excellent means for doing this is to create a very minute pit or dimple at the exact desired point of contact in the opposing stone tooth surface with the tip of an explorer tine. Closure of the articulator to form the wax will produce a very small bleb that indicates the exact location of the desired contact.

Figure 88 The second cusp cone is established.

Figure 89 Proper location of the contact is established and verified.

Figure 90 The third major centric contact of a lower molar occurs in the central fossa. This fossa receives the mesiolingual cusp tip of the maxillary molar.

Figure 91 Wax is added in position to establish a fossa that receives the upper lingual cusp. The contact is formed by closure of the upper cusp into the still warm wax.

Figure 92 The fossa thus formed should encompass the apex of the upper cusp.

Figure 93 The perimeter of the fossa is trimmed as necessary.

Figure 94 When the primary centric components are established, their compatibility with eccentric relationships should be examined.

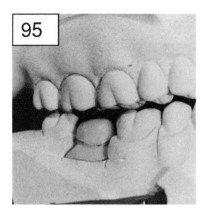 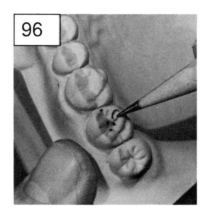 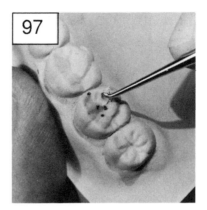 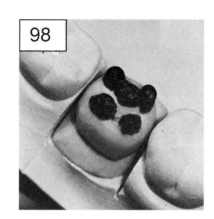

Functional interferences can be eliminated by altering either the established lower facial cusps or the opposing inclines. If the cusps cannot be altered without loss of stability of centric contact, the opposing functional inclines should be altered. The exact location of any such changes of opposing teeth should be marked for later identification so that the dentist can reproduce them clinically.

Nonfunctional interferences occur between inclines of opposing centric holding cusps—the lingual incline of lower facial cusps and the facial incline of upper lingual cusps. Elimination of these undesirable contacts can usually be accomplished by alteration of the inclines without involving the centric holding cusp tips.

Figure 95   A check of nonfunctional relationships reveals contact between the lower distofacial cusp cone and the upper mesiolingual cusp. Closer inspection shows that this contact is coincident with one of the points of centric contact on the lower cusp.

Figure 96   The contact on the opposing upper tooth is on the facial incline of the mesiolingual cusp (as outlined with pencil) and does not involve the actual area of centric contact of that cusp.

Figure 97   As a result, this incline can be relieved to eliminate the nonfunctional interference without altering the centric contacts. Nonfunctional contacts should be eliminated with clearance to spare.

On rare occasions nonfunctional conflict may occur between the centric cusp tips—the lower distofacial cusp and the upper mesiolingual cusp. In these cases one of two solutions can be employed.

First, one or both of the centric cusps may be shifted mesiodistally to bypass the conflict (usually the upper cusp distally, the lower cusp mesially). Such relocation may permit better escape of these cusps through opposing grooves, thus providing clearance during the nonfunctional excursion. This solution is often best when the dentist is adjusting natural teeth to eliminate nonfunctional contact.

The second solution is usually more effective and appropriate when developing restorations. This involves shortening one of the cusps sufficiently to eliminate the nonfunctional conflict. Obviously this means the immediate loss of a centric contact. However, if proper selection is made, the loss of one of the two facial or lingual centric contacts should not result in loss of stability of tooth position. More important, when a restoration is being developed centric contact need not be forfeited. If the cusp opposing the fossa of the restoration pattern is relieved, the fossa can be rewaxed to restore contact. For instance, if in our example the nonfunctional conflict had occurred between the centric contacting tips of the lower distofacial and upper mesiolingual cusps, which one should be relieved? If the lower facial cusps were relieved, centric would be lost without potential for reestablishing it at the new level. However, if the upper lingual cusp were relieved, the lower fossa could be rewaxed at an elevated level, thus eliminating the nonfunctional contact and maintaining centric. For such effort to be effective in providing a better service for the patient, both the technician and the dentist must understand and be aware of the changes made.

Figure 98   Once the centric contacts have been established and cleared of any eccentric interference, the other features of the occlusal surface can be established. The next additions are appropriately the noncentric

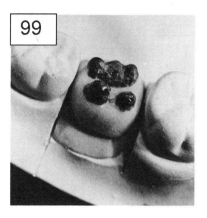
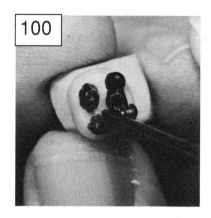
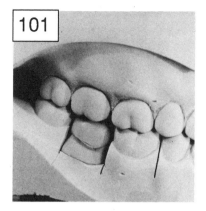
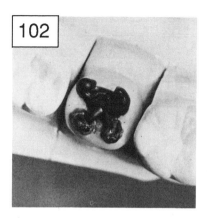

holding cusps. They are established by placement of cones in positions estimated by evaluation of adjacent and opposing anatomic features.

Figure 99   The noncentric holding cusps are always functional cusps (mandibular lingual and maxillary facial). Once established, these cusps must be checked to see if they provide the desired range of functional contact. Again, dusting can facilitate examination of these contacts. No lingual range functional contact was desired in this case, and accordingly no contact is evident on either of the lingual cusps.

Note the centric contact with the maxillary mesiolingual cusp. Noting the poor faciolingual relationship of these teeth, it is not surprising that this lingual range centric contact falls further toward the lingual than the original central groove.

Figure 100   With all cusps and the central fossa contact established, the anatomic features connecting these points can be easily created. These are, of course, the triangular or cuspal ridges. All cuspal ridges might be considered as having eccentric contact potential. To wax a pattern properly, one must have assessed this potential and decided what role it is to play in the desired occlusal plan. For example, in this case the cuspal ridges (lingual inclines) of mandibular facial cusps have nonfunctional contact potential. Because such contact is undesirable (except in abnormal circumstances), it is important that these ridges be developed with the desired clearance in the nonfunctional excursion.

Figure 101   The location and direction of these ridges can be initially estimated on the basis of ideal anatomy. Once placed, the elevation and

position of the ridges must be checked for clearance. Again, dusting would identify actual contact. However, when clearance is desired, cellophane or paper strips used like a feeler gauge are best.

Figure 102   The cuspal ridges (facial inclines) of the mandibular lingual cusps have functional contact potential. If lingual range function is desired, the elevation and location of these ridges must be established to provide the appropriate range of contact. It was mentioned earlier that lingual range function was not desired in this example. This might often be the case because of the positional relationship or bone support of the teeth. Lower molars are normally inclined to the lingual. If this inclination is excessive or bone support is poor, forces imposed on the lingual cusps might be deleterious to the stability of the tooth.

Because of the faciolingual positional discrepancy of these teeth, the central fossa and lingual cusps are being established further to the lingual of the center of the tooth than is normal. The potential effect of this relationship can be minimized by restricting the dimension of the lingual cusps and eliminating their contact in function. Certainly it is not the province of the technician to determine what occlusal relationship is appropriate, but the fact is that such considerations are not prescribed. They are seldom given specific consideration until the restoration is being developed. Much better understanding and communication regarding these factors is indicated.

Figure 103   When the cusp tips and their triangular ridges are established, the perimeter of the occlusal table must be established. The cuspal arms are waxed with consideration for their functional contact.

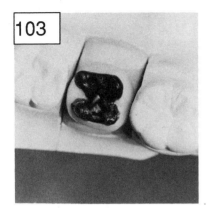

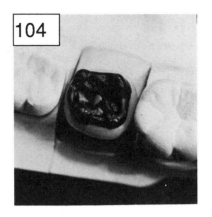

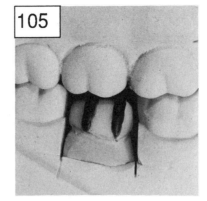

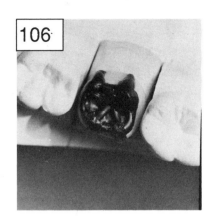

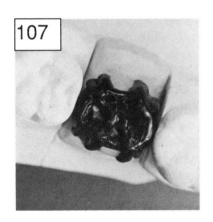

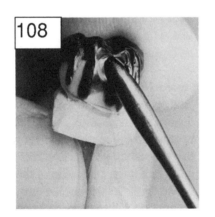

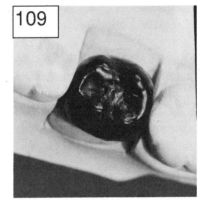

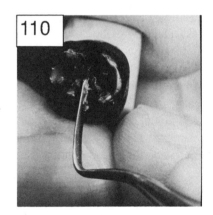

Because the facial slopes of the facial cusps are the primary functional surfaces of the lower posterior teeth, the exact functional relationship desired is established at this time. The basic consideration of whether actual contact is to occur during the functional excursion (as in the segmented-group-function concept) or whether these functional inclines will shear by the lingual inclines of the upper facial cusps with clearance (as in the canine guided concept) must be dictated by the remaining teeth or authorized by the dentist.

Figure 104   Marginal ridges are added with consideration for proper location of any indicated centric contact. Ideally, centric contact would be established between the distal marginal ridge of the mandibular second molar and the distolingual cusp of the maxillary second molar.

Figures 105 and 106   Ribs representing the facial and lingual heights

of contour may be added to guide development of proper occluso-gingival contour of these axial surfaces.

Figure 107   Marginal ridges and proximal contours are expanded to create interproximal contact and embrasure forms. Wax is also added as indicated to complete the proximal pits in proper relation to the marginal ridges.

Figure 108   Additional wax is added to the facial and lingual surfaces to complete their contour.

Figure 109   At this point the essential contours of the pattern are established. Removal of the pattern, internal adaptation, and marginal adaptation should be confirmed before proceeding with completion.

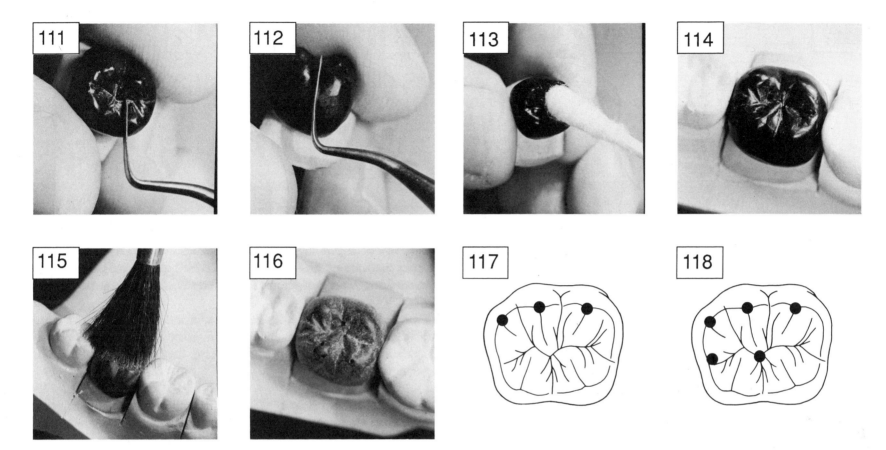

Figures 110 through 112   Refinements in occlusal anatomy are accomplished with appropriate instruments, remembering to carefully avoid the established areas of desired occlusal contact.

Figures 113 and 114   Smoothing of the pattern should be carefully accomplished. Much time can be saved when finishing the casting by a few minutes spent smoothing the pattern now. However, patterns waxed with this much care should be smoothed very carefully on the occlusal surface to avoid disturbing the established contacts.

Figures 115 and 116   When final anatomic detail and smoothing are complete, occlusal contacts should be rechecked by dusting. If zinc stearate powder is used for this purpose, there need be no concern for its removal before investing and casting, as it will burn out cleanly.

To review, the sequence described for establishing the occlusal table in this example was as follows:

1. Centric contacts
   a. Centric holding cusp tips
   b. Fossa and/or marginal ridge contacts
2. Remaining cusp tips
3. Triangular ridges
4. Cuspal ridges
5. Remaining marginal ridges, pits, and grooves

This sequence is very appropriate to generating the occlusal surface of a pattern when the opposing occlusal table is established.

The full significance of the positive waxing technique is not evident until opposing occlusal tables are waxed simultaneously, as is often

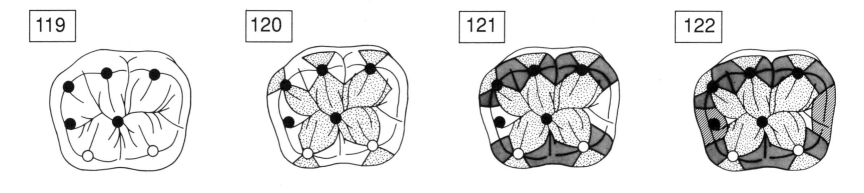

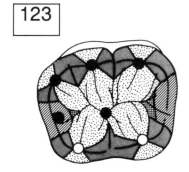

done in full mouth reconstruction cases. In this circumstance the sequence is of necessity different, as grossly illustrated by the following drawings of a mandibular permanent molar. The procedure described is known as the Payne Technique.

Figure 117   Centric Holding Cusp Tips   Facial centric holding cusp tips of the mandibular molar are established and checked for occlusal relation in all functional movements.

Figure 118   Fossa and Marginal Ridge Contacts   The centric holding contacts in the central fossa and on marginal ridges are established by the lingual centric cusp tips of the maxillary molar and checked for appropriate occlusal relation in all functional movements.

Figure 119   Noncentric Holding Cusp Tips   The noncentric holding

cusp tips of lingual cusps of the lower teeth and the facial cusps of the upper teeth are established and checked for position and height as they move through the grooves and embrasures in all functional movements.

Figure 120   Triangular Ridges   The facial and lingual triangular ridges of each cusp are established in appropriate sequences between the upper and lower teeth to permit checking the functional and nonfunctional potential of each.

Figure 121   Cusp Ridges   The mesial and distal arms or ridges of each cusp are established in appropriate sequence between upper and lower teeth to permit checking the functional and nonfunctional potential of each.

Figure 122   Marginal Ridges   The marginal ridges are waxed to establish and maintain appropriate centric contacts and compatible anatomic relationships with adjacent marginal ridges so that equal height is maintained.

Figure 123   Pits and Grooves   The remaining pits and grooves are established with special emphasis on creating and maintaining the fossae centric contacts and the excursion of cusps through grooves.

This very abbreviated and modified overview of the Payne Technique is presented for identification only. Limitations of instrumentation, time and space preclude full coverage of the special waxing techniques in this manual. Opportunities are available to experienced technicians who wish to learn this and other special waxing techniques.

REVIEW QUESTIONS

1. What are four significant advantages of the indirect technique for pattern development?
2. Why should undercut wax be removed from a wax pattern before investing, if undercut wax adheres to the pattern?
3. Explain the effects of low thermal conductivity on inlay wax.
4. Name and discuss the two ways wax may be formed into a given shape or pattern.
5. What area of the wax pattern is the most critical in the waxing procedure? Discuss.
6. List the usual sequence in waxing for establishing the occlusal table of a wax pattern.

Spruing and Investing

Once the pattern has been accurately established, one can begin to consider the process of converting it into a metal casting. This is accomplished by embedding the pattern in an investment material that is contained in a metal casting ring to form a mold from which the wax can then be removed and replaced by molten gold alloy. Thus the purpose of a wax pattern is to form a mold. The accuracy of size, form, and detail that was carefully developed in the pattern must be duplicated by the material with which the pattern is surrounded to form the mold. In addition, this investing material must be sufficiently resistant to heat and strong enough to permit burning away the wax and a somewhat forceful introduction of the molten alloy. Moreover, molten alloy shrinks as it cools to room temperature. To preserve the accuracy of the pattern, this shrinkage must be compensated by making the mold oversized by the same amount that the alloy shrinks. Present investing techniques provide for these requirements.

SPRUING

If castings are to be formed in a mold as described, an opening must be provided through which the wax can be removed and the molten gold alloy introduced. This opening is called a *sprue*. The word *sprue* (origin unknown) means "the hole through which alloy is poured into a mold." In dentistry the term is also applied to the object that forms the hole. More specifically, the hole or opening into the mold is termed the *sprue channel*, and the object forming the sprue channel is the *sprue former* or *sprue pin*.

The sprue pin is attached to the wax pattern before it is invested. Its purposes are (1) to support the pattern in proper position on the *sprue base* during the investing procedure (**Figure 1**); and (2) to form the sprue channel (**Figure 2**).

The purposes of the sprue channel are (1) to provide an escape route for molten wax and subsequent volatile residue during the wax elimination (burnout) procedure; (2) to provide a pathway for the molten alloy from the surface of the investment into the mold; and (3) to provide a reservoir of molten alloy from which the casting may draw to compensate for the loss of volume that occurs as the alloy shrinks during solidification.

Sprue Formers

Sprue formers may be made of plastic (**Figure 3a**), wax (**Figure 3b**), or metal (**Figures 3c and d**). The choice is relatively academic, provided each is used properly.

Metal sprues may be hollow (**Figure 3c**) or solid (**Figure 3d**) and are usually made from brass so that they will not contaminate the investment and subsequent casting. They were originally designed and used primarily for direct patterns—patterns waxed and sprued directly on the tooth. Hollow sprue pins provide stronger attachment to the pattern and are generally preferred over solid pins. The inside of the hollow sprue pin is usually filled with sticky wax to prevent the drawing of wax from the pattern into the hollow portion. Metal sprue pins are removed from the pattern and investment before the casting ring is placed in the burnout furnace. This is done by heating the pin and then gently twisting it out of the investment with a pair of pliers.

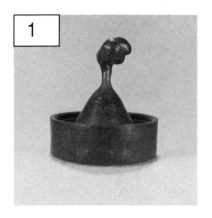
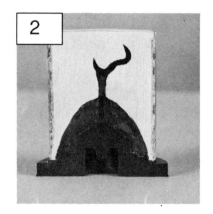
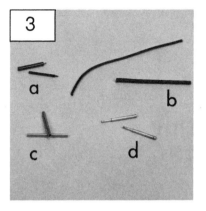
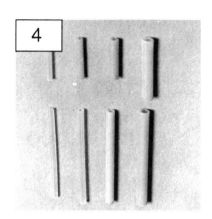

Plastic sprue pins may also be solid (**Figure 3a**) or hollow (**Figure 4**) and are widely used for indirect patterns. Although solid plastic sprue pins volatilize cleanly in the burnout process, they should be removed in a manner similar to metal pins before the ring is placed in the burnout oven. If this is not done, the sprue pin will act as a plug, because the wax pattern melts sooner than the plastic. The boiling of wax within the mold cavity may produce a rough mold surface. Also, more time is required to volatilize wax that has penetrated into the investment. Melted wax can clog the pores of the investment as it is carbonized, thereby decreasing the venting of the mold gases, which may cause back-pressure porosity in the casting.

Another reason for removing plastic sprue pins before the ring is placed into the oven is that they expand when softened and can crush or scuff the investment wall of the sprue channel. These bits of investment may subsequently be carried into the mold by the molten alloy and cause porosity in the casting due to their inclusion. A thin coating of utility wax placed over the sprue pin before investing makes removal easier.

Preformed wax rods (**Figure 3b**) of the proper diameter may be preferred as sprue formers. These are desirable because they melt at the same or a lower temperature than the wax pattern and do not need to be removed prior to burnout. They leave a clean smooth sprue channel and can be gently curved and positioned for the best flow patterns of the alloy.

Sprue Bases (Crucible Formers) and Casting Rings

The *sprue base* is the pedestal on which the sprued pattern is positioned and held in place during the investing procedure. The sprue base is also termed a *crucible former*, because it forms a depression in the investment that is used to hold the alloy during the melting procedure in the air-pressure casting technique. This depression in the investment, termed the *investment crucible*, functions as a funnel in the centrifugal casting technique. It receives the flow of molten alloy from a separate melting crucible and directs it into the sprue channel.

Several types of sprue bases are available (**Figure 5**), made of metal, rubber, resin, or various combinations of these materials. They come in a variety of sizes and shapes to fit various sizes and types of casting rings. Some are designed for one specific technique, such as the water-added hygroscopic technique. The shape of the sprue base is often varied in order to help locate the pattern in correct position in the ring.

Because investment material is mixed much like dental plaster or stone and poured around the pattern, an enclosure must be developed about the pattern that can contain the fluid investment mix until it hardens. The walls of this enclosure are provided by placing a metal *casting ring* on the sprue base.

Casting rings (**Figure 6**) are usually made of stainless steel and are available in a variety of shapes, diameters, and heights in order to accept patterns of various sizes and shapes. The diameter of the casting ring should be sufficient to allow a minimum of ¼ inch investment between the pattern and the ring liner.

If a solid metal casting ring is used, provision must be made for lateral expansion of the investment. In most techniques, the metal ring is lined with ring liner to form a cushion that permits the proper amount of setting and hygroscopic expansion (**Figure 7**). The ring liner should be at least 1 millimeter thick to accomplish this.

The liner must not extend to the end of the ring, especially if

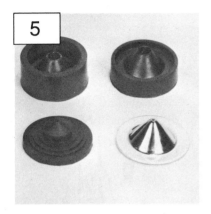

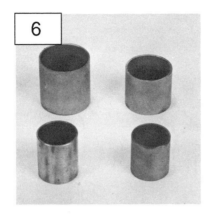

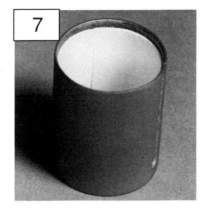

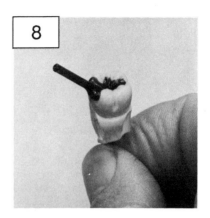

vacuum-investing or air-pressure castings are to be made. It must be cut short so that the investment forms a seal with the end of the ring, to prevent leaks from occurring through the liner and to control proper expansion of the investment.

Diameter and Area of Attachment of the Sprue

There are many variables associated with the spruing procedure. The diameter, length, and attachment of the sprue must be related to the size and shape of the pattern and the type of casting machine to be used.

The sprue former should be attached to the thickest area of the pattern, and its diameter should equal the thickness of the pattern at its area of attachment (**Figure 8**). The diameter of the sprue must be sufficient to ensure a supply of molten alloy during the period of solidification ("freezing") of the casting. When the casting is made, molten metal is introduced into a relatively cold mold (the investment mold is several hundred degrees colder than the molten alloy). As a result, the surfaces of the casting in contact with the mold walls freeze first. Freezing progresses inward until finally the inner portion of the thickest area of the casting freezes. Obviously the shrinkage associated with freezing of the alloy progresses from the thinner portions of the casting to the thickest. Thus the thickest portion of the casting will supply the molten alloy needed to compensate the progressive loss of volume resulting from solidification. Unless the sprue can in turn supply molten alloy to this thick area of the casting, *shrink spot porosity* will result.

The proper sprue diameter for a dental gold casting varies between 8 and 16 gauge, depending upon the type and size of the wax pattern and the type of casting machine to be used. When a centrifugal casting machine is to be used, a 16-gauge (1.3 millimeters) sprue former is used for small, thin inlays; a 14-gauge (1.7 millimeters) is used for most Class I and Class V inlays; a 12-gauge (2.1 millimeters) is often used for Class II inlays and onlays; and an 8- or 10-gauge (2.6–3.0 millimeters) is used for large bulky crowns. (Note that as the gauge decreases, the diameter of the sprue increases.) In general, the largest sprue consistent with the size and shape of the pattern is used with a centrifugal casting machine.

When a pressure casting machine is to be used, the largest sprue former that can be used is 14-gauge. Larger sprue formers will permit molten alloy to fall into the sprue channel during melting, thus plugging the sprue channel and preventing further ingress of alloy.

Reservoirs

As previously stated, the sprue should be the last part of the casting to freeze, so that it may act as a reservoir. An additional reservoir may be necessary if the diameter of the sprue pin is too small for a particular wax pattern or if a pressure casting machine is to be used. A reservoir is a bulk of wax added to the sprue former 1–2 millimeters from the pattern (**Figure 9**). The reservoir is usually 2–3 millimeters in length and should be larger than the thickest cross section of the adjacent portion of the pattern. The purpose of the reservoir is to prevent shrink-spot porosity. If a proper size sprue pin or a smooth, flaring junction between the sprue pin and the wax pattern can be used, a reservoir is not necessary.

Attaching Sprues

The area of attachment of the sprue former to the wax pattern is a matter of individual judgment, depending upon the shape, size, and

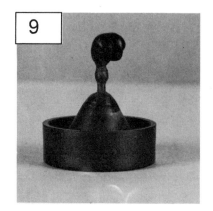

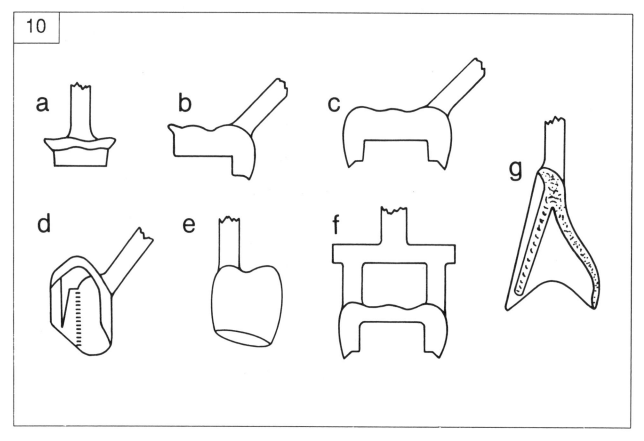

form of the pattern. In addition to the reasons cited previously, the sprue former is attached to the bulkiest portion of the pattern (usually a marginal ridge or the bulkiest noncentric holding cusp) to reduce the chance of distortion. All sprues should originate from a common orifice at the center of the sprue base.

Direct Spruing A single sprue attachment is desirable where a sufficient supply of adequately heated, free-flowing alloy is used. However, multiple units require multiple sprues. Direct sprues should be oriented so that the molten alloy has direct access to the mold cavity with no sharp bends.

In some instances, such as a large MOD inlay, one or more thick areas will exist in the pattern separated by a thin area. Multiple direct sprues, one to each thick area, should be used for these castings. Whenever multiple direct sprues are used, they should leave the sprue base from a common point (**Figure 10f**).

Class I inlays are sprued on the occlusal surface.

Class V inlays are sprued on the facial or lingual surface (**Figure 10a**).

Class III inlays are sprued on the proximal surface.

Other multiple-surface inlays are generally sprued on a marginal ridge (**Figures 10b and c**).

MOD patterns may need to have a sprue attached to each marginal ridge if the occlusal surface is thin (**Figure 10f**).

Partial crowns are generally sprued on a noncentric holding cusp tip or on the lingual surface (**Figures 10d and g**).

Full cast crown patterns are sprued on the bulkiest noncentric holding cusp (**Figure 10e**).

Indirect Spruing When multiple-unit castings are made, the indirect method of spruing is very effective. The indirect spruing system (**Figure 11**) consists of three components:

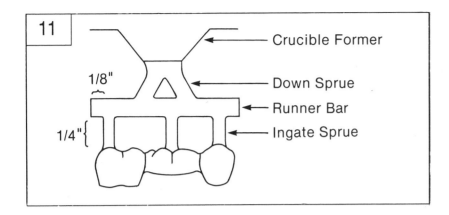

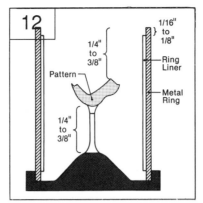

1. *Ingate sprues (feeder sprues)*, diam. 8–10 gauge. These are approximately ¼ inch in length and are attached to each of the wax patterns to be supplied with alloy.
2. *Runner bar (reservoir)*, diam. 4–6 gauge. This wax bar extends across each of the ingate sprues, with about ⅛ inch left extended beyond the two terminal ingate sprues.
3. *Down sprues (primary sprues)*, diam. 8 gauge. These sprues lead from the investment crucible to the runner bar, where they are attached so as to be staggered in between the ingate sprues on the opposite side of the runner bar.

The indirect system reduces turbulence in the mold cavity by allowing the molten alloy to collect in the runner bar and then flow through the ingate sprues into the mold cavity. The ingate sprues should be kept short to prevent placement of the patterns too close to the end of the casting ring. The ingate sprues are attached to the appropriate areas of each pattern first and are aligned perpendicular to it. Then the ingate sprues can be cut with a warm instrument to an even ¼-inch height. The runner bar is made by softening and rolling together two lengths of 8- or 10-gauge round wax. It may be curved if necessary to follow the alignment of the ingate sprues. If the runner bar is curved, the wax should be allowed to relax before being attached to the ingate sprues; otherwise the bar could distort the ingate sprues and the wax pattern alignment. The primary sprues are then attached to the opposite side of the runner bar in between the ingate sprues on the opposite side of the bar. This staggered positioning of the down sprues causes the molten alloy to pool in the runner bar before spilling into the ingate sprues.

The indirect system of spruing is especially appropriate for one-piece splints, bridges, and long-span frameworks.

Sprue Length and Venting

In length, the sprue former should extend ¼ to ⅜ inch from the sprue base to the pattern, regardless of the length of the casting ring. The minimum distance from the portion of the wax pattern most remote from the sprue base to the open end of the casting ring should be ¼ to ⅜ inch (**Figure 12**). This distance is necessary to facilitate the escape of air from the mold cavity in modern, dense investments. If necessary the height of the sprue base is adjusted to conform to these measurements. Direct sprues should not be less than ¼ inch long in order to direct the flow of alloy and to prevent splashing or turbulence within the mold cavity. It appears that the length of the sprue has little effect on filling time (time required for molten alloy to fill the mold cavity), but there is some evidence that longer, thinner sprues decrease the incidence of "subsurface porosity" (small voids located just beneath the surface of the casting), probably because of a cooling effect on the molten alloy.

The real significance of sprue length, however, is not so much the length of the sprue channel itself but the overall position of the pattern (and subsequent mold cavity) in relation to the surface of the investment. The thickness of the investment between the mold cavity and the end of the ring is critical. The time required for air and other gases to escape from the mold cavity during casting is directly proportional to the thickness of the investment. The entrapment of gases due to inadequate venting during the critical filling period will cause surface porosity, back-pressure porosity, and incomplete castings.

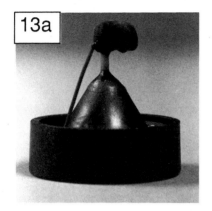

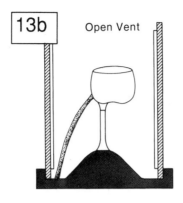

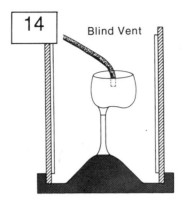

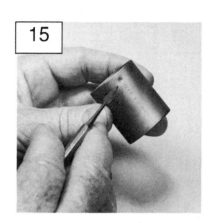

The proper thickness for this ("back-up") investment is ¼ to ⅜ inch. This distance is measured by trial placement of the casting ring over the wax pattern mounted on the sprue base. Correction is made by slightly increasing or decreasing the length of the sprue, by changing the height of the sprue base, or by partially filling the ring. (Partial filling is difficult to control when vacuum investing machines are used.)

Another method of promoting adequate venting of the mold is increased casting pressure. This may be accomplished by increasing pressure on an air pressure casting machine, or by increasing the number of wind-up turns or increasing the amount of alloy used with the centrifugal casting machine.

Specifically created vents are another way to avoid trapping gases in the mold. *Open vents*, (**Figures 13a and b**), made from small-gauge wax rods (18–24 gauge), may be attached to the pattern at the terminal flow point (the last area that the flow of molten alloy reaches as it fills the mold cavity) to provide an open channel for gas to escape. These vents extend from the pattern to the sprue base and are attached at a point as far from the center as possible, so that molten alloy does not enter them from the crucible as the casting is made. *Blind or closed vents* (**Figure 14**) are made from larger wax rods that are attached just inside the terminal end of the ring. Each rod is positioned so that its free end terminates as close to the center of the casting as possible yet ensures a 2-millimeter thickness of investment between it and the pattern, to prevent a breakthrough of the molten alloy.

Orientation of the Sprue

It has already been established that the sprue should be *attached to the bulkiest area of the pattern*. To this might be added the phrase *as far*

from the margins as possible. It is desirable to have the thinner marginal areas as directly remote from the sprue as possible, so that they are cast first, followed by filling of progressively thicker regions of the mold cavity. Another expression related to point of attachment is "keep the pattern ahead of the sprue." This means, simply, to *attach the sprue at such an area and with such direction that no portion of the pattern is closer to the sprue base than the point of sprue attachment*. Violation of this principle would require the molten alloy to flow in a direction opposite to the entry flow (and opposite to the casting force) in order to fill the mold. This rule also implies that the mold cavity should be generally "in line" with the sprue channel and not markedly displaced to one side, so as not to require an abrupt overall change in direction of flow of the molten alloy.

More particularly, the sprue should be attached to the pattern such that the alloy flow encounters no abrupt changes in the direction or cross-sectional area of the flow channel. Such changes result in turbulence, "mold washing," and aspiration of mold gases into the melted alloy. Mold washing is the erosion of a mold surface by the force of the onrushing stream of molten alloy. Certainly some mold wall always stands in the path of the molten stream; however, sharp angles and corners should be avoided, as they are weak and tend to focus the force. Obviously, mold washing results in the inclusion of investment debris and distortion of the casting surface in the area of washing. In most cases rounding of the sprue attachment so as to produce a smooth flaring of this orifice of the sprue channel is necessary to avoid a sharp break in the flow channel.

The sprue should be placed near the center of the mass of the pattern to promote a uniform filling time for all areas of the pattern. Said another way, the sprue should be so positioned as to fill all regions of the mold cavity at the same rate regardless of their volumetric differences.

Another point that deserves consideration when centrifugal casting machines are used is the relation of sprue and pattern to the direction of casting force and gravity. A "straight arm" machine creates two components of force: machine-centrifugal force and an antirotational inertia. The resultant casting force is outward and backward in relation to the counterclockwise direction of motion of the machine during the acceleration period, which is probably longer than the mold filling period. With the "broken arm" machine, however, the casting force is essentially in line with the ring, because the attitude of the arm changes progressively with acceleration. In either case the force of gravity adds a downward component of force as well. Although these forces are possibly insignficant in all but the bulkiest castings, the experienced technician will take advantage of this knowledge and orient the sprue-and-pattern arrangement to a landmark on the ring—usually a dimple (Figure 15). Then, at the time of casting, the ring can be properly oriented in the casting machine so that the bulk of the casting will not be "above" or "ahead of" the sprue as related to the motion of the machine, but rather "down" and "back" of the sprue.

INVESTMENT TECHNIQUES

Once an accurate pattern is developed and sprued, it must be invested in a suitable refractory material to form the casting mold. If metals did not expand when heated and then shrink when cooled, this procedure would be simple enough. However, because the casting alloy must be molten in order to fill the mold, the resultant shrinkage must be accurately compensated if the casting is to be an exact duplication of the pattern.

Dental gold alloys shrink on cooling from solidification temperature to room temperature by approximately 1.25 percent to 1.70 percent. To compensate for this shrinkage, the investment mold must be expanded a like amount.

All investments gain expansion in three ways: during setting, when setting in contact with water, and when heated. Each investment material has different expansion characteristics, but the total expansion should equal the amount needed to compensate for the shrinkage of the alloy being used.

Setting Expansion   As with plaster and other dental stones, this expansion occurs when the investment hardens as a result of crystallization. Depending upon the brand of investment and the water/powder ratio, setting expansion may run as high as 0.5 percent.

Hygroscopic Expansion   Although the mechanism is somewhat obscure, this expansion occurs when the investment sets in contact with water. The amount of this expansion is in addition to the normal setting expansion and may total as much as 1.4 percent depending on (1) composition of the investment, (2) water/powder ratio, (3) temperature of the water in which the investment is immersed, (4) time lapse between mixing and immersion, and (5) amount of time the investment is kept immersed. For example, under standard conditions of 15/50 water/powder ratio and immersion immediately after investing in a 100° F water bath for 30 minutes, hygroscopic investment is stated to have a combined setting and hygroscopic expansion of 1.4 percent. Exactly how effective this is in producing an expanded mold is questionable, because the wax pattern (even though softened by the 100° F water bath) inhibits expansion of the investment to some extent. To be sure, the metal casting ring would restrict some of the radial (lateral) expansion of the investment if it was not overcome by placing a liner in the ring to serve as a cushion.

Thermal Expansion   Thermal expansion occurs during the burnout procedure as the investment is heated in the furnace. Easily determined and controlled, this expansion may be as much as 1.35 percent, depending on (1) composition of investment, (2) water/powder ratio, and (3) temperature to which the investment is heated.

Two basic wax elimination (burnout) and mold expansion procedures are used:

1. *Low-temperature burnout* (850°–950° F). This procedure is designed to be used with hygroscopic investments, as thermal expansion in this temperature range is about 0.3 percent. Thus hygroscopic investment would yield 1.4 percent hygroscopic expansion and 0.3 percent thermal expansion for a total of 1.7 percent compensating mold expansion. As most dental gold alloys shrink from 1.25 to 1.70 percent, this technique would apparently result in adequate compensation for any alloy. In actual laboratory usage, it works quite accurately when controlled or slightly modified to meet the exact compensation requirements for the different types of patterns and alloys by variation of water/powder ratio and spatulation time. Evidently, however, some restriction of hygroscopic expansion by certain designs of wax patterns

reduces the net expansion to below the actual compensation requirements of certain combinations of pattern form and alloy.

2. *High-temperature burnout* (1,250° F). For use with techniques (and investments) that produce only normal setting expansion (no hygroscopic expansion involved), the high-temperature burnout procedure produces a thermal expasion of about 1.3 percent depending on water/powder ratio. From such an investment (for example, Kerr Cristobalite) a setting expansion of .35 percent (16/50 water/powder ratio) and a thermal expansion of 1.32 percent for a total of 1.67 percent compensating mold expansion can be obtained. This likewise appears adequate, but in actual practice it is sometimes insufficient, due again to the wax pattern's restriction on expansion (in this case, simple setting expansion rather than hygroscopic setting expansion).

Types of Investments

Three types of investments are recognized by the American Dental Association Specification Number 2 for Dental Inlay Casting Investment: Type I, inlay, thermal; Type II, inlay, hygroscopic; and Type III, partial denture, thermal. All of these are gypsum-bound investments that are mixed with water. Phosphate-bound investments are also available; these usually require special liquids for mixing.

Many brands of investments that meet the ADA specifications are available, each with its own particular composition and handling requirements. Specific directions are provided by each manufacturer and should be thoroughly understood before the investment is used.

Normally only the gypsum-bound investments are used for conventional gold alloy castings. The three types of gypsum investments are based on composition and technique for use.

Thermal Expansion Investment Technique Type I (thermal) investments obtain their primary expansion for mold compensation from the thermal expansion of the investment. The wax pattern is invested in a casting ring and is allowed to set on the bench top for a minimum of 45 minutes before being placed in the burnout furnace. A normal setting expansion of about 0.3 percent occurs during the setting time. The invested pattern is then placed in a cool oven (usually below 200° F) and heated slowly (during a period of 1 hour) to 1,250° F. At this temperature, a thermal expansion of approximately 1.3 percent has taken place.

Water Immersion Hygroscopic Technique Type II (hygroscopic) investments are designed to set in contact with water and to gain the major portion of their expansion in this manner. As generally used, the term *hygroscopic expansion* denotes the normal setting expansion *and* the hygroscopic expansion, as both occur simultaneously. About 1.4 percent expansion occurs as the investment sets in contact with water. Approximately 0.3 percent expansion occurs thermally during the wax elimination procedure.

Immediately upon completing the investment of a wax pattern, the casting ring is completely immersed in a 100° F water bath and allowed to remain for a minimum of 30 minutes. This procedure permits the investment to reach the maximum amount of hygroscopic expansion. The invested ring is then placed in a preheated furnace at 850°–950° F for one hour or more, where the remaining mold compensation is obtained during burnout.

Controlled Water Added Investment Technique A different type of hygroscopic investment is used for this technique. The technique is also different in that the wax pattern is invested using a special sprue base and a rubber liner within an aluminum ring. After the pattern is invested, the aluminum ring is removed and the proper amount of water is placed in a special reservoir ring on top of the investment (see **Figure 72**). The water is added with a syringe that is accurate to 0.2 milliliter. The amount of water is varied depending upon the type and configuration of the wax pattern. After the investment has set for one hour, the crucible former and rubber liner are removed. The investment containing the pattern is placed into a preheated burnout furnace (850°–950° F) for one hour or more to obtain a thermal expansion of about 0.3 percent and to eliminate the pattern.

Only one variable, the amount of water added, is necessary to control the amount of expansion in the water added hygroscopic investment technique. In contrast several variables affect the amount of expansion in the water immersion hygroscopic technique: the water/powder ratio, the mixing time, and the temperature of the water bath. The choice of an investment technique will depend on the training and preferences of the dental laboratory technician and the availability of materials and equipment.

Control of Expansion

Several factors influence the expansion of all dental casting investments. The water/powder ratio has a direct and significant effect on expansion, both setting (normal and hygroscopic) and thermal. An important rule is "the thicker the mix (that is, the less water in it), the more expansion."

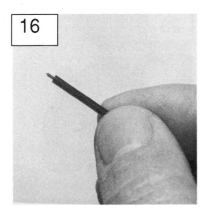 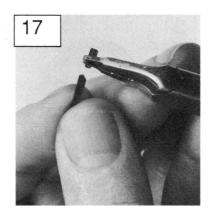 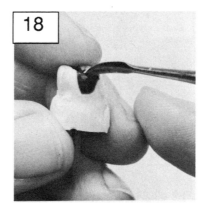 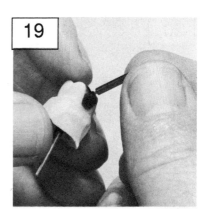

Increased spatulation, in both rate and time, results in increased expansion up to a point. Mechanical spatulation is always preferred to ensure complete mixing, and it should be timed accurately. The time is based upon the rpm of the machine. When using a hand operated spatulator, the number of turns should be counted.

Aging and hydration affect the properties of investment as well as other dental gypsum products. The proper amount of expansion will not be obtained if hydration has occurred. It is usually caused by improper storage of the investment.

TECHNICAL PROCEDURES

The remainder of this section is devoted to a step-by-step presentation of the technical procedures required to sprue and invest a wax pattern. Spruing is presented first; the thermal expansion investment procedure, the water immersion hygroscopic investment procedure, and the controlled water added hygroscopic investment technique are then discussed in turn.

Spruing

Figure 16   A sprue pin of the proper gauge is selected. A plastic sprue pin is shown here. It should be remembered that even though plastic sprue pins will burn out, they should be removed from the investment before it is placed in the oven.

Figure 17   The sprue pin may be shortened by removing a portion to permit its proper positioning in the sprue base.

Figure 18   With the completed pattern seated on the die, a drop of inlay wax is added to the pattern surface where the sprue will be attached. The wax must be of proper temperature so that it will attach securely to the pattern but not flow over its surface. The drop of wax should never be placed closer than 1 millimeter to a margin, as distortion of the pattern may result. Melting the pattern surface to receive the sprue is likewise not desirable, as it may result in distortion or alteration of contour.

Figure 19   Quickly, before the added globule of wax solidifies, the tip of the sprue pin is placed in the wax and held in proper orientation to the pattern while the wax cools.

Figure 20   Wax is added to fillet the joint between the pattern and the sprue. The fillet is a smooth, flaring (funnel-shaped) junction that directs the alloy into the mold.

Figure 21   The finished junction between the wax pattern and the sprue is smooth and flows evenly from the sprue pin to the pattern so that the junction diameter is never less than the sprue's diameter—in fact the junction diameter becomes progressively greater (flares) as it approaches the pattern. Restriction of the sprue channel at this point would have the same restrictive effect as a nozzle on a water hose. If a smooth, even sprue diameter is not present, an incomplete or porous casting may result.

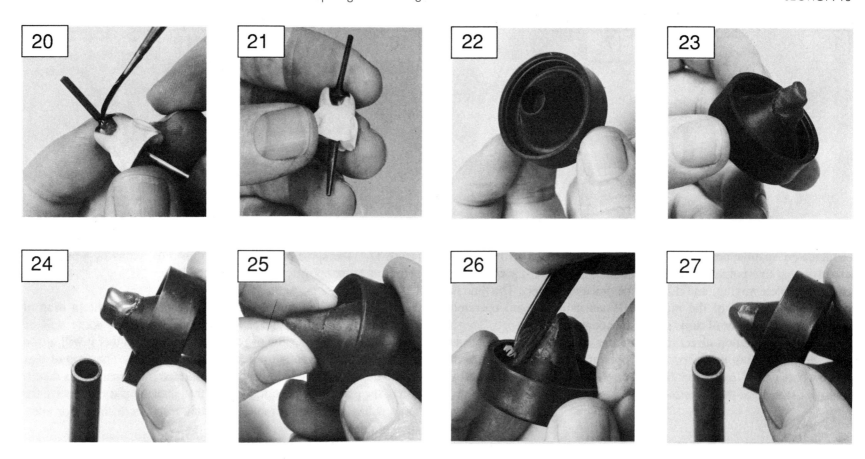

Any depression or uneven surface in the sprue or the junction will become a positive projection in the investment. The injection of molten alloy during casting may cause these projections to break and be carried into the casting as debris, resulting in a defective casting. Therefore a smooth and even surface from the sprue base to the wax pattern is essential.

Before proceeding further, one should make preparations for the subsequent steps in spruing and investing so that these procedures can be accomplished in an orderly, efficient manner. To minimize the possibility of distortion, the pattern should be invested as soon as possible after it is removed from the die. Accordingly, the liner should be placed in the ring; the investing machine (if one is to be used) should be checked to be sure it is in proper working order; the water bath should be checked; and the investment should be weighed and the water

measured. (These steps are purposely not described in detail at this point; variations required for the different investment procedures are identified at appropriate steps to follow.)

Figure 22 A sprue base (crucible former) is selected to fit the casting ring required for the pattern. The shape of the sprue base must be selected for the type of casting machine to be used. The one shown here is for a centrifugal casting machine.

Figure 23 Utility wax is pressed into the hole in the sprue base that receives the sprue pin and is grossly molded into a smooth mound with the fingers.

Figures 24 and 25 The wax is heated and further shaped with the fingers to a height that will provide for ³⁄₈ inch of sprue and a like distance between the end of the pattern and the top edge of the ring.

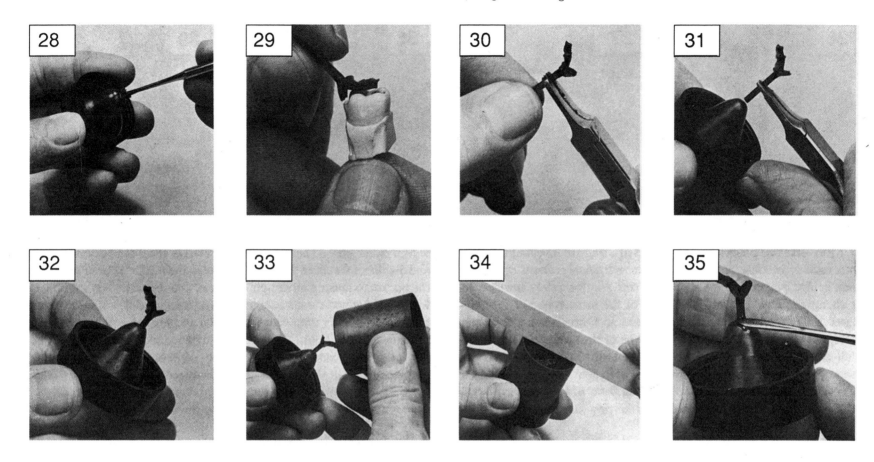

Figures 26 and 27 The wax contour is trimmed flush with that of the sprue base and smoothed by rotating in a flame. The wax should continue the taper of the sprue base to create a funnel-shaped investment crucible.

Figure 28 A hot spatula is used to make a hole in the wax on the sprue base to receive the sprue pin.

Figure 29 The die is carefully removed from the pattern. For one- and two-surface inlays this may be done by using the sprue pin as a handle. For more retentive patterns the opposed thumbs and forefingers approach is indicated. The pattern should be checked closely for any cracking or breaking of the margins.

Figure 30 The sprued pattern is transferred from fingers to pliers.

Figures 31 and 32 The sprue pin is placed into the wax portion of the sprue base.

Figures 33 and 34 The ring is placed on the sprue base and the space between the pattern and end of the ring is checked. There should be a minimum of ⅜ inch between the end of the pattern and the end of the ring. The sprue pin is seated into the sprue base until this dimension is established. If the sprue pin now turns out to be too short or long, the wax over the sprue base may be slightly altered by the trimming or adding wax.

Figure 35 When the position of the pattern in the ring is satisfactory, inlay wax is applied to stabilize the position of the sprue and form a smooth joint in the same manner as described for the junction between the sprue pin and the pattern. Heat must be kept away from the pattern as much as possible.

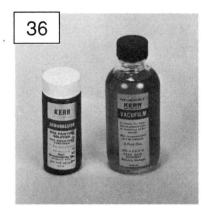

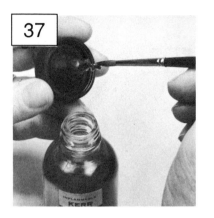

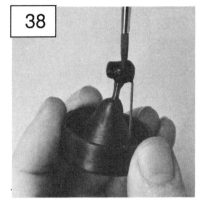

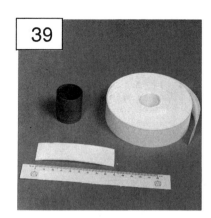

More than one pattern may be placed in a ring for investing if proper precautions are observed. Usually three individual patterns or a three-unit bridge pattern are the maximum that may be safely invested together. Individual patterns should be of the same type and design—three MOD inlays, three DO inlays, and so forth. When a three-unit bridge is invested, the retainers should be of the same configuration—full crown, partial crown, and so forth. Individual inlays or crowns should be placed no closer than ⅛ to ¼ inch apart, so that a sufficient amount of investment may surround each pattern. Each pattern should also lie at least ⅛ inch to ¼ inch from the ring liner.

Figure 36 Wetting agents are used to reduce the surface tension of the wax so that investment will flow evenly over the pattern. There are many satisfactory wetting agents on the market; each should be used according to the manufacturer's directions.

Figure 37 Wetting agent is applied to the surface of the wax pattern with a fine brush. All excess is removed by using a gentle blast of room temperature air. The remainder is allowed to dry.

Figure 38 Wetting agent is here being applied to a pattern for a full crown that has had an open vent placed in position. This vent is formed by first attaching an 18-gauge wax rod to the sprue base as close to the outer edge as possible without interfering with subsequent placement of the lined ring. The other end is then attached to the crown at what is expected to be the terminal flow point (the portion of the mold that will be filled last). This exact point cannot always be accurately estimated. For practical purposes it can be rationalized to be like filling a bucket

with a water hose. The water fills the bucket from the bottom upward and displaces the air in the bucket in like manner. If a lid were placed on the bucket to make it an airtight container and the water was introduced by a hose that had a sealed connection (no backward flow), water would enter the container until such time as the air pressure equaled the water pressure. At that point, the water would be in the bottom of the bucket due to gravity, and the air would be on top. To fill the container completely an air vent would have to be placed in the top. The investment mold is a similar container, except that top and bottom relate not to gravity but to the direction of casting force. The bottom of the mold is the portion closest to the top end of the ring. The top of the mold is the portion closest to the sprue-base end of the ring. Thus a vent for the investment mold container would have to be placed on the portion of the pattern closest to the sprue base. Of course this is also the surface to which the supply sprue is attached, and some separation must be maintained between the two.

Figure 39 A ring liner is required when either the thermal expansion or water immersion hygroscopic technique is used. The liner must be at least 1 millimeter thick and should be slightly narrower than the length of the ring.

Figure 40 A strip of ring liner the length of the circumference of the ring is measured by wrapping it around the outside of the ring. The liner is cut and then rolled and inserted dry into the ring.

Figure 41 The ends of the strip of liner slightly overlap one another. The liner is positioned so that it is just ⅟₁₆ to ⅛ inch short of the top and

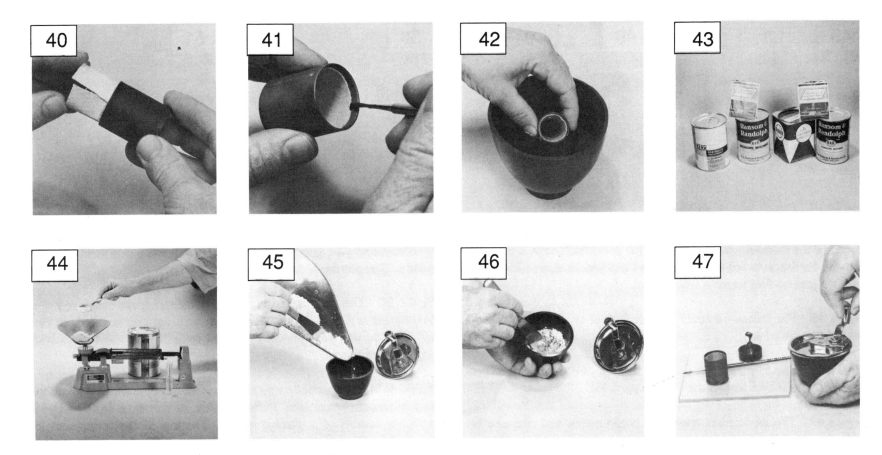

bottom edges of the ring, to permit investment to come into direct contact with the ring there. This direct contact of investment with each end of the ring helps to restrict longitudinal expansion of the mold, thus producing a more accurate casting. *It is imperative that the top edge of the wax pattern be at least ¼ inch below the top edge of the liner* if adequate expansion of this portion of the mold is to be achieved.

If a long casting ring is used, two strips of liner may be necessary to cover the inside of the ring properly.

Figure 42 *The ring liner is wetted after it is placed within the ring. This is done by dipping the ring into a bowl of water and then setting it aside so that excess water will drain off.*

Figure 43 Several types of investments for dental castings are avail-

able. For best results be certain that the investment meets ADA specifications for the casting at hand, and use it as directed.

Thermal Expansion Investment Technique

A hand operated mechanical spatulator is used to mix the investment in this example. Consistently superior results are obtained when investment is mechanically mixed on a motor-driven unit under vacuum. However, a pattern may be successfully invested using a hand spatulated technique, provided that care is used and the variables involved are understood.

Figure 44 The investment is weighed on a beam-balance. Filling the standard-size inlay ring requires 50 grams of investment. The correct amount of room temperature water is placed in a graduated cylinder. A certain additional amount of water is required to dampen the mixing

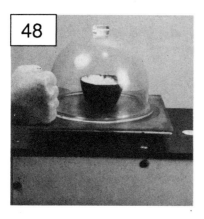
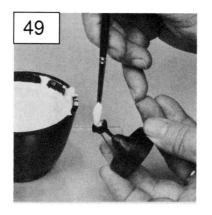
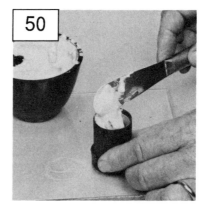
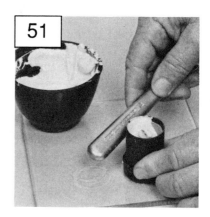

bowl and the instruments, about 0.8 to 1.0 milliliter. The best means to provide for this is to wet the mixing bowl and wipe it almost dry before use. Be sure no free water is left in bowl.

Figure 45   The measured water is placed in the mixing bowl and the investment added to it.

Figure 46   The investment is incorporated into the water with a spatula, being careful to wet all the powder particles.

Figure 47   The mechanical spatulator is assembled and operated for either a specified period of time or for a certain number of revolutions. The unit should not be operated too rapidly, or air will be whipped into the mix.

Figure 48   The investment may be placed in a vacuum machine if one is available. While in operation, the table may be jarred by hand in order to help bring air to the surface. Placing the investment under vacuum is most helpful but not essential.

Figure 49   To hand invest, the sprue base with the mounted pattern is held in one hand and the investment is applied to the pattern with a soft sable-hair brush. To prevent trapping air bubbles next to the pattern, investment is picked up with the brush and applied to the pattern by being carefully pushed ahead of the brush. The investment should be flowed onto the pattern starting from one area and expanding to cover the entire surface. To further minimize any trapped air, the excess

investment may be gently blown off so as to leave a thin film over the pattern. The pattern is then repainted.

Figure 50   The ring is placed carefully on the sprue base, and the investment is flowed around the pattern until the ring is filled. In the filling procedure the assembled ring and sprue base are held at a slight angle in one hand.

Figure 51   The assembly may be placed on top of a vibrator to aid in distributing the investment within the ring, or it may be lightly tapped with the handle of a plaster spatula. The top of the investment is smoothed with a plaster spatula after the ring is filled.

Figure 52   Thermal investment is allowed to set on the bench top for a minimum of 45 minutes before the sprue base is removed and the ring placed in a burnout oven.

Water Immersion Hygroscopic Investment Technique

A pattern may be hand invested using any type of investment as shown in the previous series of illustrations. Likewise, a pattern may be invested with a mechanical vacuum investor using any type of investment. In the present example a vacuum investment technique is shown in conjunction with the water immersion hygroscopic investment technique.

Figures 53a and 53b   Two types of vacuum investing machines are illustrated. Each consists of a vacuum pump, a drive mechanism for

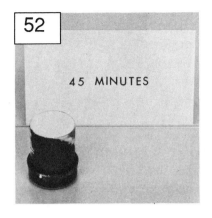

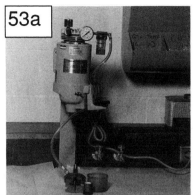

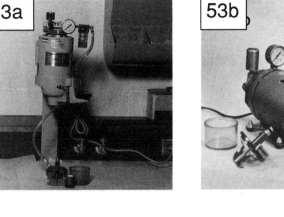

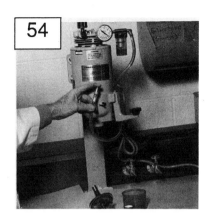

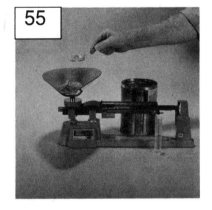

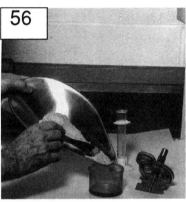

turning the mechanical spatulator, and a vibrator. These machines are basically the same except for the drive mechanism for the spatulator.

Figure 53a is a combination mixer and investor that has two drive shafts, each with a different rotational speed, so that one drive shaft can be used for mixing gypsum products and the other for investing wax patterns.

Figure 54 Before beginning, the vacuum investing machine should be checked. When the machine is running, the vacuum gauge should read between 10 and 15, but there should be a significant increase in vacuum (to at least 27 on the gauge) when the end of the hose is covered with the finger as illustrated. Lack of any change indicates a stoppage in the vacuum line. The connector filter should be checked first; then the hose and pump filter; and finally the vacuum pump itself if necessary.

Figure 55 The correct amount of investment and water is measured (see chart).

Data chart for investing
(water immersion hygroscopic technique, Whip-Mix vacuum investing machine)

Type pattern	w/p Ratio	Spatulation time	Vibration time
Full crown, inlay (I, V)	14/50	20–22 sec.	10–15 sec.
Inlay/onlay (MO, DO, MOD)	15/50	12–14 sec.	10–15 sec.
¾ Crown	16/50	12–14 sec.	10–15 sec.

Figure 56 Before the water and powder are mixed, the bowl and lid are wetted and the excess water is shaken off. The bowl should be damp, not wet, so as not to affect the water/powder ratio. The water is placed in the mixing bowl first.

Figure 57 The investment is incorporated into the water (this procedure minimizes bubbles). All the water and powder must be mixed thoroughly, so that no dry powder remains.

Figure 58a The casting ring with the sprued pattern is placed into the

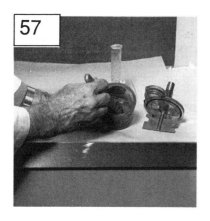
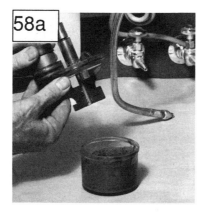
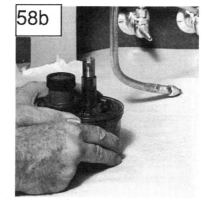
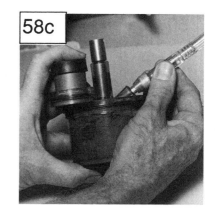
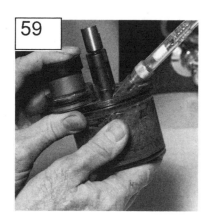
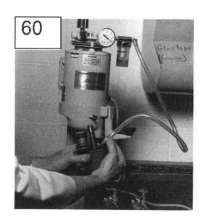
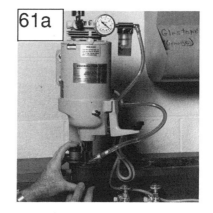
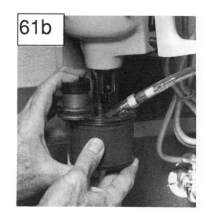

lid opening on the mechanical spatulator by gently twisting the ring until completely seated.

Figure 58b The mechanical spatulator lid with the casting ring is placed on the bowl. A gentle twisting motion will produce a tight seal between the lid and bowl.

Figure 58c The vacuum line is securely plugged into the top of the lid by slipping the metal cap trap into the opening.

Figure 59 The bowl is held securely so that the vacuum line remains in the up position during investing; this prevents investment from being pulled into the vacuum line.

Figure 60 With the assembly held firmly together, the switch is turned

on to start the motor. The gauge should rise from about 15 to show 27 to 30 inches of mercury, an indication that vacuum is established. If a leak is present, the ring-lid-bowl assembly may be wiggled and pressed together until a seal is established. Note that the vacuum line is still in the "up" position.

Figures 61a and 61b With the assembly still grasped firmly, the bowl is positioned to engage the drive mechanism, and the mix is spatulated for the recommended length of time. Motors in the various brands of investing machines turn at different speeds. This affects the amount of spatulation. For example, the Whip-Mix Investing unit (**Figure 53b**) turns at 1,750 rpm; on the mixer-investor (**Figure 53a**) one drive shaft turns at 1,750 rpm and the other turns at 425 rpm. Manufacturer's instructions should be studied in advance, as spatulation times are relatively short and must be continuous.

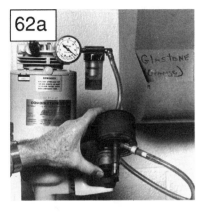
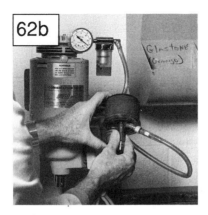
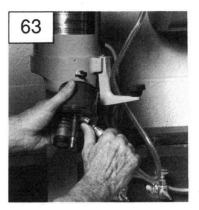
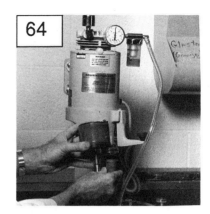

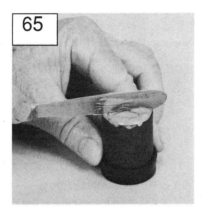
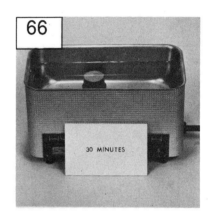

Figures 62a and 62b When mixing is completed, with the motor still running, the bowl is disengaged from the drive shaft. The bowl assembly is placed on the vibrator platform (knob) with sufficient pressure to engage the vibrating mechanism. The sprue base should rest on the platform, with the bowl and ring tilted so that the vacuum line is still in the "up" position compared to the ring. The paddle should not block entry into the ring. The investment is then vibrated into the ring for the recommended length of time. As the ring is filled, the bowl is gradually tilted to the 45° position. It is good procedure to rotate the spatulator drive wheel slowly during vibration to help feed the investment mix into the ring. *Do not overvibrate*; that may cause separation of the investment particles from the liquid, producing a water-rich, weak investment at the pattern margins that will result in ragged, lacy metal margins on the casting.

Figure 63 When vibration is completed with the motor still running and the bowl still inverted, the vacuum line is *slowly* disengaged from the bowl with a twisting motion. Allow the machine to run for about 1 minute before turning it off in order to flush the water vapor from the vacuum pump and to lubricate the investor.

Figure 64 The ring is removed from the bowl by holding the bowl still inverted and gently twisting the ring and pulling downward. If the ring is unfilled to the extent that the pattern is not covered, the vacuum line should be quickly replaced, the ring reseated in the lid on the bowl, the machine switched on and checked to ensure a vacuum seal, and the ring and bowl vibrated further. If the ring is not completely filled but the pattern is covered, the required investment may be removed from the

mixing bowl with a spatula and carried into the ring by adding it down one side with intermittent tapping on the bench top.

When the ring is filled, the lid, bowl, and hand spatula should be cleaned at once by thoroughly washing them under running water after the excess investment is removed from these items.

Figure 65 Excess investment may be removed from the top of the ring with a spatula, leaving a smooth, flat surface.

Figure 66 The ring is placed *immediately* in a 100° F water bath. No more than two minutes should elapse between incorporating the powder into the water and inserting the invested ring into the water bath. The invested ring is completely submerged. Unless the ring is securely fastened to the sprue base, the assembly must be held by the sprue base during the submerging procedure.

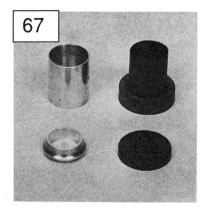
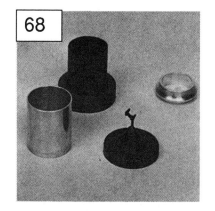
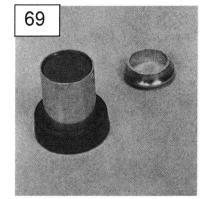
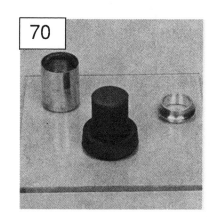

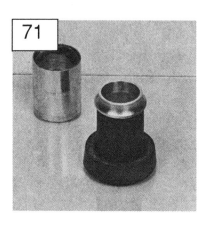
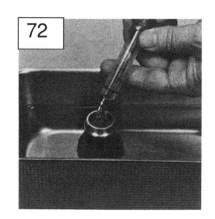
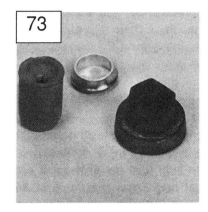
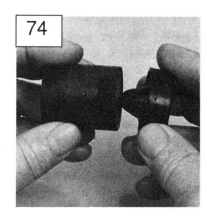

The ring must be left in the water bath for a minimum of 30 minutes. It may be left longer, even overnight. If a delay of several days is required before casting, the ring should be removed after 30 minutes' immersion and stored dry. Before a dry ring is placed in the furnace, it should be resoaked: the sprue base is removed, and the ring is placed in a bowl of water that does not allow the top of the ring to be covered; when absorbed moisture reaches the exposed top of the investment in the ring, the investment has been adequately resoaked. The purpose of resoaking is to ensure even heating and subsequent even expansion of the investment mold.

Water Added Hygroscopic Technique

Figure 67   The sprue base, aluminum ring, reservoir ring, and rubber liner required are unique for this technique.

Figure 68   An MOD wax pattern has been attached to the sprue base and checked to ensure there is proper clearance between the end of the pattern and the end of the ring.

The ring, liner, and sprue base are assembled. The pattern, previously painted with a surface tension reducing agent, is invested by one of the standard techniques, preferably a vacuum technique as illustrated in **Figures 53–66**.

Figure 69   The ring after the investing procedure has been completed. (The reservoir ring has not been used up to this point.)

Figure 70   The aluminum outer ring is carefully removed.

Figure 71   The reservoir ring is placed on the rubber liner.

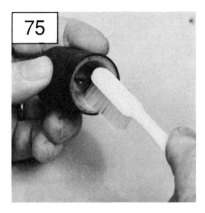 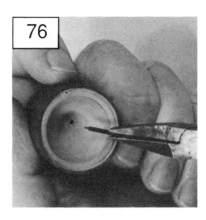

REVIEW QUESTIONS

1. What are the purposes of sprue pins?
2. What are the purposes of the sprue channel?
3. Where should the sprue pin be attached to a wax pattern, and what should its diameter be?
4. Compare and contrast the direct and indirect spruing of wax patterns.
5. Identify the components of an indirect spruing system.
6. Identify the types of vents. What is the primary purpose of venting?
7. What are the two primary methods of mold expansion investment techniques to compensate for alloy shrinkage during casting?

Figure 72   The invested pattern and reservoir ring may be placed in a water bath. The use of a water bath is optional. If used, *the water should not cover the top of the ring*.

The proper amount of water is added to the reservoir, and the investment is allowed to set for a minimum of 30 minutes.

Figure 73   The reservoir ring is removed from the assembly, and the investment block is separated from the sprue base and rubber liner. With this technique the ring is not used during the wax elimination (burnout) phase.

Removal of the Sprue Base and Sprue Pin

Figure 74   Regardless of the investing technique, the sprue base must be removed before the ring is placed in the oven. This is done after the investment is completely set.

Figure 75   Any loose pieces of investment may be removed with a soft brush before the sprue pin is removed.

Figure 76   Metal and plastic sprue pins are removed before the ring is placed in an oven. (Metal sprue pins may be lightly heated over a Bunsen burner flame to facilitate removal.) The sprue pin is grasped with pliers, slightly rotated, and removed. Note that the ring is held so that loosened bits of investment will not fall into the sprue channel.

Wax Elimination and Casting

WAX ELIMINATION (BURNOUT)

Once the process of developing the investment mold about the pattern is complete, the wax pattern must be eliminated from the mold to permit introduction of the metal. In addition, the investment mold must be conditioned to receive the molten metal. Although usually considered a simple and perfunctory step, proper burnout of the mold is vital to the success of developing an accurate casting. Failure here can produce bad effects that even care in other steps of procedure cannot overcome.

The purposes of wax elimination (burnout) are as follows:

1. To eliminate all moisture from the invested ring.
2. To eliminate from the mold cavity the volatile portions of the wax or plastic used to form the pattern.
3. To eliminate from the mold cavity, or from the interstices of the surrounding investment, the carbon residue remaining from the wax.
4. To raise the temperature of the mold to the proper level to receive the molten gold when the cast is made.
5. Through temperature rise, to produce the necessary expansion in the investment to compensate for the shrinkage of the gold after casting and cooling, and so produce a nicely fitting casting.
6. Through proper control of temperature, to prevent damage to the investment through overheating, which can lead to a coarse grain structure and weaknesses in the gold, rough surfaces resulting from breakdown of cavity walls, and sulfur-contaminated gold.

It is essential to use a good furnace to eliminate the wax pattern. In the past burnout was accomplished by open flame or gas furnaces, but these techniques are now obsolete. All modern burnout furnaces employ electric muffles (heating chambers) and are designed to provide relatively uniform heating throughout the muffle chamber (**Figures 1, 2, and 4**).

It is also vitally important that the muffle create an oxidizing atmosphere. This is accomplished by providing an open vent hole—usually located high in the back wall of the furnace. When the wax pattern melts and burns, it leaves a residue of carbon in the mold cavity and interstices of the investment surrounding the cavity. At elevated temperatures this carbon residue combines with oxygen to form carbon monoxide and carbon dioxide gas, thus effecting its complete removal from the mold. This process requires time. Thus, *complete elimination of the wax is a result of time and temperature*. Control of these two factors is essential yet simple.

Temperature

All modern burnout furnaces are equipped with a pyrometer that indicates temperature of the muffle chamber. As with all such measuring instruments, accuracy of the pyrometer must be verified. This can be done by test melts of pure silver (1,762° F) or gold (1,945° F), or more appropriately some of the manufactured indicators designed for this purpose that melt at about the temperature at which burnout will be executed (usually, 1,000° F).

Figures 3 through 6 illustrate the proper method for checking the temperature of the muffle chamber. A test pellet (usually metallic

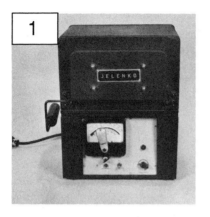

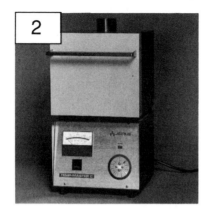

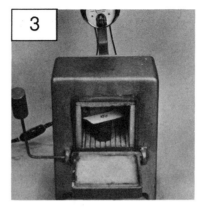

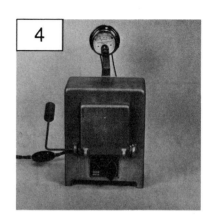

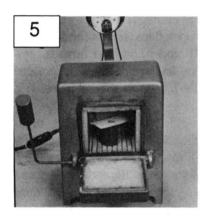

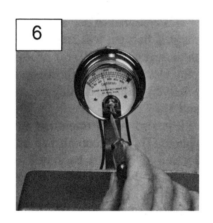

oxides) with a known melting point near the required burnout temperature is placed in the center of the oven on a ring liner resting on a casting ring (**Figure 3**). The furnace door is closed and the temperature is raised gradually until the pyrometer registers about 100° F below the melting point of the test material (**Figure 4**). The sample should be inspected after every 10° F rise in temperature until it melts. When the test material melts, the reading on the pyrometer is noted (**Figure 5**). The pointer needle on the pyrometer is adjusted to the correct melting temperature of the material by means of the screw adjustment (**Figure 6**). The adjustment is checked by cooling the furnace and repeating the test.

Once the pyrometer reading is verified and correctly adjusted, or at least identified as an indicator with a known quantity, burnout can be accomplished at a specified temperature. It should be understood that because of change in resistance of the dissimilar wires forming the

thermocouple, periodic rechecking of the pyrometer is mandatory. Thus, control of burnout temperature requires a furnace with an accurate pyrometer and a temperature control capable of effecting the exact temperature desired.

The temperature at which the pattern is eliminated is dictated by the investment technique that has been used. If the thermal expansion investment technique has been used, the casting ring containing the wax pattern is placed in a "cold furnace," that is, at room temperature. The investment assembly (commonly referred to as the "ring") is raised to a temperature of 1,250° to 1,275° F over a period of one hour. The ring is then kept at this temperature ("heat soaked") for 15 to 30 minutes before casting to be certain that the investment is heated uniformly throughout.

If gypsum-bound investments are being used, burnout temperatures should never exceed 1,275° to 1,300° F, as rapid breakdown of these investments occurs at higher temperatures. This breakdown produces sulfur gases that may cause brittle castings. Physical roughness of the mold walls may also occur as a result of investment breakdown and, if present, will cause rough surfaces on the casting. Higher investment temperatures may also produce coarse grain structure in the casting because of slow cooling during the solidification period. Because very little additional thermal expansion is to be gained above 1,250° F, higher temperatures should not be used. Instead, expansion is controlled by the water/powder ratio to produce the correct setting and thermal expansion at 1,250° F burnout.

Hygroscopic expansion investment techniques dictate a different burnout procedure. The invested pattern (ring) is placed in a preheated furnace at 900° to 950° F. The amount of thermal expansion is minimal

(0.3 percent), so there is little danger of the investment cracking. The ring must be left in the furnace for not less that 60 minutes, and preferably for nearly 2 hours, in order to obtain the proper amount of thermal expansion (even though it is minimal) and to ensure wax elimination. The invested ring should not be left in the furnace longer than 8 hours, or the mold will tend to break down and cause sulfur contamination. In this case the breakdown is more the result of time rather than temperature alone.

Time

Adequate time must be permitted for complete burnout. Regulation of time requires only a reasonably accurate timepiece and understanding. The most important fact to be understood is that, regardless of furnace temperature (as indicated by pyrometer), it takes time to bring the investment in the ring up to proper burnout temperature. Time-heating curves charting temperature increase in the investment show a relatively rapid rise up to about 240° F. The curve flattens out at this temperature for a period of about 20 minutes before it continues to rise—regardless of furnace temperature. This lag is readily explained by the physical transformation that occurs at this point. Investment temperature will not rise much above the boiling point of water until all the water in the ring is transformed into steam. This physical transformation requires energy in the form of heat. It takes maintenance of an elevated temperature over an extended period of time to provide the energy necessary to drive off all the water in the investment. This time cannot be reduced, as the presence of water is essential. Raising furnace temperature or placing the ring in a preheated furnace will have little affect on this time requirement.

Drying the ring prior to insertion into the furnace would obviously reduce the burnout time, but such drying requires more time than the routine furnace burnout. Moreover, investment must be wet when placed in the furnace—especially a preheated furnace—to ensure uniform heating and thus prevent distortion and cracking of the investment.

Other factors related to time and conditions of burnout are critically important. A furnace loaded with more than one ring requires more time for burnout than one loaded with a single ring. A ring placed in a furnace containing partially or completely burned-out rings will contaminate the other rings with carbon residue, requiring additional burnout time for all. A safe rule is to time burnout on the basis of the last ring inserted into the furnace and add 10 minutes for each additional ring present. Additional rings should not be added when using the high-temperature burnout technique. One should remember that it matters little whether the ring is placed in a cold or preheated furnace as far as the time required for adequate burnout is concerned.

Minimum burnout time
(Low-Heat technique, 900° F, hygroscopic investment)

Ring size	Time*
Small inlay	1 hour
No. 1½ (regular inlay)	1 hour, 20 minutes
Medium	1 hour, 45 minutes
Large	2 hours

*Add 10 minutes for each additional ring. Cast no ring until the last ring inserted has been in place for the full burnout period.

The times recommended on the minimum burnout time chart supplied are for wet investment rings. If for any reason the investment has been allowed to dry, the ring should be soaked in a bowl of water as previously described (see Section 13) before it is inserted into the furnace. *A dry invested ring is never placed in the burnout furnace.*

Placement of Ring in Furnace

The ring should be placed inverted (crucible end down) on the furnace tray (**Figure 7**). If the furnace is not provided with a tray, strips of ring liner may be placed on its floor, as some cover should be present to prevent molten wax from soaking into the floor (**Figure 8**). The tray should be grooved to provide for an airway beneath the end of the ring, to encourage exchange of gases (**Figure 7**). When flat metal furnace trays are provided, an airway may be established by propping the ring up on one edge of the tray, or by seating it on separated strips of ring liner (**Figure 9**). By whatever means, air must get into the ring so that oxygen will be present to combine with the carbon residue, permitting its removal in the form of carbon monoxide or carbon dioxide gas. When possible, the ring (or rings) should be placed in the back center of the furnace under the thermocouple (**Figure 9**).

Technicians who use the water-added hygroscopic investment tech-

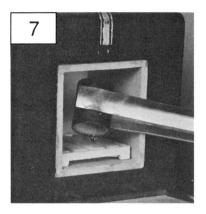
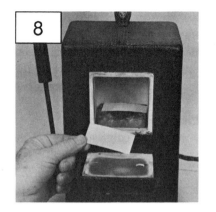
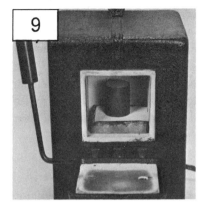
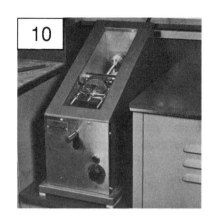

nique advocate placing the invested pattern in the oven with the sprue hole down for the first 30 minutes, so that the major portion of the wax, which soon liquefies, may drain out. The investment mold is then inverted with the sprue hole placed upward; this improves air circulation, so that remaining wax elimination will be completed quickly. All invested patterns may be burned out following this procedure, but care must be exercised not to allow loose pieces of investment or other debris to fall into the sprue channel. After complete burnout, when the ring is being removed to make the casting, many technicians give it a light tap or two against the bench top (crucible end down) to dislodge any loose particles of investment. Once removed from the furnace, the ring should not be allowed to cool unduly before the cast is made.

CASTING

The casting procedure involves two pieces of equipment: a device for melting the dental gold alloy, and another to execute the transfer of the molten alloy into the mold. Basically, two types of equipment are available for each procedure. Melting is accomplished by a gas-air or gas-oxygen torch (**Figure 12**), or by an electric muffle (**Figures 25 through 36**). The actual "casting" of the alloy into the mold is accomplished by either an air pressure or a centrifugal casting machine. Some air pressure machines also employ a source of vacuum to pull the alloy into the mold at the same time that positive air pressure pushes it into the mold. The most simple centrifugal machine is a sling—a cradle with a length of small chain or rope attached—that the operator swings by hand. Although some technicians still use slings and others prefer air pressure and/or vacuum machines, the majority of castings are now made in centrifugal machines. These machines are simply a rotating arm mounted on a spring-loaded shaft.

Melting Dental Gold Alloys

Gold alloys must be melted quickly and in a clean environment. One method of melting gold alloys is to use a casting machine with an electric muffle (**Figure 17**). Some casting machines available today use an induction melting process that reduces a dental gold alloy to its molten state in a matter of a few seconds (**Figure 10, and, close-up, Figure 11**).

The other means of melting the casting alloy is by use of a blowtorch—usually gas-air or gas-oxygen. Gas-air torches are adequate for melts up to about the 1,900° F range. Above this, the gas-oxygen torch becomes necessary. The limiting factor is not flame temperature, but heat transfer. Rate of combustion of gas-air mixtures under normal pressures is too slow to effect a heat transfer sufficient to raise a casting alloy to a temperature equal to the flame temperature. Thus, although actual flame temperature of the gas-air torch is much higher than 1,900° F, heat transfer limits its effective use to melting alloys below that heat.

The blowtorch must be adjusted properly and the proper portion of the flame used to melt dental gold alloy. **Figure 12** illustrates the four zones commonly described in a properly adjusted torch flame. The dark blue or almost black zone adjacent to the tip of the blowpipe nozzle is called the *inner cone* and contains unburned gas and air and conse-

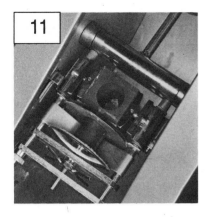

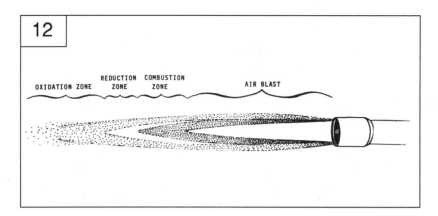

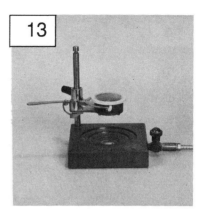

quently generates no heat. This portion is also referred to as the *air-blast zone* because of its high concentration of air.

The next cone is the area of combustion and is thus called the *combustion zone*. It is light blue in color and immediately surrounds the inner cone. Gas and air are in partial combustion here, so this zone is an oxidizing area. This zone should not contact the alloy during the melting procedure.

The *reducing zone* lies just beyond the combustion zone and surrounds the tip of the combustion cone. The reducing zone is the hottest part of the flame and is dim blue in color. This portion of the flame should be large enough to cover the gold and should be the only portion contacting it.

The fourth or *outer zone* is not a cone but rather an outer sheath composed of waste products of combustion, burning gas, and air. Combustion also occurs with oxygen in the air in this zone.

Oxidizing areas of the flame (the inner zone, the combustion zone, and the outer sheath) should not contact gold alloys during melting or soldering procedures.

When properly adjusted, the reducing zone of the flame has a slightly reducing atmosphere and thus not only supplies heat but also prevents oxidation of the alloy. To provide this atmosphere, the flame should be gas-rich, that is, it should have a supply of gas greater than the air supply can burn. However, the air supply must be sufficient to support combustion to the extent that there is adequate heat transfer.

The correct type of flame is also important. It has been described as a nonluminous brush flame with the different zones clearly defined. A very short, pointed flame does not provide an adequate reducing zone to cover the gold, whereas a large, luminous brush flame does not concentrate the heat sufficiently to accomplish the melt in a short

period. The air supply for the flame should not be excessive, and a roaring sound is to be avoided. Incomplete combustion, lower temperature, and excessive oxidation result with an air-rich type of flame.

Many types of blowtorches are available. The one used should be compatible with the type of gas being used. It should also be provided with a tip large enough to develop a reducing cone that will cover the melt.

It is best to ignite a blowtorch with a gas supply only, then add the air or oxygen supply. The supply of either or both may then be adjusted until the proper flame is obtained. The objective is a gas-rich flame that is large enough to cover the melt, yet forceful enough to effect a rapid melt.

Casting Machines

There are many types of casting machines available; some examples are briefly described here. The use of a conventional centrifugal machine is described in detail later in this section. Electronically controlled programmable combination burnout ovens and casting machines are available. Whatever machine one elects to use, the manufacturer's instructions should be carefully followed.

Figure 13 illustrates a simple casting machine that operates by vacuum alone. It consists of a brass base with a vacuum outlet, and a ceramic crucible on the post above the base. The outlet is hooked to a vacuum line, and the gold is melted in the crucible illustrated. The ring is then transferred from the oven and placed on the rubber-lined base. When ready to cast, the vacuum is applied, the molten gold is dropped in the crucible of the casting ring, and the gold is drawn into the mold by the vacuum.

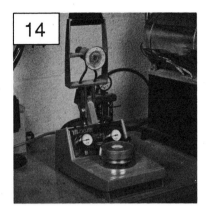
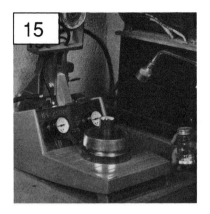
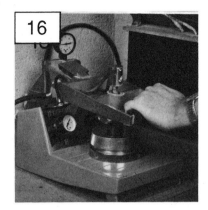
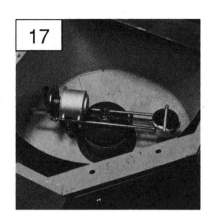

In a vacuum casting technique, it is actually the normal pressure of the atmosphere that forces the molten gold alloy into the mold. Thus a vacuum casting machine might be considered a type of air pressure casting machine.

Air Pressure Casting Machine Increased air pressure is used to force molten gold into the mold when using this type of machine. At least 10 pounds per square inch of gauge air pressure is required to use the machine illustrated in **Figure 14**. This machine can also be supplied with a vacuum source to provide a combination pressure-vacuum casting force.

Figures **15 and 16** briefly illustrate the use of this machine. The casting ring is removed from the oven and placed in the preheated base of the machine. The gold alloy is placed in the crucible formed in the investment and melted using a gas-air blowtorch (**Figure 15**). When the gold is melted, the upper arm of the machine is brought down rapidly onto the ring (**Figure 16**), thus activating valves that introduce air pressure to the top of the ring and vacuum to the bottom. This combination of pressures forces the molten alloy into the mold with greater efficiency and without problems of back pressure porosity.

Centrifugal Casting Machine Although a few centrifugal casting machines rotate in a vertical plane (see **Figures 10 and 11**), most rotate in a horizontal plane. Centrifugal machines basically consist of an arm with the casting mechanism at one end and a counterweight at the other. The casting mechanism consists primarily of a platform to hold the crucible in which the gold alloy is melted and some type of cradle to hold the heated casting ring. The cradle is designed so that the ring, when placed in the machine, will be oriented to the end of the crucible such that the molten gold is slung out of the melting crucible and into the open end (crucible) of the ring.

Some centrifugal machines have a straight arm (**Figure 17**); others have a "broken" arm (**Figure 18**). The obvious advantage of the latter is that the direction of force (the direction in which the gold is being slung) is more directly in line from the melting crucible into the ring crucible and sprue channel, especially during the initial moment of rotation before the arm has accelerated enough to have a significant centrifugal force. In the straight arm machine, this initial force is oriented toward the side of the melting crucible and does not come in line with the ring crucible and sprue channel until the rotational speed is sufficient to produce a significant centrifugal force. The importance of this difference is questionable, as both machines produce acceptable castings under normal conditions.

The casting arm is supported at its center on a rotating shaft that is either spring-loaded or motor-driven. In spring-loaded arms, the spring is placed under tension by winding the arm a specified number of times. Most machines rotate counterclockwise and are thus wound clockwise. Better machines have a lock nut that tightens the rotating arm to the spindle. Release of this lock nut permits the arm to be easily balanced by addition or removal of counterweights when different size rings are used.

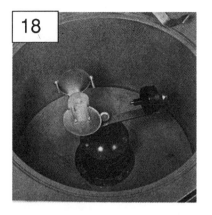
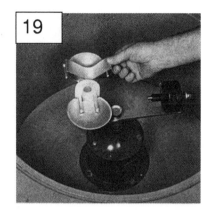
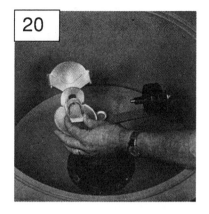
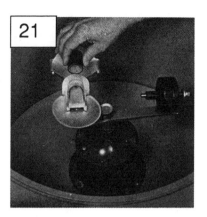

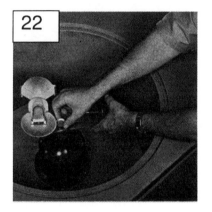
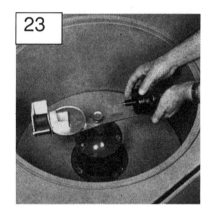

Figure 22   The lock nut that holds the arm tight on the shaft is loosened to check the balance of the machine.

Figure 23   Counterbalance weights are adjusted and/or added or removed with the broken arm placed in a straight line. When the arm balances, the lock nut is tightened and the dummy ring removed. The machine is now ready for use.

Casting Accessories

Several instruments are necessary for routine casting procedures. A *torch ignitor* is not essential but is good to have in the event that the flame is lost during the melting procedure. A lighted Bunsen burner close to the casting machine is the best source for reignition.

Laboratory tweezers are used to place the alloy ingots or buttons in the melting crucible. They may also be used to carry the melting crucible when it is preheated, on a Bunsen burner, to the casting machine.

A *flux dispenser* such as a salt shaker is used to apply flux during the melt.

Ring tongs are used to transfer the heated casting ring from the oven to the casting machine.

Shaded glasses may be an advantage if the casting is being conducted in a light environment or if higher-fusing alloys are being melted with a gas-oxygen torch. These glasses also provide protection.

PREPARATION FOR CASTING

Balancing the Centrifugal Casting Machine

Figure 18   A broken arm casting machine with various cradles that are used with different sizes of casting rings.

Figure 19   The cradle that will allow proper alignment of the hole in the casting machine with the sprue hole in the casting ring is selected and put into place.

Figure 20   The melting crucible is placed in the casting machine.

Figure 21   A cold investment or "dummy" ring is placed in the cradle.

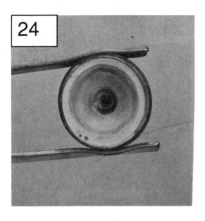
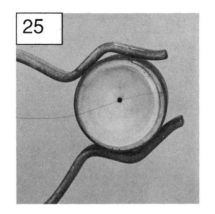
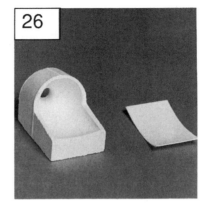
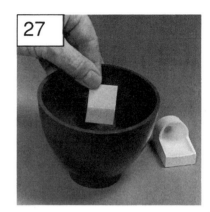

USING A CENTRIFUGAL CASTING MACHINE WITH A GAS-AIR BLOWTORCH

The following series of illustrations demonstrate the procedures to be followed when making a dental casting using a broken arm centrifugal casting machine and a blowtorch. The principles apply to all casting procedures.

Figure 24 Be sure that the casting ring has been left in the furnace a sufficient time to effect a complete burnout. This photo shows the crucible end of a ring in which the wax has *not* been completely eliminated. Note the dark carbon residue about the sprue hole.

Figure 25 This ring has had the wax completely eliminated, as evidenced by the clean investment. All casting investment should have this appearance before the casting is made.

Figure 26 Although a melting crucible may be used without a liner, most careful technicians use a liner in the crucible when melting regular gold alloys. If a liner is not used, a different crucible should be available for every different type alloy used. If a liner is used, it should be made from a chemically and physically clean strip (as supplied by a *dental* manufacturer) and should be replaced for each melt (unless immediately successive melts of the same type of alloy are being made). The liner is placed by cutting a strip slightly longer than the crucible.

Figure 27 The ring liner is wetted.

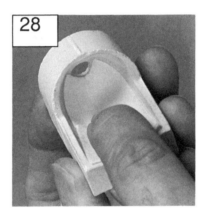
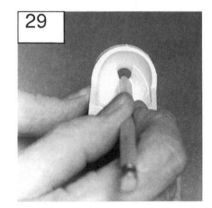

Figure 28 The ring liner is adapted to the crucible.

Figure 29 A suitable instrument or side of a pencil is used to adapt the liner around the orifice of the crucible spout. A close fit is necessary.

Figure 30 Whether or not a liner is used, crucibles should be freed of any dust and debris before each use, by an air blast or even washing if necessary.

Measuring the Gold The amount of gold to be used is naturally determined by the size of the casting to be made. Twice the volume of gold necessary to fill the mold is used, so that there will be as much alloy in the sprue and button as in the casting proper. This is necessary to avoid casting defects.

Experienced technicians can make reasonably accurate estimates of the amount of alloy necessary to cast a given wax pattern. Small inlay

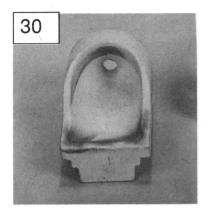
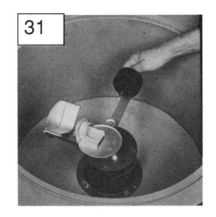
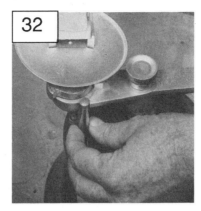
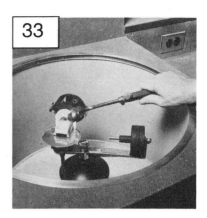

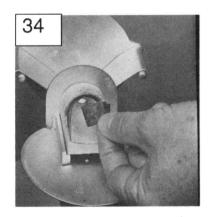
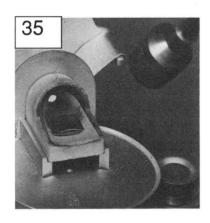

castings require 3 to 4 dwt. Large three-surface and cusp-capping onlays require 4 to 5 dwt. Premolar crowns require 3 to 5 dwt.; 4 to 6 dwt. may be used for molars. (These are the total amounts needed for the casting, including sprues and buttons.) Very large molar crowns may require as much as 6 to 8 dwt., but this is most unusual.

Another approach is to weigh the wax pattern and multiply the weight by 17. An accurate gram scale may be used to weigh patterns and used gold. (1 gram = ⅔ dwt. or 18 grains.)

Use of all-new gold is preferred but hardly practical. Sprues and buttons that are properly cleaned may be reused by adding an equal amount of the same brand of new gold. *Do not mix gold alloys,* either brand or type. Buttons should be carefully cleaned and pickled (See Section 15) before reuse.

Figure 31   The casting machine is balanced and wound the correct number of turns, usually four.

Very thick crowns requiring a large volume of gold may require only three to three and one-half turns, because the large volume of gold increases casting pressure due to its weight, and the large mold cavity affords unrestricted filling and slow freezing. Thin castings may require maximum winding—four and one-half to five turns—in order to fill the thin mold cavity before freezing occurs. The sluggish high-fusing alloys also require maximum casting pressure.

Figure 32   When properly wound, the machine is held in place with the lock pin.

Figure 33   A cold melting crucible will prolong the time required to accomplish the melt. Thus the prepared crucible should be preheated before the melt is made. There are three ways in which this can be done: the crucible may be placed over a Bunsen burner flame, placed in the burnout furnace with the ring, or heated with a torch before the alloy is placed. The third method is illustrated here.

The torch can be properly adjusted during the crucible preheating procedure. Most torches have at least one control valve, many have two. If only one is present, it usually controls the gas supply. Before ignition, one should make sure the supply lines are attached to the proper source. These are marked on the inlet nozzles of the torch. The torch is ignited with gas supply only, then air or oxygen supply is added. The supply of gas, air, or both is then adjusted until the proper flame is obtained. A proper flame is gas-rich but large enough to cover the melt and forceful enough to effect a rapid melt.

Figure 34   The proper amount of alloy is placed in the crucible.

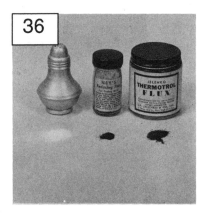
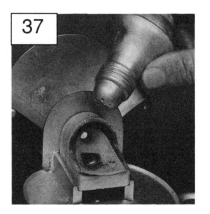
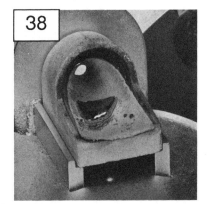
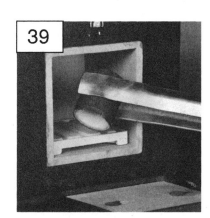

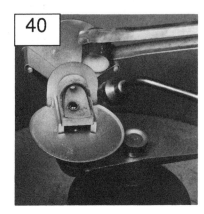
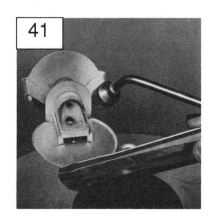

Figure 35 The flame is applied while viewing it obliquely so that it can be seen that the reducing cone encompasses the alloy, producing a bright, shiny surface on the alloy.

Figures 36 and 37 If necessary, a very small amount of flux may be added to reduce the formation of oxides on the surface of the melt. Specially prepared fluxes are available from dental manufacturers, but borax is commonly used as a casting flux for regular gold alloys. The use of borax is not recommended by some gold manufacturers as it slags off oxides, thus removing them from the alloy and thereby changing its composition. Prepared fluxes containing reducing agents supposedly reduce these oxides to the pure metal, permitting the base metal components to return to the alloy solution. (In any case, *never add flux after the ring is placed in the casting machine*. The flame blast may blow flux into the sprue channel and mold cavity, causing it to be included in the casting.) Continue heating with a gentle, slow circular movement of the flame.

Figure 38 If the flame is correctly adjusted and positioned, the ingots and buttons will soon begin to slump and coalesce into a molten pool. If an oxide film appears, correct the torch position or flame adjustment. Oxidation results from the flame being either too close to or too far away from the alloy, or a change in flame adjustment such that it is no longer gas-rich.

Figure 39 When the gold reaches the consistency shown in **Figure 38**, the ring is promptly removed from the furnace. Many technicians give

the ring a gentle tap or two, with the crucible end down, to remove any loose particles of investment or other debris. The time lapse between the removal of the ring from the oven and making the casting should not exceed 30 seconds and is usually only 5 to 10 seconds.

Figure 40 The ring is quickly placed in the casting machine. If the ring has been marked to take advantage of the sprue-mold cavity relation to casting forces, correctly align it in the cradle.

Figure 41 When the ring is properly positioned, the tongs are placed against the front edge of the melting crucible and it is pushed snugly against the ring. By this time, the alloy should be fluid and about ready to cast.

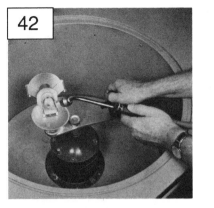

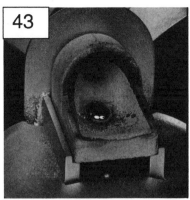

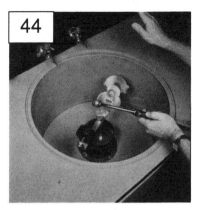

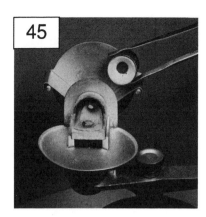

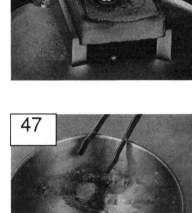

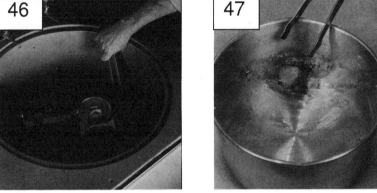

Figure 42 The counterweight end of the casting machine is grasped and pulled gently to release the tension on the lock pin so that it will drop.

Figure 43 The exact time to make the casting is determined by the appearance of the molten alloy. Slight jiggling of the casting arm should produce ready mobility in the alloy. The surface of the melt should appear *bright and mirror-like* and present a radiant light orange color.

Caution: do not overheat the alloy, as evidenced by sparks flying or "boiling" of the melt. However, the more common error is to underheat the alloy rather than overheat it. Proper heating is indicated when the alloy displays adequate mobility in response to flame movement or "jiggling" of the casting arm.

Figure 44 As soon as the alloy is ready to cast, the arm is released. The flame is kept on the melt until the arm starts to move. If the torch is properly positioned, it will be above the path of travel of the machine and thus will not interfere with rotation. One must learn to assure this position.

Allow the machine to spin until it stops.

Figure 45 When the machine stops spinning, the ring is removed.

Figure 46 The button end of the ring is observed in subdued light. The ring should not be quenched until the button looses its red color. Quenching leaves the gold alloy in a softened, easily adjusted state. Some gold manufacturers suggest a cooling period between the time of casting and quenching to harden their gold. Type I soft and Type II medium golds are not affected by hardening heat treatment procedures. However, when harder golds are used, hardening heat treatment may be accomplished in accordance with the manufacturer's instructions if desired. The casting is quenched without heat treatment if a subsequent soldering procedure or burnishing of the margins is planned, as heat treatment may be accomplished during soldering or after the burnishing is completed.

Figure 47 The ring is quenched in cold water.

Figure 48 After quenching, the liner will usually permit the investment to be pushed from the ring. A few light taps of the side of the ring against the sink wall or bench top may facilitate removal.

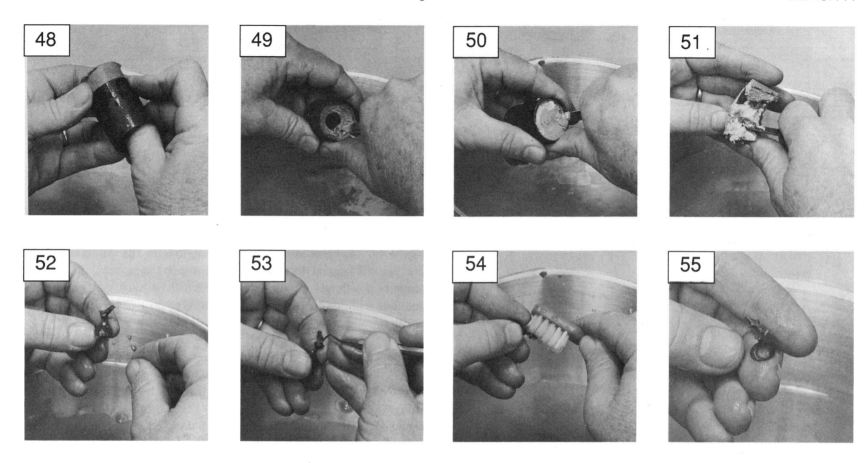

Figures 49 and 50   Some investment may need to be removed from the ends of the casting ring before the entire investment block can be pushed out.

Figure 51   The investment is broken away from the casting. It is best to work from the region of the button and sprue toward the casting to avoid damage to the critical margins of the casting.

Figure 52   The gross investment has been removed.

Figure 53   A small instrument may be used to remove investment remaining in less accessible areas.

Figure 54   The casting is then thoroughly scrubbed with a stiff bristle brush under running water to assure that all investment is removed. The casting may be cleaned in an ultrasonic unit containing an investment remover solution.

Figure 55   The casting is now ready to be pickled and finished.

USING A CENTRIFUGAL CASTING MACHINE WITH AN ELECTRIC MUFFLE

The Jelenko Thermotrol illustrated in **Figure 17** is an example of a centrifugal machine that employs an electric muffle. It is a straight arm centrifugal machine. Instead of a platform to receive an open melting crucible, it has an enclosed electric muffle that contains a carbon crucible.

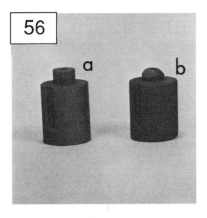

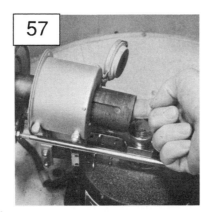

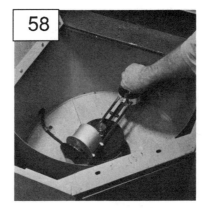

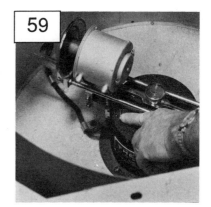

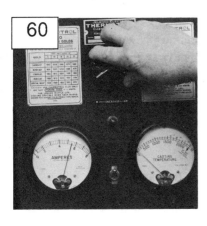

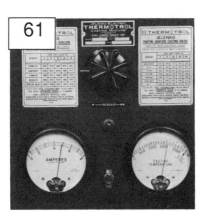

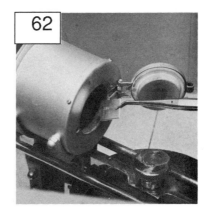

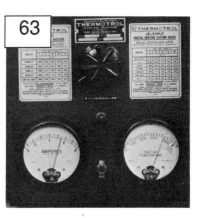

Figure 56   When the tip of the carbon crucible (a) becomes rounded from use (b), the crucible should be replaced.

Figure 57   The carbon crucible is placed in the casting machine. Dust and debris are removed from the crucible with an air blast before beginning the melt.

Figure 58   The casting arm is wound appropriately and held in position by elevating the lock post so that the arm can rest against it.

Figure 59   Electric contacts are provided on the lock post and the casting arm such that contact is made when the machine is wound and stopped against the post.

Figure 60   The contacts shown in **Figure 59** are connected by a cable to the control unit, which contains a pyrometer, ammeter, and rheostat. The principle of operation is simple. Current is supplied to the muffle to bring it up to a temperature of 200° to 300° F below casting temperature. This is done by periodically adjusting the rheostat to provide a current of 5.5 amperes. The amount of current being supplied to the muffle is shown on the ammeter; the temperature of the muffle is shown on the pyrometer.

Figure 61   The muffle is now at a temperature 200° to 300° F below casting temperature of the particular alloy to be used.

Figure 62   The casting alloy is placed into the muffle, and the temperature increase is continued until the alloy is melted.

Figures 63 and 64   About 50° below the casting temperature, the dummy ring is removed from the casting machine.

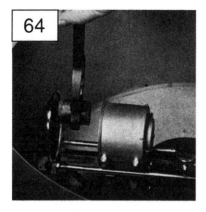

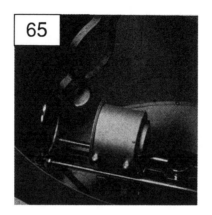

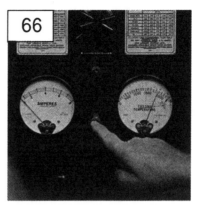

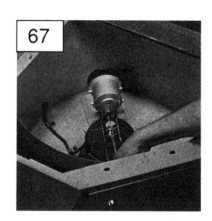

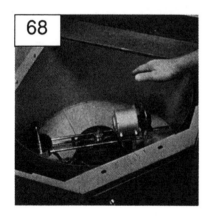

The advantages of this machine are obvious. The melt is made in a controlled environment—the reducing atmosphere of a carbon crucible—and is accomplished relatively quickly and uniformly to exactly the desired temperature.

Figure 65　The casting ring is placed in the machine. If the ring has been marked to take advantage of the sprue-mold cavity relation to casting forces, it is aligned correctly in the cradle.

Figure 66　When the pyrometer indicates that the casting temperature has been reached, the muffle door is opened momentarily to verify the condition of the melt. When ready, the switch on the control panel is turned off.

Figure 67　The casting arm is backed off from the lock post, which must be lowered so that it will not interfere with rotation of the arm.

Figure 68　The machine is released and the casting is made.

REVIEW QUESTIONS

1. List four purposes of wax elimination (burnout).
2. Complete elimination of wax is the result of two factors. Discuss.
3. What are the two basic types of burnout procedures? Compare and contrast procedures concerning expansion of the mold.
4. What are the reasons for placing a wet invested ring in a burnout furnace?
5. Discuss two methods of melting gold alloys, including the advantages and disadvantages of each.
6. Identify the zones of a properly adjusted flame when used to melt dental gold alloy. What are characteristics of an overheated alloy?

SECTION 15

Finishing the Casting

After a casting is recovered from the investment, the following sequence of procedures is necessary to bring about its proper finishing.

1. Cleaning and pickling
2. Inspection
3. Test fitting the casting on the die
4. Sprue removal
5. Swaging and burnishing
6. Machining and surfacing
7. Correction of occlusion
8. Polishing

The rationale and technique for these procedures are the subject of this section.

CLEANING AND PICKLING THE CASTING

Cleaning the Casting

All gross deposits of investment should be removed by the "digging out" process and subsequent scrubbing with appropriate brush and water.

Figure 1 If available, an ultrasonic cleaner with the proper variety of solutions can be most useful in the process of finishing a casting. A stone and investment remover bath such as potassium citrate can effectively dislodge any residual investment debris.

Pickling the Casting

Pickling is the process of cleansing products of oxidation and other impurities from metallic surfaces by immersion in a strong acid solution. Dental castings are pickled with the sprue and button still attached, so that this portion of the alloy will also be cleaned and ready for reuse.

Pickling requires considerable care because the solutions used may cause physical injury if they come in contact with the skin. Their fumes may also cause personal injury and may damage equipment. Noncorrosive pickling solutions that significantly reduce the dangers caused by fumes are commercially available. Even so, all pickling procedures should be done in a well-ventilated area, if possible under a vent hood.

A 50-percent solution of hydrochloric, sulfuric, phosphoric, or nitric acid may be used for pickling. Nitric acid is indicated whenever there is a possibility that the casting has been contaminated with a low-fusing base metal alloy. This is usually due to the use of low-fusing base metal dies. Such base metal contaminants on a casting must be removed by boiling the casting for one minute in nitric acid before it is subsequently heated (such as for soldering) or finished. This is to prevent the infusion of the base metal into the gold alloy.

Improper pickling may cause a gold restoration to tarnish in the mouth. This is because acids are electrolytic solutions and can cause a plating of the casting if the solution is contaminated. When a casting is placed in a contaminated pickling solution with metal tongs, an electric cell is formed. The tongs serve as one electrode and the gold casting as the other. The result is a flash plating of the casting—usually copper, as this is the most common contaminant of pickling solutions.

Although most of this copper plating can be removed when polish-

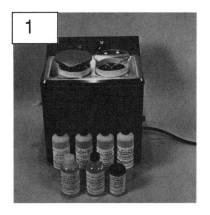 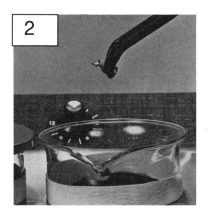 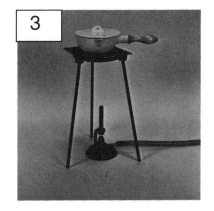 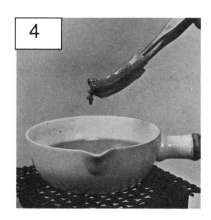

ing, small pits will remain plated. When the restoration is placed in the mouth, with saliva serving as the electrolytic solution, another electric cell is formed between these residual areas of copper and the surrounding gold surface. Subsequently, corrosion will occur about the pit. Such bimetal or galvanic corrosion will also result from heterogeneous gold castings or a very low-carat solder in contact with a higher-carat casting alloy. These causes of electrocorrosion and other problems related to pickling can be eliminated in the laboratory by observing the following rules:

1. Never use unprotected metal tongs to place or remove castings from a pickling solution. Plastic-coated and glass-beak tweezers are available commercially. If these are not at hand, the beaks of regular laboratory tweezers can be covered and extended with autopolymerizing resin to provide protection.
2. When pickling solutions become contaminated or discolored, discard and replace with fresh solution.
3. Use a noncorrosive pickling compound if possible. If regular acids are used, store carefully, use them in an area remote from other equipment, and exhaust the fumes. Do not mix one type of pickling solution with another.
4. Never mix different gold alloys in one casting.
5. Store pickling solutions in appropriate, well-stoppered bottles, and observe precautions when handling acids.

Figure 2   With the correct solution in an appropriate beaker, the ultrasonic unit may be used to pickle a casting. Note here the commercially available plastic-tipped tweezers that are used to prevent contamination of the pickling solution.

Figure 3   Conventionally, a ceramic "pickling dish" is used to contain the acid solution and is warmed over a Bunsen flame or electric heating element.

In the past castings were often held in a Bunsen flame until red hot and then dropped into the acid solution. This is *not* recommended, because the rapid cooling may result in warpage of the casting. It is true that at times castings will have a gray-black discoloration that will not remove in the warm acid bath. This film is due to a carbonized wax residue and can be removed in a warm acid bath if first oxidized. Oxidation of the film is most readily accomplished by heating the casting in a Bunsen flame. However, the casting should then be slowly cooled and subsequently pickled in a warm acid bath, rather than plunged into acid while still hot from the flame.

Figure 4   Pickling is continued or repeated until all apparent oxides are removed. Note that the beaks of the tweezers shown here have been covered and extended with autopolymerizing resin to avoid contaminating the acid solution.

Figure 5   These three castings have been thoroughly cleaned and pickled.

INSPECTION

Figures 6 and 7   The castings are dried and carefully inspected. Good lighting and magnification are essential.

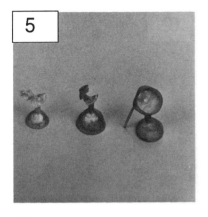
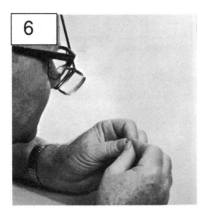
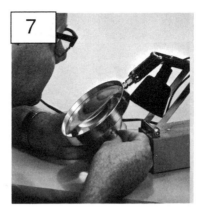
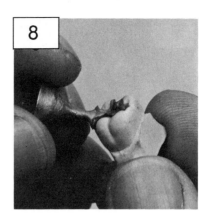

The casting is systematically checked for:

1. *Positive defects*. Positive defects protrude from the casting. Blebs and projections from the casting may result from air bubbles trapped in the investment or from excess moisture that collected on the pattern surface during investing. Fins result from cracks in the investment.

At times a fine lacy, fin-like excess may be present as a result of moisture collecting usually along the margin most remote from the sprue. Concentration of moisture results in a weak area in the investment. When the molten alloy hits such a weak area, it tends to crush or crack the investment, leaving a light, lacy, fin-like excess of alloy along the marginal edge. The source of the excess moisture may be a wet pattern, incomplete mixing of the investment, or, most likely, separation of the mix due to excessive vibration during the investing procedure.

In this instance "excessive" relates to the quality of the vibration rather than the quantity. For example, 30 seconds of smooth oscillation seems to produce no ill effects, whereas 10 to 15 seconds of sharp, jarring vibration at the same frequency causes the investment to separate. Correction of this "lace defect" involves controlled vibration during investing and reduction of casting pressure. The casting may need to be redone if the lacy margin cannot be corrected during the finishing procedure.

2. *Negative defects*. Voids in the casting are generally referred to as *porosity*. Most larger defects of this kind occur as a result of inclusion of debris. Although the cause of this condition is obvious, it is well to trace the source of debris to prevent recurrence of such defects in subsequent castings. Porosity from other causes may be due to incorrect spruing (see Section 13).

One other negative defect is an incomplete casting that is due to incomplete filling of the mold. This may result from insufficient alloy in the melt, premature freezing of the alloy, inadequate venting, incomplete burnout, or insufficient casting pressure. Again the cause should be determined to prevent recurrence.

Although marginal defects must be either positive or negative, the importance of this region of the casting warrants particular attention to its inspection. It should be scrutinized carefully under magnification.

Regardless of cause or type, positive defects must be removed. If this cannot be done without damage to the margin, the casting must be rejected and another made. Excess alloy involving the edge or external aspects of the margin can usually be removed successfully using a true-running flame-shaped finishing bur or similar instrument (see **Figure 19**).

Negative defects involving the marginal edge usually mean rejection of the casting unless they can be corrected by soldering.

Additional information regarding casting defects and their causes is presented in the chart at the end of this section.

TEST-FITTING THE CASTING ON THE DIE

Figure 8 After methodical inspection and correction of any significant discrepancies in the casting, it must be test-fitted on the die. *Do this carefully.*

Figure 9 The casting should go into place with little or no pressure. It

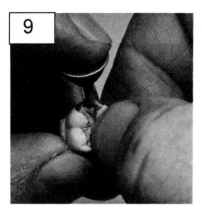
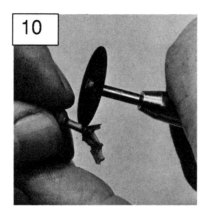
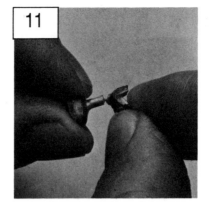
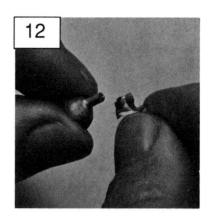

should have the same feel or fit when it is placed on the die as did the wax pattern. If the casting seems to bind or fits poorly, a decision must be made immediately regarding progress: one must chance forcing the casting into place and possibly ruining the die, or decide to forfeit the casting and rewax the pattern. Difficulties in seating the casting on the die are usually due to casting errors and indicate that the casting should be remade. *Avoid damage to the die if at all possible.*

An alternative at this point is to duplicate the die and seat the casting on the duplication. Often a second die can be obtained from the original impression. If it is determined that the casting will in fact seat, or if the error is found and corrected, the casting can then be returned to the original die for completion. It might be well to take advantage of such a second die for polishing procedures. This alternate approach is desirable whenever possible.

REMOVAL OF THE SPRUE

Figure 10   Once the casting is accepted, it is removed from the die and the sprue is sectioned away. A true-running separating disc is used for this procedure. If necessary, the disc can be trued after it is firmly mounted by running it against an old diamond instrument (see **Figure 22**). To conserve gold alloy the section should be made as close to the casting proper as possible.

Figure 11   The sprue should not be cut completely through: a small uncut portion should remain in the center. To prevent binding, the cut should be made about twice as wide as the thickness of the disc. If the

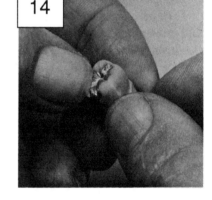

sprue is cut completely through, control of the disc is sometimes lost, which results in damage to the casting or the fingers.

Figure 12   The uncut portion of the sprue should be so small that it will break in two easily when bent back and forth with light finger pressure.

Figures 13 and 14   After the sprue is removed, the casting is replaced on the die. Complete seating of the casting is ensured by firm pressure.

BURNISHING AND SWAGING

Figure 15   *Burnishing* is related to abrading and polishing, the difference being that in burnishing, the surface of the alloy is smoothed to a greater depth. In burnishing, a hard metal point, usually steel, is firmly

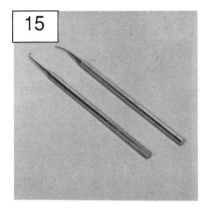

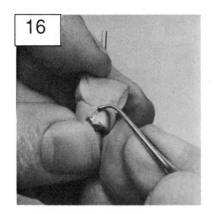

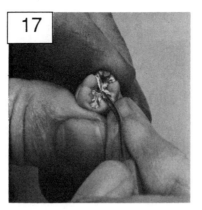

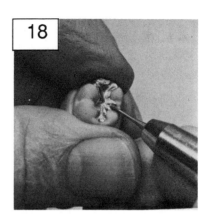

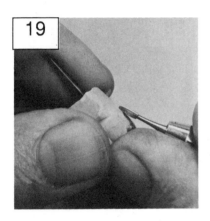

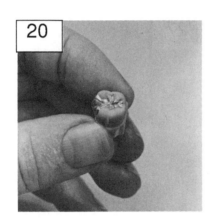

rubbed over the surface of the thin marginal areas of a casting to better adapt it to the die or tooth. Through this same effort small spaces between the casting and the die may be closed. This bending of the casting to provide closer adaptation is known as *swaging*. Finishing burs and special stones may also be used as burnishers. In any event, a suitable type of metal must be used in a burnishing instrument. Gold and copper are not used, because they will rub off on the surface of the casting and contaminate it. This illustration shows hand burnishers that are made of stainless steel.

Figures 16 and 17 The marginal alloy is burnished in an area about 1 millimeter wide immediately adjacent to the entire length of the margin. Note that the pressure rubbing effort improves marginal adaptation by swaging and begins the smoothing process by almost imparting a polish to the burnished surface. Care is exercised not to injure the die at the margin; this can occur if the burnisher touches the die or if excessive pressure is used. When burnishing is complete, marginal openings should not be detectable even under magnification. Burnishing will usually improve retention of the casting on the die so that it will not come loose during subsequent polishing procedures. Burnishing is particularly indicated for inlay/onlays and three-quarter crown castings.

Figure 18 A *dull* flame-shaped finishing bur may also be used to burnish and smooth the margin. Care must be exercised not to injure the adjacent die surface or cut the gold short of the margin. Note that the tip of the finishing bur shown here has been removed.

Figure 19 In burnishing margins with a dull finishing bur, the blunt bur tip should be carried just to the margin but never over it. The bur is rotated at modest speed with firm pressure. It must not cut the alloy. A further safeguard against cutting is obtained by rotating the bur backwards.

Figure 20 The burnishing is complete. Note the excellent marginal adaptation.

MACHINING THE SURFACE OF THE CASTING

Figure 21 Any remaining portion of the sprue stump can be ground away and contoured with an appropriate stone or disc.

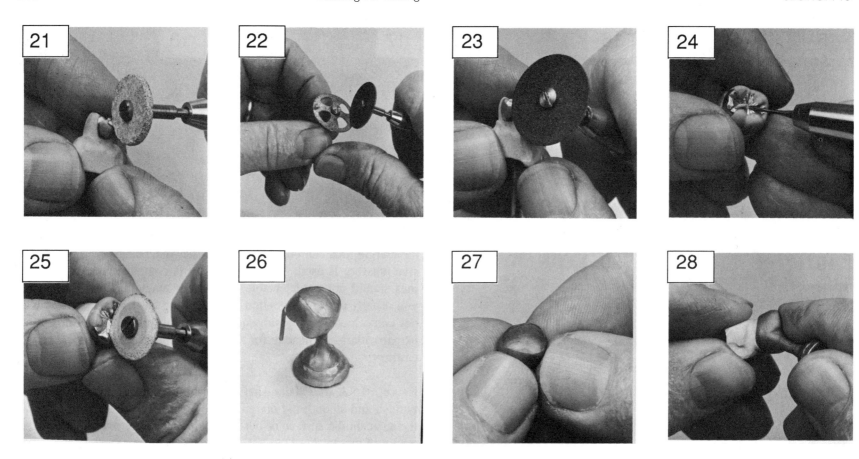

Figure 22   All rotating instruments used to finish dental castings must run true. Abrasive instruments that rotate eccentrically may be trued by rotating them against a harder abrasive. In this instance an old diamond instrument is being used (see also **Figure 38**).

Figure 23   The sprue stumps are further smoothed with separating discs, sandpaper discs, and other suitable instruments.

Figure 24   The occlusal grooves are accentuated by using a slightly dull, small round bur or a flame-shaped finishing bur. The point of the finishing bur has been removed.

Figure 25   All accessible casting surfaces are next smoothed with a rubber polishing wheel. Rubber wheels are available in several grades of abrasiveness. The finest grade that will smooth the surface should be used, to avoid the removal of alloy. These wheels can be "lathed" by running them against a stone or diamond wheel to generate the form most suitable for access to various surfaces of the casting. The wheel pictured here has been lathed to a knife edge.

Figure 26   A pickled full crown casting, ready for polishing. The next six figures briefly illustrate the initial procedures used in polishing a full crown. The procedures are basically the same as those shown in **Figures 8–25** except that a dental lathe is being used.

Figure 27   The casting is carefully inspected.

Figure 28   The casting is placed on the die to check fit.

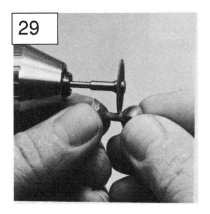

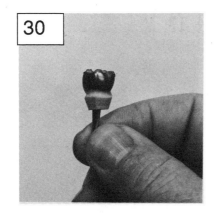

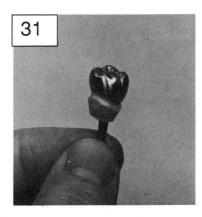

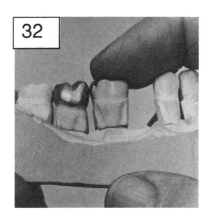

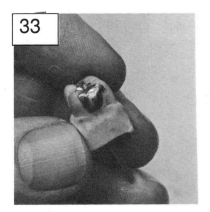

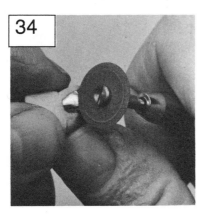

Figure 29   The sprue and vent are removed. (All rotating instruments on a lathe should be trued as illustrated in **Figure 22**.)

Figure 30   After the sprue is removed, the crown is replaced on the die and the margin again checked for fit. The margins may be burnished with a hand instrument or dull flame-shaped finishing bur in a handpiece if this is deemed necessary.

Figure 31   The surface of the crown is smoothed with suitable rubber abrasive wheels as described previously.

Many technicians use a lathe to polish full or partial crown restorations. However, a handpiece is more suitable for surfacing inlays and onlays due to the length and position of the margins.

ADJUSTMENT OF PROXIMAL CONTACTS

Figure 32   Proximal contact areas are adjusted *one tooth at a time*. A decision is made each time regarding which contact area is to be relieved. This judgment is based upon the potential of creating ideal proximal contours on each restoration. Note that in this illustration the inlay and its die are being placed in the working cast together. If the dowel pins have been placed parallel to each other with the correct direction of draw in relation to the die, this procedure is relatively simple. If, however, the dies have an incorrect draw, it may be necessary to remove the casting from the die, reseat the die in the cast, and gently place the casting on the die rather than seating the die and its inlay together.

Note that the first molar inlay restoration and its die do not seat completely into the cast because of the overcontoured contact area.

Figure 33   A shiny spot on the proximal area indicates the exact location of the excessive contacting contour.

Figure 34   The shiny spot is removed with a medium-grit rubber abrasive wheel. The die is again test-seated, and this procedure is repeated until the die and inlay seat properly.

Figure 35   The inlay and its die now seat in the cast with the correct pressure and contour of the proximal contact. Only light occlusal pressure should be required to seat the die and casting.

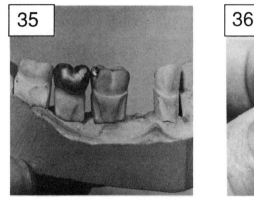

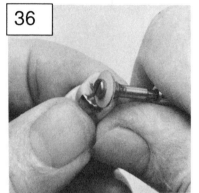

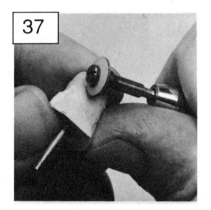

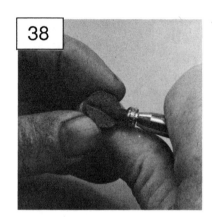

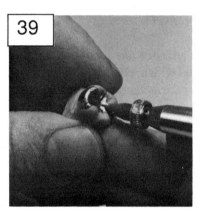

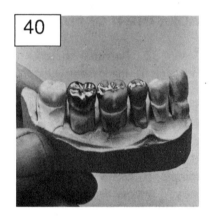

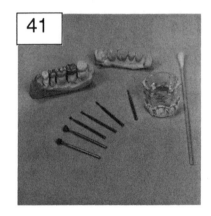

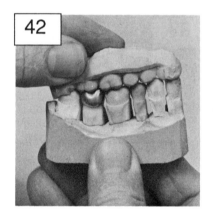

Figures 36 and 37 Smaller, fine-grit rubber abrasive wheels are useful in areas not accessible to larger-sized discs. Such areas are the 1 millimeter of alloy immediately adjacent to the margins and the grooves within the occlusal surfaces.

Figure 38 Rubber abrasive points may be used to further refine the occlusal anatomy. These points are trued, smoothed, and sharpened by rotating them against an abrasive stone.

Figure 39 The sharpened rubber abrasive points reach many areas inaccessible to other instruments.

Figure 40 These three restorations have been surfaced and the contact areas adjusted. They are now ready to have the occlusion checked and then to receive the final polish.

CORRECTION OF OCCLUSION

The following nine illustrations demonstrate the technique for refining occlusion when using an occlusal core—either a functional core, a centric occlusion core, or an anatomic core.

Figure 41 shows the working cast, a centric occlusion core, a disclosing solution in a Dappen dish, and the instruments used to refine the occlusion.

Figure 42 If the opposing core does not seat perfectly onto the die and cast, the interference must be located.

Figure 43 A disclosing solution such as zinc stearate, Mercurochrome, Prussian blue, or white shoe polish is applied to the opposing core and allowed to dry.

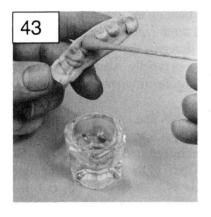
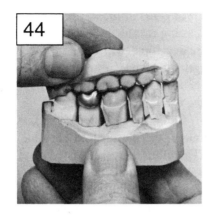
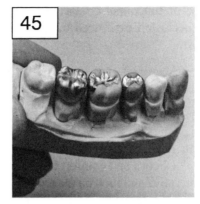
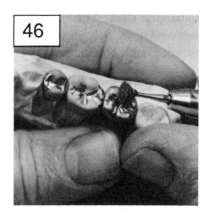

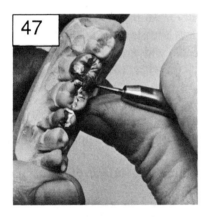
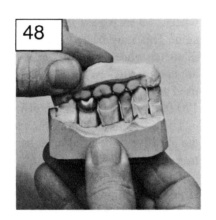
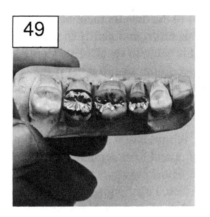

Figure 44   The core and cast are pressed together.

Figure 45   The disclosing solution (Mercurochrome was used in these illustrations) will identify the high spot by marking the casting.

Figures 46 and 47   The interference is reduced using suitable rotating instruments. This procedure—applying disclosing solution to the core, assembling the core and working cast, and then relieving the interferences—is repeated until the core can be accurately seated on the working cast.

Figure 48   The core can now be placed on the working cast with no discernible interference.

Figure 49   The occlusal surfaces of the castings are now compatible with the centric occlusion core.

This same technique may be employed to identify and correct the occlusion of restorations being developed on working casts mounted in any type of articulator. In addition, many other indicators may be used. Gross discrepancies are most easily identified by the use of conventional articulating paper. As such corrections near completion, errors may be more discretely identified with ribbon or disclosing solutions. Very thin cellophane strips or shim stock may also be used between the opposing casts at appropriate points to determine areas of actual contact. This is especially helpful in locating and checking for continuity of functional and nonfunctional contact in excursive movements on adjustable articulators.

Regardless of technique, one must *always* properly locate centric contacts on the centric holding cusp tips and stable areas of the opposing central groove or marginal ridge. The adjustment of centric occlusion does not simply eliminate contact, but properly locates the points of contact and times them to be coincident with the contact of the remaining teeth. The amount or range of functional contact will be determined by the type of functional occlusion evidenced by the remaining teeth or indicated by the dentist.

SURFACING AND POLISHING

All restorations placed in the mouth must be smooth and highly polished. Polishing is not only good for esthetics and comfort but also prevents the accumulation of debris from saliva and food on the restoration, with less chance of resultant tarnish, corrosion, and recurrent decay.

The artistic effort and ability devoted to the development of the wax pattern must be preserved by comparable effort and ability in machining and polishing the casting. Perhaps it is better to speak of *surfacing* a restoration rather than machining and polishing, as surfacing is the act of conditioning a surface so that it reflects light in a regular manner at any angle. Thus surfacing includes both machining and polishing.

Surfacing is accomplished through the use of abrasive substances that scratch the surface of a restoration. A succession of abrasives from coarse to fine are used, which leave finer and finer scratches until the scratches are scarcely visible to the eye. Polishing agents are then used that remove very little, if any, of the surface. Polishing agents redistribute the surface atoms rather than scratch. Even so, the distinction between an abrasive and a polishing agent is not critical, as the difference is usually one of particle size rather than of material.

There are many types of abrasives, some natural and some manufactured. They range in hardness from diamond and silicon carbide (Carborundum) to calcium carbonate (prepared chalk) and tin oxide. These materials are available in several sizes of particles.

Three factors affect the rate of abrasion: particle size, applied pressure, and the speed with which the particles are moved across the material being abraded.

The choice of abrasives is primarily based on particle size. The initial abrasive used in a polishing sequence is selected according to the condition of the surface to be polished and/or the amount of surface to be removed. In any event an orderly, step-by-step procedure and choice of abrasives is indicated, as a fine abrasive used on a coarse surface requires an excessive amount of time to produce desired results. Selection of abrasives is a matter of exercising good judgment in order to effect the best economy of time and material.

In general, greater pressure used in holding the abrasive against the casting results in deeper scratches and more rapid abrasion. However, heavy force will tend to dislodge or fracture the particles so that a grinding wheel used in this fashion is worn rapidly. Also, because more heat is generated with heavy forces, light, intermittent pressure should be used.

Similarly, in general, the faster the wheel that contains the particles turns, the more times per unit time the particle contacts the surface. Therefore increased speed results in increased rate of abrasion. In this context speed is not only the rotation (rpm) of the machine being used but also the linear speed of the particle as it crosses the object being abraded. Thus a larger polishing wheel at a given rpm moves an abrasive particle across a given surface more quickly than a smaller wheel. An increased linear speed results in an increased rate of abrasion. This may be reduced by using less pressure. In general, large-diameter wheels are used at lower speeds, and small wheels and burs are used at higher speeds. A large-diameter wheel (3 inches) should be used at a speed of about 6,500 rpm; a ³⁄₁₆-inch wheel should be used at 120,000 rpm in order to be efficient.

The decision regarding the size of wheel, the speed of rotation, and the abrasive to be used must be based on an intelligent appraisal of the task at hand.

The procedural sequence for smoothing the surface of a casting requires attention to several considerations.

The first is stepping of the abrasive. As suggested, the most coarse abrasive needed should be used first: stones and discs to shape and smooth the sprue attachment and any other rough areas, and burs to redefine and shape the occlusal surface. The scratches left by these instruments should be reduced by a finer abrasive, but the difference in fineness should not be so great as to make the procedure inefficient. Each succeeding series of scratches is removed with abrasives and polishing agents of increasing fineness.

Second, the direction of the abrasion should be changed with each change of abrasive. If possible, after each change to a finer abrasive, the new scratches should be at right angles to the coarser scratches for more uniform abrasion to occur.

Third, the work must be thoroughly cleaned with soap and water between each change in size of abrasive.

Fourth, particle size should not be changed until the entire casting surface reflects a uniform scratch size for the particle in hand. When the scratches are so fine and uniform that they are no longer visible, a polishing agent is used.

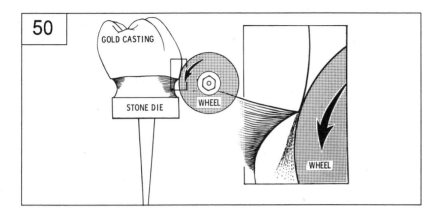

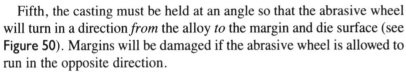

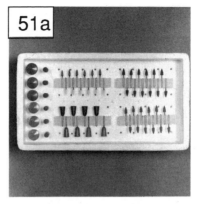

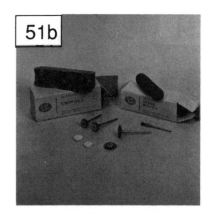

Fifth, the casting must be held at an angle so that the abrasive wheel will turn in a direction *from* the alloy *to* the margin and die surface (see **Figure 50**). Margins will be damaged if the abrasive wheel is allowed to run in the opposite direction.

The following outline is presented to aid in selecting instruments and abrasives used in finishing gold castings:

1. *Gross corrections* (changes in contour, sprue removal, etc.). Carborundum (silicon carbide) discs, flame or wheel stones, coarse sandpaper discs.
2. *Gross smoothing*. Medium sandpaper discs, coarse rubber wheels, and burs (both finishing and regular). Because burs are most useful in refining and smoothing occlusal anatomy, both round and flame shapes are listed here:
   Flame finishing (numbers 242, 245)
   Round finishing (numbers B, C, and D)
   Round regular (numbers 2, 4, and 6)
3. *Final smoothing*. Fine sandpaper discs, fine rubber wheels and points, wet fine or flour of pumice on brush or rag wheel.
4. *Polishing*
   a. *Tripoli*. Fine brush wheels, very small felt or rag wheels.
   b. *Rouge*. Small felt wheel, fine brush wheel, or a chamois wheel.

Figure 51a Commercial polishing points and kits are available for polishing metals and ceramics. These types of polishing devices are more costly initially but may save time and money in use. However, care must be exercised in the use of any polishing procedure not to

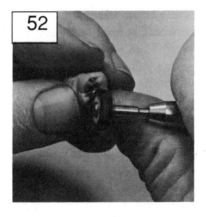

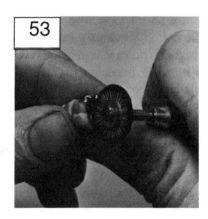

overheat the piece being polished. Care also must be taken not to explode these polishing points by using too high speed.

Figure 51b The supplies and equipment needed for final polishing. Tripoli, a very fine abrasive, and rouge, a fine polishing agent, are used in these steps. Small felt wheels and bristle brushes are most commonly used with them.

As in all polishing procedures, the largest suitable instrument should be used first. Tripoli is applied to a small felt wheel by rotating the wheel against the polishing agent.

Figure 52 The felt wheel with tripoli is used on the proximal and other accessible surfaces. Because the casting has been smoothed previously, a luster will appear shortly after using tripoli. The luster will improve if some pressure is applied.

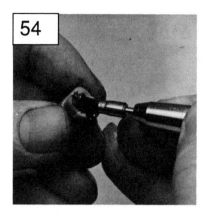
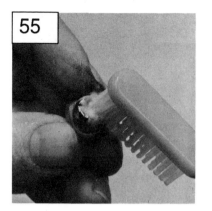
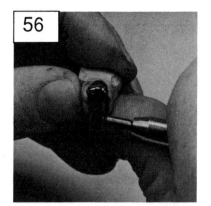
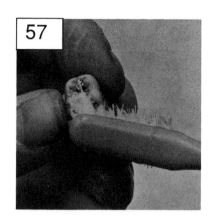

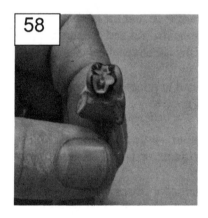
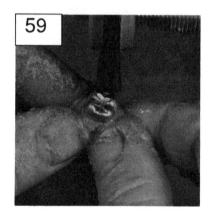

Figure 53 Tripoli is applied to a soft-bristle brush wheel in the same manner as previously stated. The brush wheel is used to polish the irregular occlusal surface (pits and grooves). High speed and frequent changes in brush position and pressure are indicated to permit the bristles to negotiate all of the grooves with sufficient polishing effect.

Figure 54 A pointed type of bristle brush may also be used to apply tripoli to the occlusal surface. A toothpick with cotton applied to it may similarly be used in a straight handpiece to polish the pits and grooves.

Figure 55 The castings are thoroughly scrubbed with soap and water and inspected. The entire surface should demonstrate a uniform luster before proceeding to the next step. If roughness or scratches are still present, repeat the step or return to the rubber wheel, if necessary, to eliminate them. It is pointless to proceed to the final polishing step until all visible scratches are removed.

Figure 56 Rouge is applied to a felt wheel in the same manner as tripoli. This wheel is then used to polish the restoration. All polishing agents should be used with high speed, being careful not to overpolish the margins. A small chamois wheel may also be used with rouge. A brilliant luster will result.

A separate wheel should be used for each polishing agent—one for tripoli, one for rouge, and so forth—and they should not be mixed. In addition, wheels used for polishing resins should not be intermixed with those used for polishing metal. Furthermore, wheels used for polishing different types of metals (for example, chrome-cobalt-nickel alloys and gold alloys) should also be kept separate.

Figure 57 The casting is again thoroughly scrubbed.

Figure 58 The casting is removed from the die. No tripoli or rouge should be present on the cavity side of the casting or on the prepared walls of the die. The presence of residual polishing material indicates that the marginal adaptation of the area is not satisfactory.

Figure 59 Full crowns are often more easily polished on a lathe. A brush wheel and wet pumice may be used to polish the occlusal surface, using slow speed and light pressure.

Figure 60 The casting may then be polished with a rag wheel and tripoli.

Figure 61 A felt or chamois buffing wheel and rouge are used to provide the final polished luster to the crown.

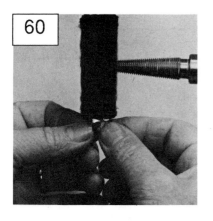 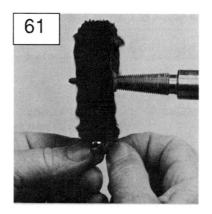 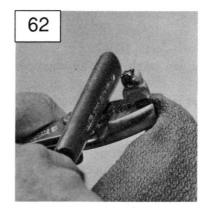 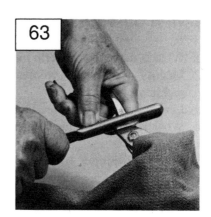

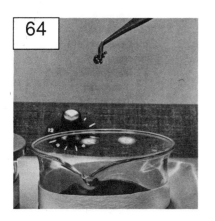 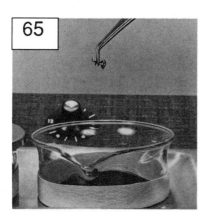 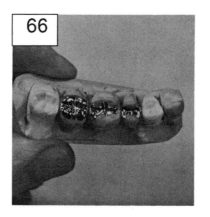

SEPARATION OF CASTING AND DIE

Figure 62   When the casting is well adapted to the die, sometimes it is not easily removed with finger pressure. When this occurs, the dowel pin may be wrapped in a cloth towel for protection and then gripped with slip-bolt pliers. The pin should be perpendicular to the beaks of the pliers. The die is held with the occlusal surface of the casting facing upward.

Figure 63   A portion of the towel is placed over the restoration, but the pliers are left uncovered except for the beaks. A small hammer or the metal handle of a plaster spatula is used to tap sharply on the bolt-head side of the plier. One tap is usually enough; the towel is then unfolded to see if the casting has been displaced. If the first tap does not remove the die from the casting, the procedure may be repeated, using a slightly

heavier tap each time until the casting is unseated. Caution must be used, or the die may fracture.

Figure 64   In lieu of scrubbing, the casting may be placed in an ultrasonic cleaner with a solution designed to dissolve polishing agents.

Figure 65   The ultrasonic cleaner removes the polishing agent thoroughly and quickly.

Figure 66   The restorations are now finished and ready for delivery to the dentist.

REVIEW QUESTIONS

1. What is meant by the term *pickling* of a dental alloy?
2. Identify and discuss problems that can result from an improper pickling process.
3. List and discuss the three factors that affect the rate of abrasion.
4. What is meant by the "stepping" of the abrasive in the finishing process?
5. When polishing a gold alloy on the die, the casting is held at an angle so that the abrasive wheel will turn in what direction?

Analysis of Casting Defects

Type of Defect	Description	Probable Cause
Gross Defects		
Incomplete castings		
Miscast	Casting entirely or almost missing	Pattern off sprue due to excessive vibration
		Pattern fractured, separated during investing
		Gold too cold
		Incomplete burnout
	(Air-pressure casting)	Frozen sprue—sprue too big
Short margins	Short, rounded margins	Temperature:
		Mold too cold
		Gold too cold
		Pressure:
		Inadequate casting pressure
		Trapped air—pattern position
		Trapped air—nonporous investment
	(With smooth, shiny surface)	Incomplete burnout
Holes	Rounded edges—near sprue	Gold too hot
		Mold too hot
		Improper spruing
	Rounded edges—between multiple sprues (*see also* Dirt, below)	Gold too cold
		Mold too cold
		Improper spruing
Fit		
Size	Undistorted but too large or too small	Spatulation
		Water temperature
		Burnout temperature
		Water/powder ratio
		Cristobalite/control powder ratio
		Immersion time (hygroscopic)
		Water-added (hygroscopic)
Distortion	Local lack of fit	Wax too hot
		Wax too cold
		Insufficient pressure in waxing
		Heating during spruing

Analysis of Casting Defects (continued)

Type of Defect	Description	Probable Cause
Rocking	Casting will not seat, rocks when seated as far as possible	Delayed investing Heat plunge pickle Soldering heat Investment erosion (*see* Bump, below) Pattern distorted

Surface Defects
Excess metal

Type of Defect	Description	Probable Cause
Bubbles	Large	Poor painting and investing technique Mix too thick
	Small, on flat surfaces, esp. bottom and sides	Air mixed into investment Overvibration of ring Loss of vacuum
	Small, on top, grooves, reentrant angles	Overvibration of ring Poor painting technique
Roughness	General, sharp feel	Mixing technique (*see* Bubbles, small, above) "Green" mold Too rapid heating
	General, mossy, lacy	Thin mix plus overvibration
	Local, bottom, mossy, lacy	Very thin mix Thin mix plus overvibration
	Local, exterior, mossy, lacy	Too much surface agent
Fins	Thin, sheetlike, extensions from casting surface	Heating ring too fast Dry, cold ring in hot oven (hygroscopic) Heating too long Weak investment Too much casting pressure Ring cooled before casting
	(Partial dentures)	Differential expansion of cast and mold
Bump (*see* Rocking, above)	Rounded projection opposite sprue Usually on large castings Often associated with "dirt"	Weak investment Too much pressure Improper spruing

Analysis of Casting Defects (continued)

Type of Defect	Description	Probable Cause
Shortage of metal		
Pits	General depressed roughness	Green ring; salts deposited in mold, noncristobalite investment
	Marginal, angular edges	Inclusion washed to margin by gold
	Marginal, rounded edges	Flux inclusion
	Local, near sprue	Shrink-spot
	Local	Green mold Incomplete burnout
Voids	Large, saucer-shaped	"Back-pressure porosity" Inadequate venting Inadequate pressure Too thick mix Incomplete burnout Mold too cold
Shrinkage (localized)	Depressions on flat surfaces near hot spots (rare in dental castings except opposite sprue)	Mold too hot Gold too hot
Dirt	Solid imbedded in metal anywhere on surface; most common near margins and sprue	Dirty sprue or crucible former
	Investment	Rough handling withdrawing sprue Green mold Heat too fast
	Flux	Too much flux in casting crucible
	Carbon (accompanied by pits or shiny surface)	Incomplete burnout
	Oxide	Insufficient fluxing Uncleaned gold Improper flame adjustment Improper flame manipulation
	Miscellaneous	Anything small enough to fall down the sprue hole or be mixed with the wax
Discoloration	Shiny, in nonreducing investments	Incomplete burnout

Analysis of Casting Defects (continued)

Type of Defect	Description	Probable Cause
	Black, removed by HCl	Normal in Cristobalite
	Black, not removed by HCl or H_2SO_4	Sulfur contamination Mold too hot Gold too hot

Internal Defects

Porosity

Type of Defect	Description	Probable Cause
Gas	Small, rounded voids below surface ("pinhole porosity")	Dissolved gas Gold too hot Flame poorly adjusted
	Large round voids reaching surface	Incomplete burnout Gas from wax
	Medium rounded voids below surface	Gold too cold
	Small round voids near surface only	Incomplete burnout H_2O vapor from green mold
Shrink-spot	Irregular voids, spongy structure	Sprue too small
	Near sprue and in thick section	Sprue not in thickest section
	Broken sprue	Too little pressure
Microporosity	Small, irregular voids throughout	Mold too cold Gold too cold
Subsurface porosity	A layer of semirounded, medium voids just below surface	Mold too hot Gold too hot Sprue too short Sprue too large

Inclusions

Type of Defect	Description	Probable Cause
Local	Investment	Dirty equipment Rough handling Inadequate trimming Improper spruing Too much pressure
	Flux	Too much flux in casting crucible—not removed
	Carbon	Incomplete burnout
	Metallic	Contamination with an insoluble metal such as aluminum
Intergranular	Metallic	Partially soluble metal such as lead, tin, or bismuth Gold exposure to mercury

Analysis of Casting Defects (continued)

Type of Defect	Description	Probable Cause
	Nonmetallic	Sulfur contamination (if extreme, the casting will exhibit very rough, blackened surface)

Mechanical Properties

Type of Defect	Description	Probable Cause
Brittleness	Contamination Sulfer	Overheated investment in casting or soldering Poorly cleaned used gold
	Base metal	Pb, Sn, Bi, Hg, Al from scrap, or contact with dies, instruments, or equipment
	Treatment	Failure to anneal wires or clasp Unintentional hardening Hot short-blue brittle
Lack of burnishability		Contamination (see above) Treatment (see above) Composition (normal in Type III or IV hard gold, hardened wires, chrome alloys)
Discoloration in surface	Surface deposit removable with brush and nonabrasive soap	Inadequate care and cleaning
	General black corrosion	Copper deposit from used pickling solution Galvanic corrosion, oxidized metal
Melting characteristics	Dull surface when molten	
	Reducible on charcoal	Oxidation
	Nonreducible	Base metal contamination
	Nonmeltable	Contamination with high-fusing metal Flame out of adjustment Extreme oxidation
	Sluggish	Burnt gold Contamination with oxide-former such as aluminum

Source: Courtesy of Dr. Duane Taylor.

SECTION 16

Soldering

Soldering is the joining together of two pieces of metal by flowing onto their surfaces a lower-fusing metal, the solder. Although welding (the direct uniting of two pieces of metal by pressure or heat) is used in dentistry (gold foil, "spot" welding, and the like), soldering is the principle means of uniting components of cast or wrought dental appliances. "Freehand" soldering is suitable for some procedures, such as orthodontic appliances and simple additions to cast structures (for example, building up proximal or occlusal contact areas). However, uniting components of a multiunit fixed restoration requires the precision of investment soldering.

Figure 1 The relationship of the components to be joined is established and maintained throughout the soldering operation by the soldering investment.

Regular soldering investments are similar to gypsum and quartz casting investments. They must meet requirements for strength and expansion (both setting and thermal). Accurate compensation for the thermal expansion and shrinkage of the cast segments is as critical to the precision soldering operation as to the precision casting procedure. Ideally the setting expansion and thermal expansion of the investment should equal the shrinkage of the soldered assembly as it cools from work temperature to room temperature.

Figure 2 Joint space must be considered when assembling the segments to be joined. Solder will not flow between pieces in tight contact; thus some space must be present in the joint areas. The setting and thermal expansion of the investment will tend to separate the pieces, leaving a spaced joint. However, thermal expansion of the gold alloy pieces causes them to expand toward one another (each expands from its own center) and close the joint space. Assuming that increase of the joint space due to thermal expansion of the investment will equal the decrease in joint space caused by thermal expansion of the metal parts, the proper joint space must be present before either occurs. A joint space of .005 to .01 inch (two to three thicknesses of notepaper) is recommended.

SOLDERING INDEX

Once the pieces to be joined are accurately related, either on the working cast or in the mouth, this relationship must be transferred in a manner that permits proper investing. This is accomplished by making either a plaster or a self-curing resin index.

PLASTER INDEX

Figures 3 and 4 The plaster index is developed with quick-set plaster carried into place freehand or in, or on, a suitable conveyor (plaster impression tray, tooth carding tray, tongue blade, or spatula blade). The plaster should encompass only the occlusal one-third of the castings.

Figures 5 and 6 When set, the index is removed and inspected for accuracy. Any overextension is carefully removed. When relationships are being established in the mouth, the dentist will often take two

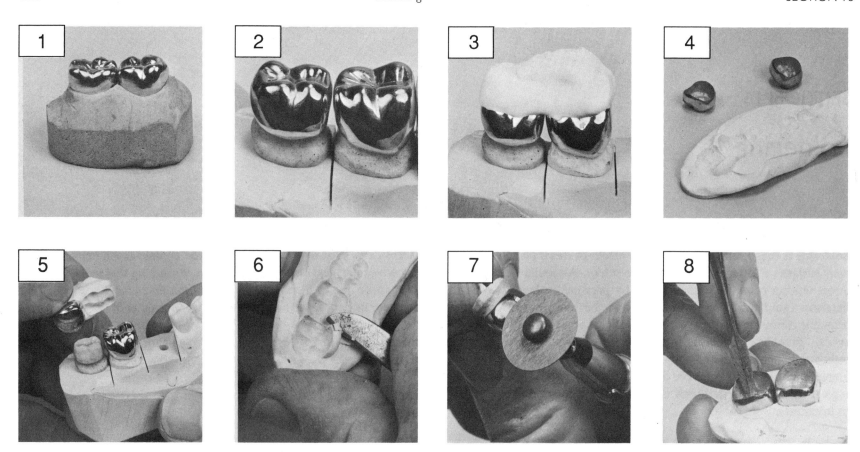

indexes to ensure a duplicate in case one is broken or the soldering operation must be aborted. If only one index is provided by the dentist, the established relationship may be duplicated by the laboratory technician in the event that the original index must be destroyed in the soldering process. First, with the castings accurately seated in the index, dies are seated in the castings, undercuts blocked out, and a cast poured about the assembly in the same fashion as for a coping transfer impression. This provides a corrected working cast from which repeated soldering transfer indexes can be taken if needed. A second technique is to take a plaster index of the components after they are invested for soldering. Of course such an index will record any change in relationship caused by setting expansion of the investment.

When the index is completed, the castings are prepared for investing.

Figure 7 Joint space is evaluated as the castings are seated in the index. This space may be established as the joint surfaces are prepared for soldering. *The surfaces must be machined smooth* (discs, burs, and rubber wheels) *and lightly coated with flux*. One must remember at this point that *cleanliness is the key to success in soldering*.

Figures 8 and 9 The cast pieces are carefully positioned in the index and maintained by sticky wax. To prevent displacement due to contraction, each casting is held firmly in place until the sticky wax cools.

Figure 10 When all pieces are positioned, the joint areas are sealed with wax, built up to sufficient dimension to provide room for the soldered joint *plus* an airway under the joint. A convenient means of accomplishing this is to position a rope of utility wax so that it extends from the joint area to the facial and lingual. *Do not permit wax to*

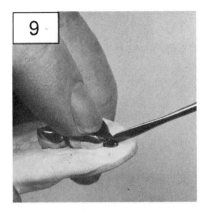
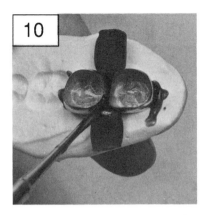
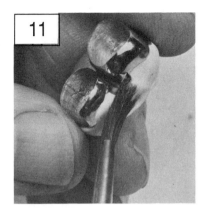
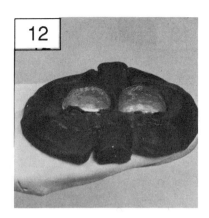

contact a margin. The wax buildup will prevent investment encroaching on the joint area and maintain an airway.

Figures 11 and 12   Suitable separation may be developed by application of gypsum separator (Super-Sep, soap, petroleum jelly, etc.) or by adapting soft boxing or rope wax to the exposed plaster surface. The use of wax as a separator also permits control of the amount of surface area of the castings that is left exposed. Maximum exposure of casting surfaces is generally desired. However, consideration should be given to having a relatively equal exposure of alloy on either side of the joint area. At this point the work is ready to be invested.

AUTOPOLYMERIZING RESIN INDEX

When transferring pieces to be soldered by indexing them with resin, joint space corrections and preparation of joint surfaces must be completed first if the pieces are to be joined by the resin. The joint areas must be cleaned, but no flux is applied, as this would prevent locking of the resin. When these preparations are complete, resin may be mixed and applied like plaster to form an index, or the resin may be applied in the joint areas by the "brush-on" technique. For the brush technique, a small quantity of Duralay monomer (4 to 6 drops) is placed in one small glass dish and a comparable amount of powder in another. Monomer is applied to the surfaces to be joined. The brush is wetted and then touched to the powder. The available monomer in the brush will cause a quantity of powder to adhere. This globule is then carried to place and

caused to flow into the joint space. (The wet brush must not touch or come too close to the surface of the dish containing the powder, as surface tension will draw the monomer from the brush to the dish surface and wet the powder.) This procedure is repeated until the joint is adequately filled. When all necessary resin has been placed, it is allowed to harden completely. A final check should make certain that all parts are rigidly united. The work is now ready to be invested.

INVESTING

Figure 13   A suitable volume of soldering investment is prepared. Water/powder ratio is measured as per the manufacturer's directions.

Figure 14   The internal portion of all units is carefully filled, using a small spatula (no vibration), and the entire assembly is covered.

Figure 15   A bulk of investment is placed on a slab, and the investment-covered pieces are placed on this base. If the investment mix is too thin to stand up on the slab, it may be placed in a paper towel and blotted before forming the base.

Figures 16 and 17   A better technique is to place a strip of boxing wax about the edge of the plaster index or wax separator layer. Once the pieces are filled and covered, the box is simply filled with investment. This ensures adequate thickness of the investment block (about ½ inch) by preventing slumping and flow of the investment. The investment is

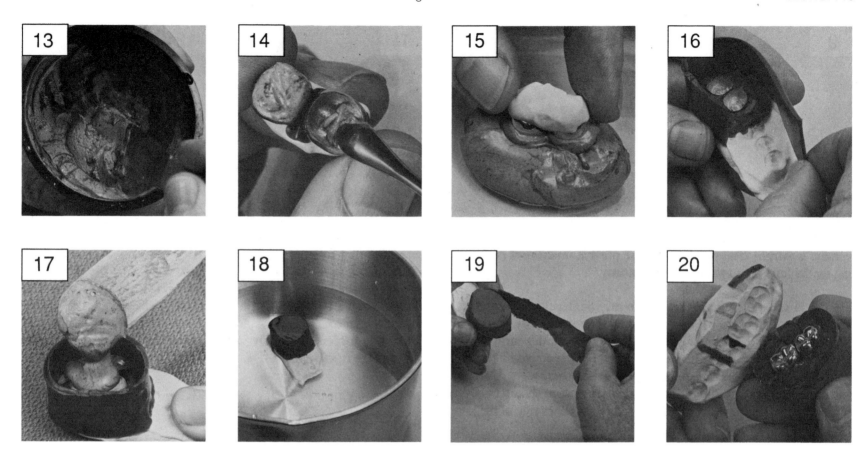

allowed to set thoroughly, to ensure strength and complete setting expansion (see manufacturer's directions).

allowed to set thoroughly, to ensure strength and complete setting expansion (see manufacturer's directions).

PREPARATION OF THE INVESTED ASSEMBLY

Figures 18 through 21   After the investment is set, the plaster index must be removed. Application of warm water will soften the sticky wax and may release the index. *Do not pry off the index*, as the investment may fracture. If locking is evident, the plaster index may be scored completely through with a sharp knife and removed in segments as necessary.

Resin can be softened for removal by open flame heat, or, if preferred, it can be burned away completely.

TRIMMING

Figure 22   The investment block is trimmed (especially in the joint regions) to permit maximum flame access and to keep investment as remote from the joint as possible. To facilitate the soldering operation, sufficient airway under the joint to permit encompassing by the flame is highly desirable. It is also important to have the investment as remote as possible from the joint, so that it will not be overheated by the torch flame and release contaminating sulfur gases. *Second to cleanliness, access to the joint area is the most important key to success in soldering.*

Trimming of excess dimension of the investment block is also important to permit adequate heat transfer. Though a poor conductor, investment acts as a "heat sink": it draws heat away from the embedded gold alloy castings. Said another way, the more investment present, the more

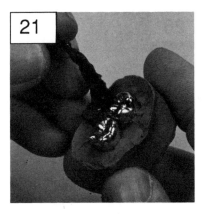 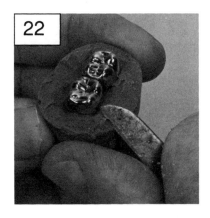 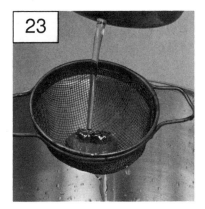 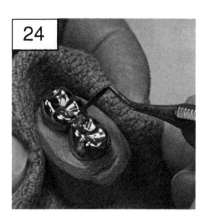

heat required to maintain the assembly at working temperature. If the investment block is approximately ½ inch thick as suggested, it need be only about ¼ inch wide about the castings. The bottom of the block should be trimmed flat to provide a stable base. The angle of the base may be adjusted to establish the faciolingual inclination suitable for the particular situation. Such gross trimming may be accomplished on a cast trimmer or with a knife. *To prevent contamination by debris, all trimming should be completed prior to boil-out or other removal of the wax protecting the joint areas.*

BOIL-OUT

Figure 23 If wax has been used in quantity to seal the joint area, it should be removed prior to burnout to avoid possible contamination from the residue. This is best accomplished by carefully digging out accessible wax and then flushing the assembly with boiling water—or, if more convenient, with a relatively forceful stream of hot (140° to 160° F) water from a spigot—until clean.

FLUX AND ANTIFLUX

Figure 24 While the work is still warm from the boil-out procedure, excess water is blown off and flux applied conservatively so that it flows over the warm joint surfaces.

The proper application and use of flux is important. Flux covers the joint surfaces and protects them from oxidation. Thus it is obviously desirable to have flux present during the burnout procedure. It is best applied prior to heating so that it may flow smoothly over the joint surface. At elevated temperatures flux dehydrates so rapidly that it has little opportunity to flow properly. Most technicians also lightly flux their solder—either strip or cubes. Some manufacturers now offer prefluxed solder. Remember that the purpose of flux is to cover and protect the alloy surfaces from oxidation, and that the solder flows between the flux and the alloy. Hence an excess of flux offers no advantage, but does increase the possibility of flux inclusions in the joint, which may well render it unacceptable.

Antiflux may be used effectively to confine the flow of solder to the joint area. A good antiflux can be made of rouge softened with chloroform or whiting and alcohol. The antiflux is *carefully* applied about the perimeter of the area where solder is desired. Solder will not flow across the antiflux; thus its judicious use may save time by eliminating the necessity of grinding away excess solder and reestablishing contour (see **Figure 74**).

SELECTION OF APPROPRIATE SOLDER

Proper selection of the solder to be used for a given procedure depends on the alloy used for the castings and the function of the soldered area. The best means of selecting an appropriate solder is to follow the recommendation of the manufacturer of the alloy used for

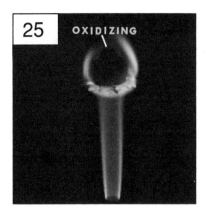 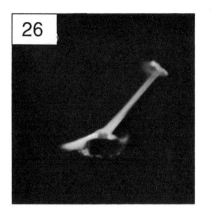 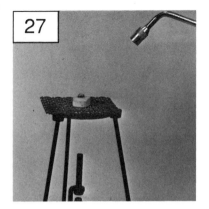 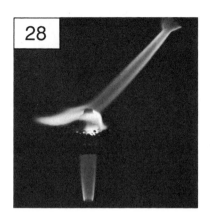

the castings. The reputable gold companies produce solders that are compatible with their alloys in fusion temperature, strength, color, and nobility.

PREHEATING (BURNOUT)

As with casting, proper burnout is an important step in the soldering procedure. Essentially, purposes are the same for both, although the relative significance may be different. Purposes of soldering investment burnout are as follows:

1. It removes water from the investment. Presence of water will hold down temperature increase and might also create steam pressure sufficient to dislodge a crown or crack the investment block if heated abruptly with a torch.
2. It produces thermal expansion to match the expansion and contraction of the alloy castings.
3. It eliminates wax or resin residue present in the joint area.
4. It promotes uniform heating of the entire investment assembly to bring it up to working temperature without excessive oxidation or distortion.

The best means to ensure uniform, controlled preheating of an investment assembly would be to place it in a burnout furnace. However, burnout furnaces produce an oxidizing atmosphere that can cause significant oxidation of the joint surfaces unless they are protected by flux.

In addition to this undesirable risk of oxidation the time required for furnace burnout is excessive for many procedural needs. As a result, furnace preheating is usually reserved for large, complicated appliances where uniform heating of the investment is especially critical. When used, furnace preheating should be initiated in a cold muffle and carried to 800° F over a 20-minute period. The case should then be promptly soldered. All joints must be properly fluxed *before* preheating in a furnace.

Figure 25   Preheating is commonly done over an open Bunsen flame. Such procedure is not recommended, however, as it produces markedly uneven heating of the investment block. This not only results in distortion due to unequal expansion but may also create spot-heating to temperatures well above 1,300° F. As with plaster-bound casting investments, the calcium sulfate in soldering investments begins to break down at about 1,300° F, producing sulfur gases. These gases produce embrittlement of castings and/or solder and cause the latter to flow poorly.

In addition to these disadvantages, it is difficult if not impossible to produce a reducing environment over a Bunsen flame. In fact, because the flame is deflected as it contacts the base of the soldering block, wire grid, etc., the environment of the castings is likely to be strongly oxidizing.

Figure 26   A better approach to soldering is preheating with the torch. Carefully done this technique is quite effective. A properly adjusted (gas-rich) torch flame offers excellent control of the environment of the

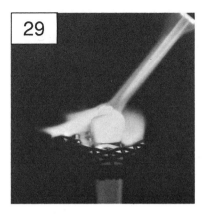 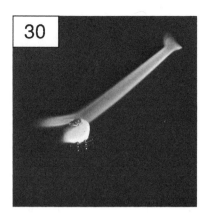 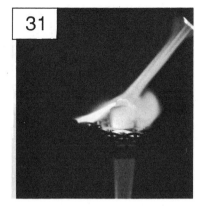 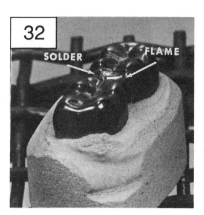

castings and can produce fairly uniform heating of the investment. However, as shown here, use of the torch alone may leave the base of the investment block cold in relation to the portion exposed to the flame.

Figures 27 and 28   With care, the disadvantages of open flame preheating can be overcome. This is accomplished by using a properly adjusted torch in conjunction with a Bunsen flame. The gas-rich torch flame imposes a reducing environment on the castings, while the Bunsen flame heats the base of the investment block. The investment block is thus completely enveloped in flame and has good potential for uniform heating.

It has been stated that cleanliness is the key to success in soldering. This statement includes the concept of a *clean flame* (nonoxidizing). Meticulous care in maintaining physical cleanliness of the joint area, maximum access, and even ideal burnout will not prevail against a poorly adjusted soldering flame. As with melting alloy for casting, sufficient heat is necessary but a reducing atmosphere must be maintained. The flame must be slightly gas-rich, and the proper portion applied to the work. Careful observation of the flame and its effect on the castings immediately indicates the nature of the flame. It should be promptly adjusted to provide sufficient heat transfer with a reducing atmosphere.

Figure 29   A hard-pointed flame is dangerous especially for the novice, as it may overheat the castings before the assembly has been uniformly elevated to working temperature. In addition the oxidizing

potential of such a flame can quickly affect both castings and solder, preventing fusion and flow of the solder.

Figure 30   With patience the soldering of units that have ample exposure of surface area (such as the two crowns in this example) can be effectively accomplished with a rather soft, gas-rich flame. The rate of temperature increase is slow, offering excellent safety. Control of the environment is assured. This approach is recommended for the novice, as it permits more time for placement of solder and observation of the work without real danger of overheating. Such a flame is shown here. Note that this flame has the investment block "at temperature," and the castings are just glowing. (The Bunsen flame has been extinguished to permit clear illustration of the torch flame). All that would be needed here to bring about fusion of the solder is to gently play the flame on the castings to elevate their temperature a few more degrees.

Figure 31   General heating of the cast segments should proceed until their color (cherry red) indicates that their temperature is approaching the melting range of the solder. If cubes or cut segments of strip or wire solder are being used, the first piece is placed in position over the joint crevice at this time. Continue heating the casting surfaces about the joint area.

If strip or wire solder is being used, the castings should be heated to a temperature sufficient to just melt the solder (bright cherry red). With the flame directed beneath the joint, the strip or wire is fed directly into the occlusal aspect of the joint space. The amount of solder must be quickly evaluated and the strip quickly removed when the joint is properly filled.

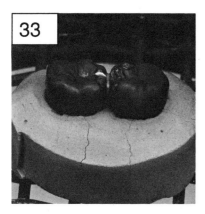
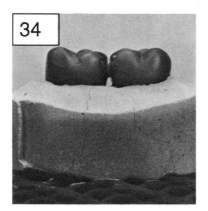
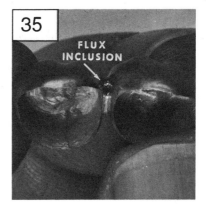
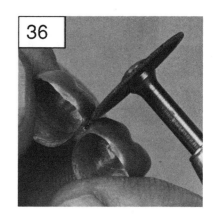

Do not heat the solder directly, but rather the parts to be joined. In all soldering operations the ideal joint is obtained by heating the parts to be joined (in a proper environment) so that they cause the solder to melt and wet their surfaces. If the solder is heated directly, or if the castings or solder are oxidized or otherwise contaminated, the solder will ball up and not flow. Should this occur, the torch flame should be checked immediately to be sure it is gas-rich (reducing); another segment of lightly fluxed solder is added immediately adjacent to the first; and *the proper portion of the flame is redirected to the proper area*—the castings, not the solder! Proper heating is continued until this segment of solder flows. If it melts and flows properly, it will superheat the first segment and melt it too. If the second segment of solder also balls up, the corrective routine may be once again repeated, but if this does not prove promptly successful, the operation should be aborted and the investment assembly quenched. The castings must be repickled, the joint areas *thoroughly cleaned*, the castings reassembled and reinvested, and the entire soldering operation repeated.

Because soldering seems to be such a critical operation to the novice, a few more observations about the actual heating procedure are useful here. Obviously the fear involved is that of overheating and thus melting or distorting the components. True, only experience will overcome this, but a few minutes (or an hour) spent adjusting a torch and observing the effects of a gas-rich soldering flame on solder and casting alloy (or a copper penny) can produce a great deal of understanding and feeling for this operation. It is important to remember that the appropriate solder should have a melting range with an upper limit 100° F below the lower limit of the melting range of the cast alloy.

Figure 32   With these thoughts in mind, consider the mechanics of the operation. The parts to be joined must be heated to a temperature that will melt the solder. This requires exposure of sufficient surface area of each piece to permit adequate heat transfer. Solder flows toward heat, but this flow is also affected by gravity and capillary attraction. Thus the solder should be placed at a high, remote portion of the joint and made to flow down and through the joint toward the heat source.

Finally, the objective of the soldering technique is to flow solder where it is needed as quickly as possible and at as low a temperature as is consistent with the operation.

Figures 33 and 34   Once conditions for proper flow are established, the addition of solder is continued until full contour of the joint is a certainty.

When the soldering operation is successfully completed, the investment assembly is quenched; or if a Type III or Type IV alloy amenable to heat hardening is being used, it may be bench cooled in accordance with manufacturer's directions and then quenched. All investment is removed by scrubbing and pickling. If available, an ultrasonic cleaner is effective.

Figure 35   When thoroughly clean, the soldered assembly is carefully inspected. Attention must be especially focused on the soldered joints. Usually the joints are partially covered by flux and they must be completely surfaced with an abrasive disc or stone. The fused flux is glass and cannot be effectively ground with burs or rubber wheels.

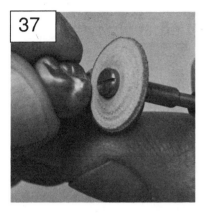

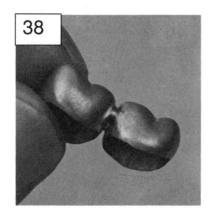

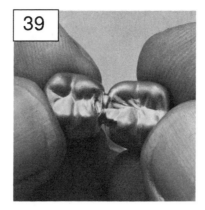

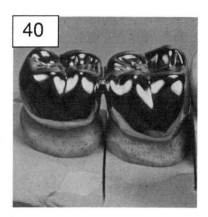

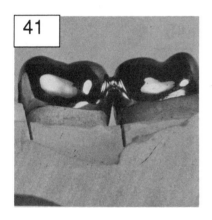

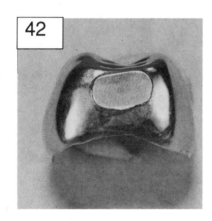

rounded surface with no sharp crevice or angles. In cross section the joint should be generally D-shaped, the flat surface along the occlusal and the curving surface forming the facial, gingival, and lingual contour of the joint. The dimensions of the joint should be directly related to the load to be imposed.

Figure 42 This photograph illustrates the maximum joint contour needed for bridge retainers. Joints for splinting adjacent units (as in the previous example) might well be appropriate at about one-half this size.

When surfacing is completed, the joint is carefully inspected for voids, debris, or flux inclusions.

DESOLDERING

Figure 36 If any pits are present, they must be pursued to their termination with either disc or bur. If such excavation destroys proper joint contour, it must be resoldered.

Soldered joints that are deficient in contour may usually be corrected by surfacing the deficient area, reinvesting, and adding more solder. However, when access for such an addition is inadequate or the joint relationship is incorrect, the units must be completely separated for resoldering. Two methods of separation are available: sectioning and desoldering.

Figures 37 through 39 When the joint is sound and properly contoured, the assembly is carefully seated and inspected on the master cast. If relations are accurate, the soldering operation may be considered successful and complete. If not, the joint must be sectioned or desoldered, a new index made, and the assembly reinvested and resoldered.

Sectioning a solder joint is accomplished with a Carborundum separating disc, either of standard thickness of one of the newer thin discs. Because of speed and directness, this approach is usually preferred for the straight solder joint. However, sectioning a joint between closely adjacent margins (inlays, onlays, partial crowns, faced pontics, and the like) can be quite critical and may place the integrity of the adjacent margins in jeopardy.

Figures 40 and 41 Finished joint contour should present a smoothly

Separation of critical joints and those that incorporate a lug-rest

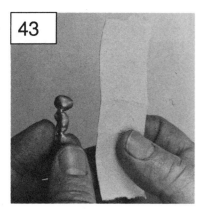

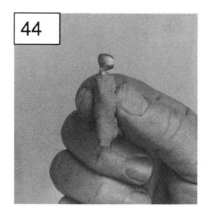

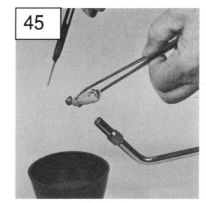

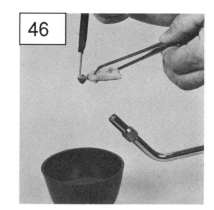

design may best be done by desoldering. An organized technique makes this procedure simple and safe.

Figures 43 and 44   If soldered joints other than the one to be desoldered are present, they are protected by a generous wrapping of wet casting ring liner or by investment. The wrapping can be molded into a firm mass with the fingertips. An ample, and relatively equal, surface area is left exposed on either side of the joint to be desoldered.

Figure 45   A torch is positioned on the bench top so that its fairly pointed but slightly reducing (gas-rich) flame is directed upward at about a 30° angle. (Most torches are designed so that this occurs when the handle is placed flat on the bench top.) A plaster bowl about two-thirds full of water is placed under the flame.

The wrapped portion of the bridge is gripped with laboratory tweezers, and the exposed joint is held in proper position in the flame. A soldering pencil (carbon rod or regular lead pencil) is held ready in the other hand. With the bridge held such that the tip of the reducing cone of the flame is encompassing the joint to be desoldered, the plaster bowl should be centered under the free segment of the framework.

Figures 46 and 47   Just as the solder begins to melt on its surface, the free segment may be gently pushed loose (not touching it near a margin) such that it falls into the bowl of water and is immediately quenched. The wrapped segment is also dropped into the water for quenching.

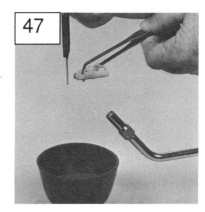

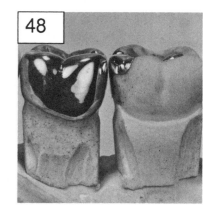

After recovery and pickling in conventional manner, the joint areas are surfaced in preparation for resoldering. Adequate joint space must be assured.

SOLDERED CORRECTIONS AND REPAIRS

Proximal Contact

Figure 48   The most common soldered correction is an addition to a deficient proximal contact. The location and amount of contour deficiency should be visualized on the working cast. In this example the distal contact of the inlay in the mandibular first molar is deficient.

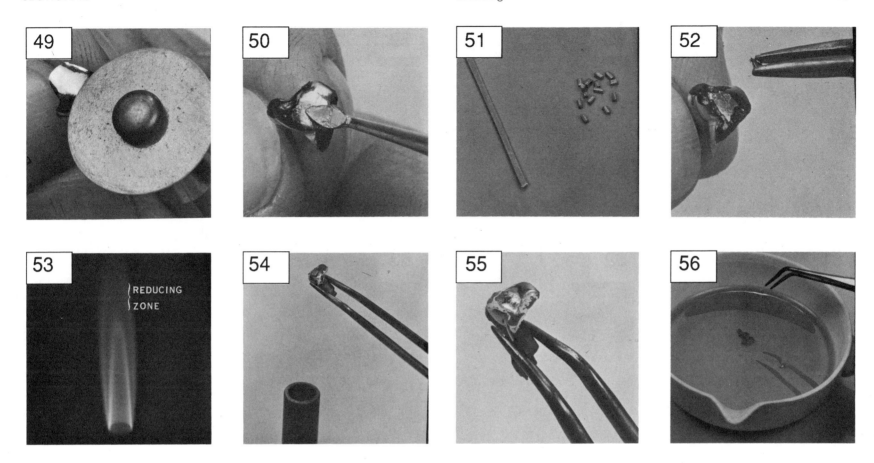

Figure 49 The proximal surface of the casting in the area to be soldered is surfaced with a disc or rubber wheel.

Figure 50 A film of paste flux is applied to the area to be soldered. Excess is wiped away.

Figure 51 The freehand addition to contact is normally accomplished using segments of solder. These are available from the manufacturer as cubes or may be cut from strip or wire solder of correct fineness.

Figure 52 An estimated correct quantity of solder is placed in proper position on the casting. Antiflux may be used if desired.

Figure 53 A Bunsen burner or blowtorch flame is properly adjusted. Note the reducing zone of the flame.

Figure 54 With soldering tweezers positioned so that they do not touch a margin, the casting is held in the proper zone of the flame at such angle as to let gravity help direct proper flow of the solder.

Figure 55 The instant that the desired flow occurs, the casting must be removed from the flame. Depending on the contour desired, the solder can be merely rounded or slumped, or caused to flow in a thin layer over a broad area. Care must be taken not to permit it to reach a margin.

Figure 56 When flow and bulk are correct, the casting is gently dropped into pickling solution. *Do not permit the metal tweezers to contact the acid.*

Figure 57 The casting is recovered from the acid bath with appropriate nonmetal-tipped tweezers. (Metal tweezers will contaminate the

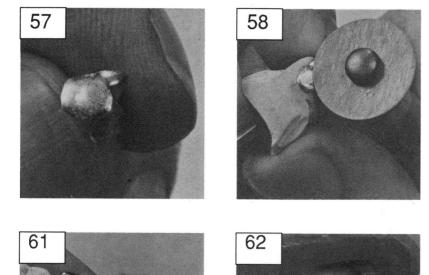

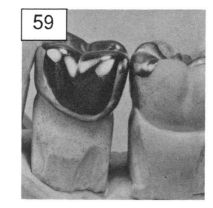

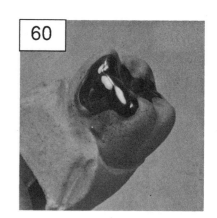

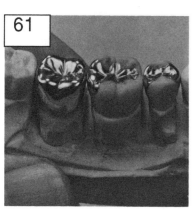

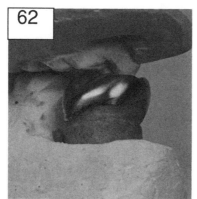

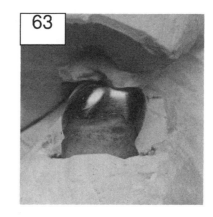

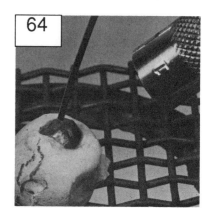

acid and may cause the casting to tarnish in the mouth.) Fused flux will no doubt be evident on the casting surface.

Figure 58   Surface smoothness and contour is reestablished with discs and rubber wheels.

Figure 59   Appropriate area and firmness of contact is established by trial-and-error adjustment.

Figure 60   When contact is correct, the surface is smoothed and polished so that no junction is evident between solder and casting. If proper contour cannot be established or porosity is present, the surface will have to be surfaced and resoldered.

Figure 61   The corrected contact should present ideal form, and there should be no evidence of soldered addition.

Occlusal Contact

A less frequent soldered correction is an addition to provide occlusal contact. This is also a relatively simple correction and may be accomplished freehand. However, if the addition required is rather large, and a cusp needs to be built up, the procedure is easier to manage with the crown invested so that both hands are free to manage the solder and blowtorch.

Figures 62 and 63   Note the lack of centric contact on the mesiofacial cusp of this mandibular molar crown.

Figure 64   The crown is invested, leaving the entire occlusal and most of the facial surface exposed. The deficient cusp is surfaced and fluxed.

When normal preheating has brought the crown to proper temperature, solder of appropriate fineness is added to excess. For gross addi-

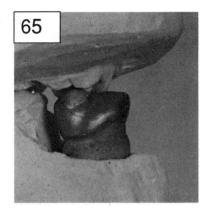

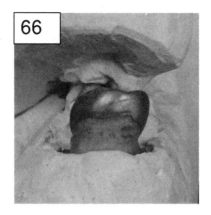

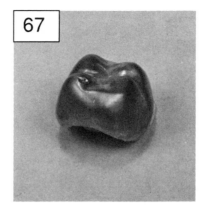

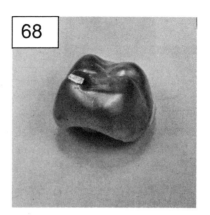

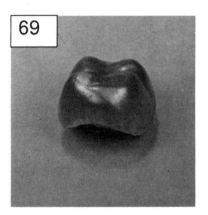

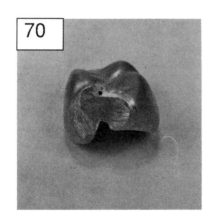

tions such as this, strip solder is best used. Experience soon teaches the importance of flame control in such built-up additions. When it is desirable to stack the solder, the flame may be focused directly on the solder just as it flows, causing it to tend to ball up or stand on the surface.

Figures 65 and 66 The soldered addition is occluded, contoured, and polished. The deficient casting has been corrected to restore centric occlusion. As with soldered contact areas, there should be no evidence of a soldered addition after finishing.

Repair of Holes

The most common soldered repair is for a hole in the occlusal surface. These occasionally result from the "suck-back" at the point of attachment of the sprue, or from the inclusion of debris in the casting. Most frequently they are the result of machining to establish anatomy or occlusion. When this occurs, the thickness of the casting adjacent to the perforation must be carefully evaluated. If a significant area is too thin and cannot be made thicker due to occlusal contact, the situation should be explained to the dentist, so that the dentist may alter the preparation and have the casting remade. If the area is quite thin but can be made thicker, a soldered repair may well suffice.

Large-diameter perforations require the adaptation of platinum foil to provide a base or floor across which the solder can flow. Solder has no affinity for an investment surface and no ability to wet it, and thus will not flow across investment.

Small-diameter holes do not require a foil base, as surface tension of the molten solder will cause it to bridge the space. It is this very phenomenon that makes the procedure for soldering holes unique.

If the diameter of the hole is small enough, solder placed on its surface will simply bridge the space. It will not flow down into the hole and fill it completely. An example best demonstrates this point.

Figure 67 A small hole is present in the mesiolingual cusp tip.

Figure 68 A cube of solder is placed across the hole.

Figure 69 The solder is fused, apparently filling the hole.

Figure 70 A section through the crown reveals the unfilled hole.

The solution to this problem is quite simple; the hole must be filled from the bottom up. There are two possibilities for doing this: to make the hole large enough to receive the solder, or to make the solder small enough to fit into the base of the hole. Either approach is effective.

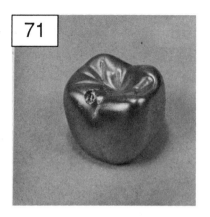

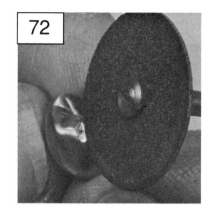

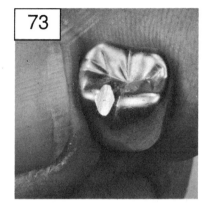

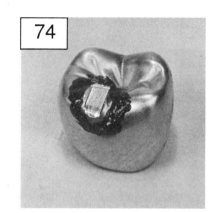

Enlarging the hole offers greater control and is thus the recommended choice. Another example clearly demonstrates the procedure.

Figure 71   Attempts to remove porosity and debris inclusions have led to a perforation in the facial groove of this full crown.

Figure 72   The area is surfaced and access established with a Carborundum disc.

Figure 73   Note that adequate access for placement of solder has been established.

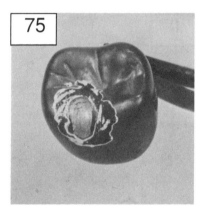

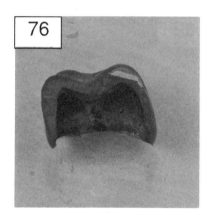

Figure 74   Antiflux (chloroform and rouge) has been placed about the defect. The defect and the solder are fluxed. A cube of solder is positioned such that it rests in contact with the floor of the defect.

Figure 75   The solder has been fused freehand in a Bunsen flame.

Figure 76   A cross section through the defect shows a marked contrast in result as compared with the previous example.

Marginal Repair

One of the more critical soldering procedures is repairing a margin. Generally a casting with a defective margin is best remade. However, there are occasions when the marginal defect occurs on a unit that would be difficult to remake—for instance, a retainer in a large bridge, a crown containing a precision attachment, or the retainer for a removable partial denture that has already been cast. In these instances a great

deal of time, work, and expense may hinge on the success of a marginal repair soldering procedure.

An example is the large porcelain-fused-to-metal bridge shown in **Figures 77 and 78**. During the final polishing of the bridge, the facial margin of the canine retainer was accidentally destroyed. Instead of removing all porcelain, sectioning the bridge, making a new reatiner casting, soldering the joints, and rebuilding the porcelain, it was possible to repair the margin very accurately by soldering. Though not nearly so sophisticated, the following example involving a single crown demonstrates the technique.

Figure 79   The lingual margin of the casting is short. This situation often arises as the result of an inaccurate impression. The casting made from it fits the die, but during trial insertion the dentist discovers that the crown has a short margin. *Before the margin can be corrected, an accurate impression and die must be obtained.*

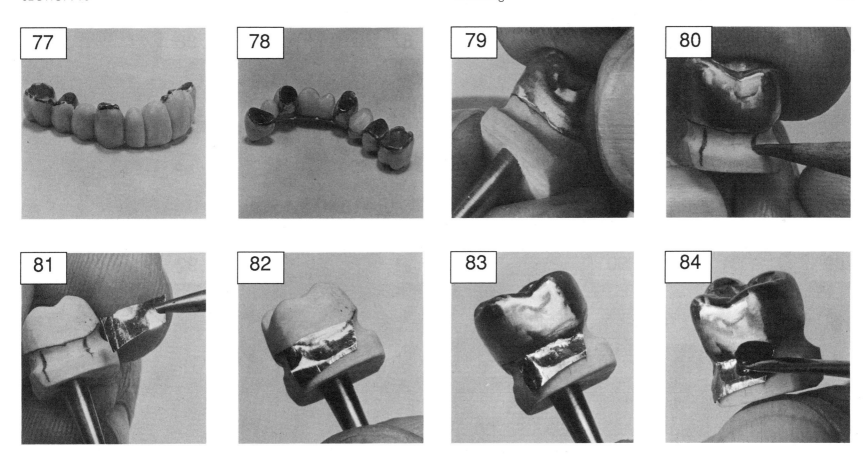

Figure 80 The region of the short margin is marked on the new, accurate die. Note that the die has been lightly ditched.

Figure 81 A strip of platinum foil longer than the area of the defect is placed on the die.

Figure 82 The foil must be carefully burnished onto the die across the involved marginal area.

Figure 83 The adjacent area of the crown is surfaced, and the crown is firmly seated on the die. The platinum foil is again lightly burnished so that it accurately fits the die. *This is imperative*.

Figure 84 A brittle sticky wax is flowed onto the foil and crown so that they are united. The wax is allowed to harden completely. If the room temperature is warm, it is wise to chill the wax.

Figure 85 The crown with foil attached is removed from the die. The removal must be carefully observed to make sure that no displacement or deformation of the foil occurs. If a brittle sticky wax was used and allowed to become completely hard, any deformation that occurs will cause it to crack. Displacement of the foil will be due to the undercut beneath the margin. One of two procedures may be followed to overcome this problem.

An experienced technician will burnish the foil just over the cavo-surface angle of margin without locking it into the undercut beneath the margin. This, of course, permits removal of the crown and foil without distortion. The foil must be accurately adapted to the margin, however.

Figures 86 through 88 A second approach (and probably more reliable for the novice) is to block out the submarginal undercut. This is done by flowing impression compound (preferably green or black stick

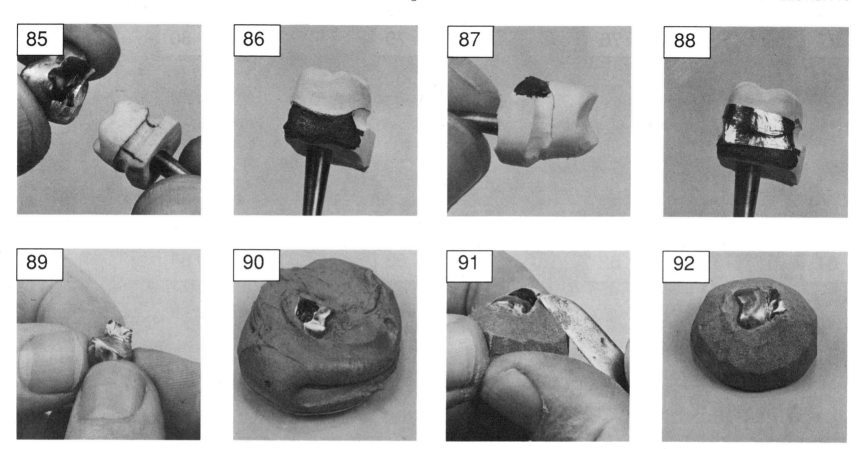

compound) into the undercut and smoothly carving it to a level barely short of the marginal angle. When chilled, the compound is hard enough to permit burnishing the foil against its surface. The contour of the compound should be such that the marginal angle is distinctly evident in the burnished foil, but with the foil not locked into a submarginal undercut. The crown is seated, sticky wax applied, and the assembly removed as before.

Figure 89 Once the crown is separated from the die, it is critically observed to see that the wax has not been fractured or displaced. The crown must be handled very carefully to avoid deformation of the foil. Note in this view of the internal aspect of the crown that the platinum foil is smoothly and tightly adapted to the inner surface of the casting, and the cavosurface angle of the margin to be soldered is clearly evident in the foil.

Figure 90 The crown is invested by filling its core using a small spatula and then gently teasing the crown into a mound of investment, leaving the involved surface exposed. Because the sticky wax was added in quantity sufficient to extend beyond the involved area, investment can be pulled over the exposed edges of the platinum foil to lock it into position. The investment is allowed to set completely.

Figure 91 Before the sticky wax is removed, the investment block is trimmed to remove excess bulk and provide access to the exposed surface. Note how the surface to be soldered is prominently exposed.

Figure 92 The wax is removed by flushing with hot water, and the involved area of crown and foil is *lightly* coated with flux.

Figure 93 Preheating is accomplished in a conventional manner, and

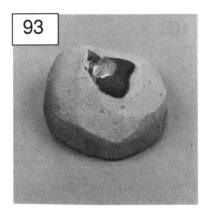 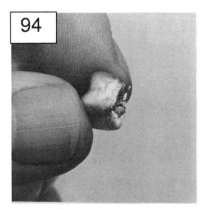 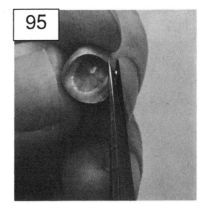 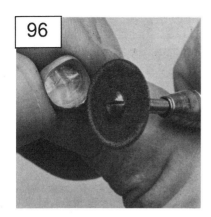

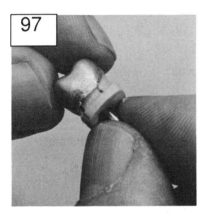 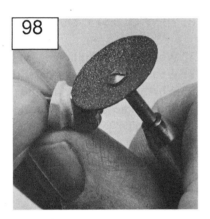 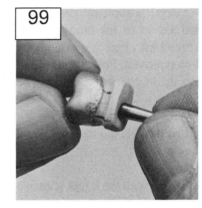 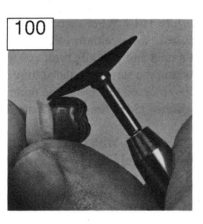

solder is placed and fused as desired. Note that the solder has been extended well up onto the surface of the crown, so that there will be no break in contour at the junction of the casting and soldered repair.

Figure 94 The crown is quenched, recovered, and pickled in routine manner.

Figure 95 Excess foil may be trimmed with scissors.

Figure 96 By visualizing the marginal angle on the internal surface of the foil, gross overextension of the soldered margin is corrected with a disc or stone, rotating from inside out.

If compound was used to block out a submarginal undercut on the die, it should be removed before the crown is reseated. If the die was left unditched to facilitate adaptation of the foil, it should be carefully

and definitely ditched before the crown is reseated. The cavosurface angle of the margin should be marked by tracing with the side of a red or blue pencil point.

Figure 97 The crown is carefully seated on the die.

Figure 98 Excess length is adjusted using a disc or stone. A true-running cup-shaped Carborundum disc is appropriate. The disc is used to surface the crown such that the margin is carefully and progressively shortened. The disc must never touch the die.

Figure 99 By lightly unseating and reseating the crown on the die, the excess length of margin can be recognized.

Figure 100 Discing of the surface is continued until proper contour and length of margin are established.

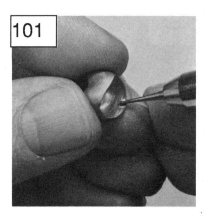
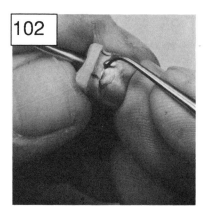
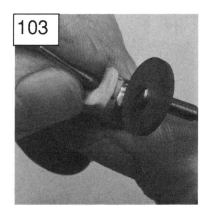
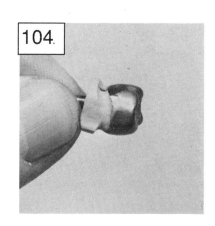

Figure 101   When correct length of the margin is approximately established, the platinum foil on the internal aspect of the crown can be thinned and partially removed using a round bur. Foil that extends up within the surface of the casting should be removed. Foil that is behind the soldered repair may be thinned above the margin but should not be touched along the marginal angle.

Figure 102   With the crown fully seated on the die, the margin should be thoroughly burnished. *Do not abrade the die.*

Figure 103   Gross smoothing is accomplished with the larger abrasive rubber wheels.

Figure 104   Final smoothing and finishing to the margin are accomplished with smaller, finer rubber wheels that have been lathed to produce a true-running leading edge. The restoration is now ready for final polishing.

REVIEW QUESTIONS

1. What is the definition of soldering?
2. What is the key to successful soldering?
3. What is the purpose of a flux?
4. Should the solder be heated directly in a soldering procedure? Explain.
5. What are the two types of soldering procedures used in dentistry?
6. Explain how desoldering is accomplished.

Summary of Technique for Individual Cast Restorations

WORK AUTHORIZATION AND PREPARATION OF DIES AND CASTS

Figure 1 The technician should first read the work authorization and examine the materials provided. The dentist may have provided a working cast with an already prepared die and supplied some form of opposing cast or appropriate occlusal record. If only an impression has been provided, it must be poured to provide an appropriate working cast for development of the restoration.

Figure 2 Band impressions are best poured using a root-form extension made by wrapping masking tape about the band. Whether some form of tape, or sheet wax, is used to form the extension, its application must not distort the band or any impression material that might extend above the margin of the band. The stone root form thus developed should be about ⅜ inch long and should receive the dowel pin.

Figure 3 If a band impression or single die is involved, some type of relationship impression must of course have been provided. This may be a wax, rubber, or zinc oxide–eugenol impression into which the die is to be seated and then the cast poured.

Figure 4 In such cases exceeding care must be taken to assure complete seating of the die. All undercuts must be waxed out, and separating medium must be applied to the die before pouring the working cast. These same precautions apply to the handling of a coping transfer impression.

Figures 5 and 6 Tray impressions can be poured by either the stripping or double pour section technique. Appropriate provision must be made for removable adjacent teeth.

Figure 7 Careful mixing and pouring of the die stone is essential to the development of a dense, accurate die, regardless of the type of impression.

Figure 8 Once the die and working cast are developed, they should be carefully trimmed and readied for establishing the occlusal relationship.

Figure 9 Most single crowns, inlays, and onlays are made using some rather simple form of occlusal record: a centric occlusion bite, a functional chew-in or core, or an anatomic core.

Figure 10 Opposing anatomic casts, or casts developed from a centric occlusion bite, should be related by means of a simple hinge articulator.

Figure 11 Anatomic cores and cores developed from functional chew-ins may be related by a hinge articulator or indexed so as to permit hand articulation. Once the occlusal relationship has been established from materials provided, the occlusal and proximal relationships should be carefully studied.

Figure 12 According to the work authorization and the need to eliminate undercut areas, the die is blocked out if necessary. Unless specifi-

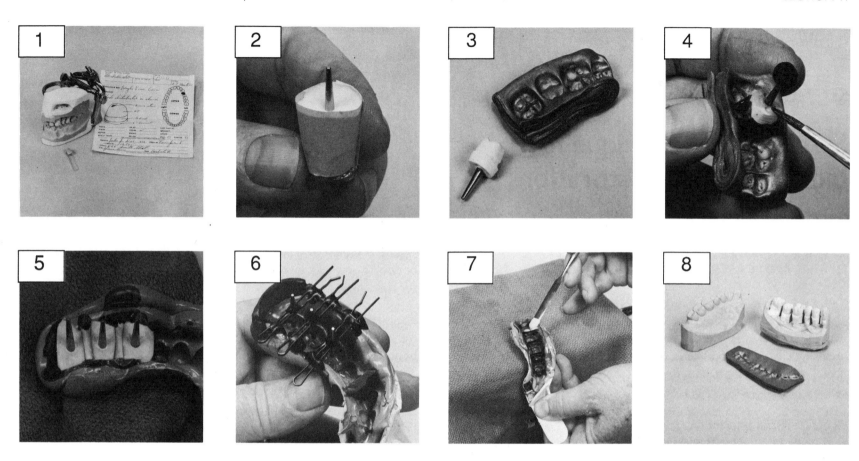

cally authorized, grooves or boxed excavations that might provide additional retention should not be blocked out.

Figure 13 The margin of the die is reexamined with accessibility for carving in mind. The prepared marginal form in conjunction with appropriate trimming should leave the margin of the die quite distinct. If this is not the case, one must decide whether or not to proceed with the case. If there is any question about the accuracy of the die, the dentist should be advised of the problem. Any other questions regarding relationship, design, or material should be resolved accordingly. In most cases the care with which the dentist has developed the various records and the work authorization will leave no question as to how to proceed. In turn, care in evaluation and development of the restoration should leave no question as to the accuracy of the technician's work. Once the die is prepared and properly related to the working and opposing casts, and all questions have been resolved, the technician may begin development of the restoration.

DEVELOPMENT OF THE PATTERN

Figure 14 Observation of the die in relation to the opposing occlusal surfaces will determine the correct position of centric contacts. If helpful, these should be marked on the opposing cast.

Figure 15 When the die has been appropriately lubricated, wax is added to form the core of the pattern (if an inlay), or to form a thimble-like coping (if a three-quarter or full crown). If a centric holding cusp is involved, wax is added to form the cusp tip such that it is in contact

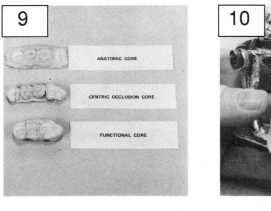

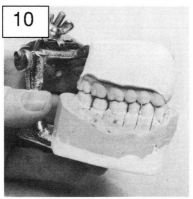

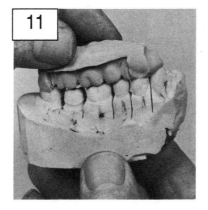

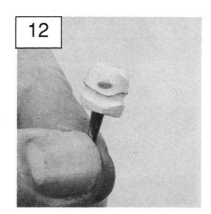

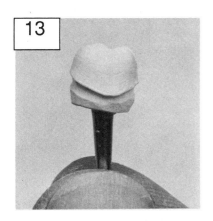

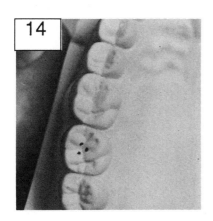

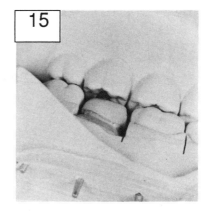

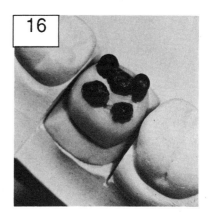

with the desired opposing centric location. If more than one centric holding cusp is involved, the other cusps are developed in like fashion.

Figure 16 When the centric holding cusp tips have been carefully located, wax is added to develop the fossa or marginal ridge that receives the opposing centric holding cusp or cusps.

Figure 17 Wax should now be added to develop the remaining features of the occlusal surface. With practice and experience the occlusal surface may be almost completely developed by the careful addition of wax.

Figure 18 However, if necessary or desired, the occlusal additions may be made slightly excessive, molded while still soft by closure of the opposing cast or core, and ultimately carved to final form.

Figure 19 The facial and lingual surfaces are added to and/or carved to develop their proper contour. Other than the dictate of occlusal relationship on the occlusofacial of lower posteriors and the occlusolingual of upper posteriors, only the contour of adjacent teeth and tissue and personal knowledge of dental anatomy can identify the contour of the facial and lingual surfaces.

Figure 20 If both proximals are involved, the contacts should be established one at a time. However, the initial contact must be correctly established before proceeding to the second proximal contact. This is most easily done when one adjacent tooth is removable. In such a circumstance contact is established with the nonremovable adjacent tooth first, then wax is added to the other proximal and the removable adjacent tooth is seated to form the contact.

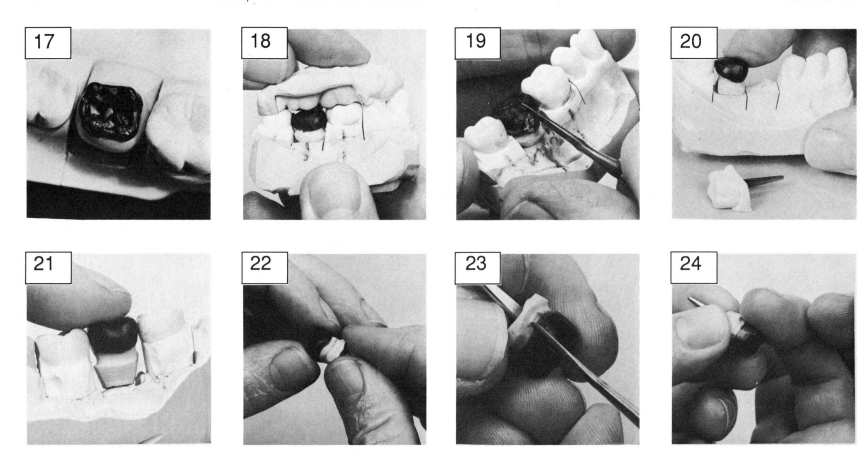

Figure 21 The addition of wax should be extended to develop contour of the involved axial surfaces. Wax is added to a proximal surface sufficiently to mold the contact by seating the die and pattern while the wax is still soft. The proper location and size of this contact is established by carving of the excess.

Figure 22 When the axial surfaces have been grossly developed, the pattern is removed to check internal adaptation. If discrepancies are present, they should be corrected now, so that finished contours will not have to be altered or destroyed. Once internal adaptation is verified, the die is lightly relubricated and the pattern is fully reseated on the die before proceeding.

Figure 23 Wax is added about the margin of the pattern, to a slight excess both in contour and extension beyond the cavosurface angle. The added wax must join thoroughly with the established pattern.

Figure 24 To ensure excellent marginal adaptation, this wax should be added to one surface at a time and followed by finger pressure as it cools.

Figure 25 The excess wax is wipe-carved with a warm instrument, using the ditched surface or the recorded unprepared tooth surface beyond the cavosurface angle as a guide. It is imperative that the die not be altered by scraping it with a sharp instrument. By carefully using a rubbing-carving technique with a smooth instrument warmed to just the correct temperature, the margin of the pattern can be formed and smoothed to exact final contour. It is extremely important that this area

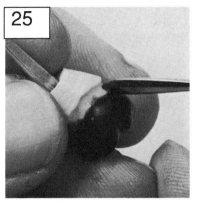

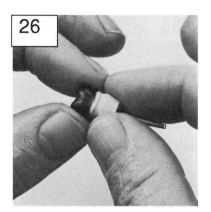

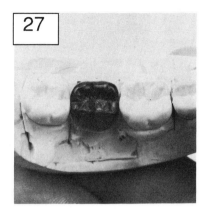

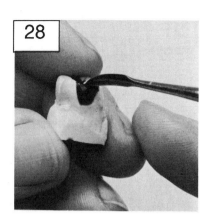

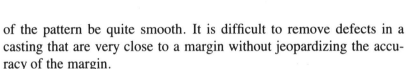

of the pattern be quite smooth. It is difficult to remove defects in a casting that are very close to a margin without jeopardizing the accuracy of the margin.

Figure 26   The pattern is removed to verify its separation from the die and the accuracy of marginal adaptation. If discrepancies exist, they are carefully corrected by repeating the marginal waxing procedure as necessary.

Figure 27   All aspects of the pattern—occlusal contacts, proximal contacts, and marginal adaptation—are then rechecked.

SPRUING AND INVESTING THE PATTERN

The appropriate size of sprue may be determined by assessing the greatest thickness and overall bulk of the pattern. If in doubt as to proper size, one should select the larger sprue pin. Sprue diameter should equal or approach the greatest cross-sectional thickness of the pattern, and the sprue should be so directed as to permit an equal flow of molten alloy to all portions of the mold cavity. If the pattern presents bulky areas separated by a thin area, as in an MOD inlay with large proximals separated by a narrow isthmus, it may be appropriate to use a double or Y-sprue. On cusp-capping onlays and crowns the sprue is attached to the bulkiest noncentric cusp; one should not involve an area of centric contact.

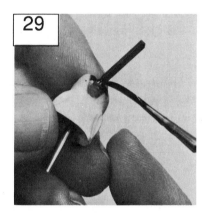

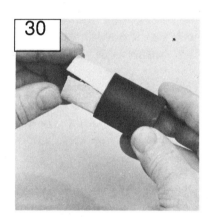

Figure 28   Once selected, the proper area for sprue attachment is touched with a drop of wax of such size and temperature that it will form a ball or cone into which a wax or plastic sprue pin may be promptly placed.

Figure 29   A strong attachment and smooth flow pattern of the sprue may be assured by adequate filleting. Again, it is essential to avoid centric contact areas.

Before the pattern is mounted on the sprue base, the equipment and materials for investing should be prepared. For the water immersion hygroscopic technique the procedure is as follows.

Figure 30   Ring liner of the appropriate size is cut and placed inside

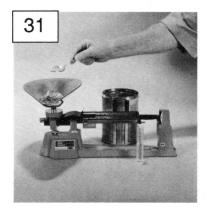

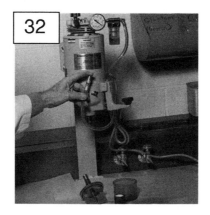

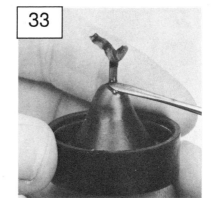

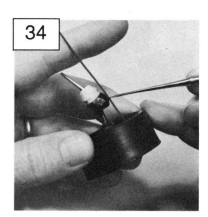

the casting ring. The ends of the ring liner may be sealed to the ring with wax if desired. The ring is dipped in clear water to saturate the liner and set aside to drain.

Figure 31 The appropriate amount of investment powder is weighed out; or, if prepackaged investment powder is being used, the proper size of envelope is selected. The mixing bowl is wetted and wiped dry. The proper quantity of water, carefully measured, is placed in the mixing bowl.

Figure 32 If a vacuum investor is to be used, its operation should be pretested. The open line reading should be low, less than 15 inches of mercury; the closed line reading should be at least 27 to 28 inches of mercury. (If necessary or desirable the efficiency of the vacuum pump may be checked by establishing vacuum in a transparent container partially filled with water. Adequate vacuum will boil the water.)

The water bath should be checked to see that the water level is adequate to cover the ring and that the temperature of the water is at the prescribed 100° F.

Figure 33 When all equipment is ready, the pattern is mounted on the sprue base. The sprue length is adjusted as necessary to provide proper back-fill dimension. The pattern should be a minimum of ¼ inch below the top edge of the ring liner. Sprue length should be about ¼ to ⅜ inch. If necessary the height of the wax portion of the crucible former (sprue base) may be modified. When the pattern is properly positioned, the sprue pin is filleted to the sprue base with appropriate wax. If the sprue pin is plastic or metal, inlay wax may be used. If a wax sprue pin

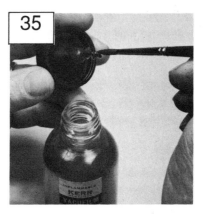

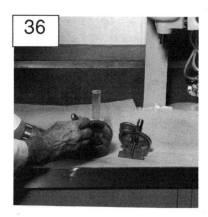

has been used, sprue wax or utility wax should be used instead, as inlay wax has a higher melting temperature than the wax sprue pin.

Figure 34 If an open vent is desired, it should be placed at this time. The point at which it should be attached to the pattern should be as close to the periphery of the sprue base as possible without interfering with placement of the ring. With a warm instrument, one end of a length of 18-gauge round wax is tacked to the sprue base below the region of the pattern to which the vent is to be connected, then gently pushed against the pattern to provide contact at the point of desired attachment, letting the resultant molten wax fix it to the pattern. If it becomes necessary to add wax to this union, it is essential to use sprue wax, as molten inlay wax will melt the vent rod.

Figure 35 A surface tension reducer is applied according to directions for the particular material being used.

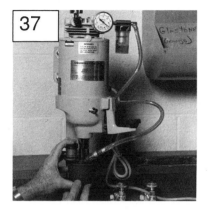

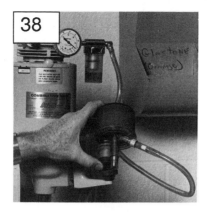

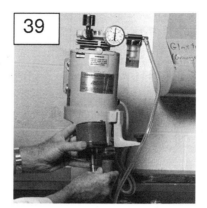

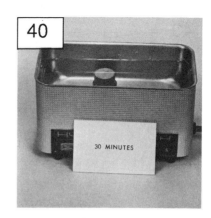

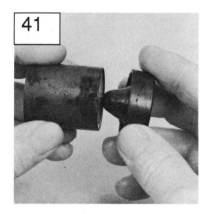

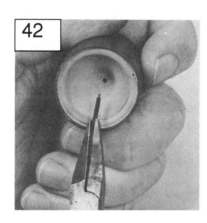

The lined casting ring is placed on the sprue base. If the sprue base does not have a rubber lip that seals about the end of the ring and holds it in position, the ring may be sealed to the sprue base with utility wax.

Figure 36 Investing may then proceed by appropriate hand or machine technique. If a machine is used, the proper sequence is to add the investment powder to the water in the bowl and hand-spatulate until the powder particles are completely wetted. The ring is placed into position on the bowl top. Next the top is placed on the bowl, and the vacuum line is plugged into the top of the bowl (the bowl is held so that the line is up). The bowl assembly is held firmly together while the vacuum pump is switched on; if necessary the bowl-ring assembly may be wiggled or pressed together until a seal is established. Once a seal is established, vacuum will hold the assembly together.

Figures 37 and 38 The mix is spatulated for the prescribed number of seconds for the type of pattern being invested, then vibrated for the minimum amount of time necessary to fill the ring.

Figure 39 The assembly is firmly held while the vacuum line plug is slowly removed from the bowl. The bowl is then tipped away from the ring and the amount of investment in the ring is checked. If the pattern is grossly *not* covered by investment, the bowl is repositioned, the vacuum line plugged in (the pump is still running), and, when vacuum seal is reestablished, the assembly is returned to the vibrating platform and given additional vibration to fill the ring. After what is judged to be sufficient additional vibration, the recovery procedure is repeated as just described.

If upon removal of the bowl the pattern is adequately covered with investment, the bowl is set aside and investment is added as necessary to fill the ring completely.

Figure 40 The invested ring assembly is immediately placed in the water bath. The investing machine is cut off after 1 minute and the investing equipment is cleaned.

WAX ELIMINATION AND CASTING

Figure 41 After a minimum of 30 minutes in the water bath, the ring is removed and separated from the sprue base.

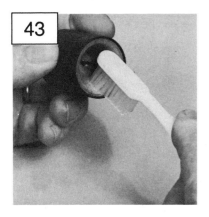

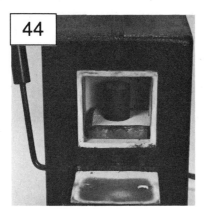

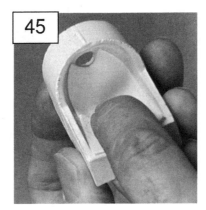

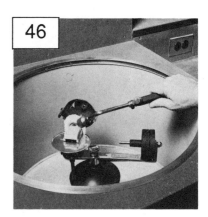

Figure 42 If a solid plastic or metal sprue pin has been used, it is removed with a slow, steady twisting pull.

Figure 43 The sprue channel is carefully washed out to remove any particles of loose investment that might have been created by this procedure. .

If for any reason transfer to the burnout furnace must be delayed so long that the investment dries out, the investment must be thoroughly resoaked before the ring is placed in the furnace. Adequate resoaking is accomplished by placing the ring in a bowl of water that does not cover the top of the investment; the water must soak through until the exposed investment at the top of the ring is moistened. If the investment is not thoroughly wet when heating for burnout is begun, it may crack.

Figure 44 The ring is placed in the burnout furnace, preferably in the back center of the muffle directly under the thermocouple. Provision must be made for adequate venting under the bottom (crucible) end of the ring, either by design of the furnace tray or by placement of ring liner strips on the floor of the furnace. The furnace is set to execute a burnout at 900° to 950° F. The ring is left in the furnace for a minimum period of burnout of 60 minutes. If there is any doubt, it is better to extend the burnout period—even overnight—rather than restrict this important procedure.

Figure 45 The melting crucible is prepared by thoroughly cleaning away any debris and attaching a new ring liner. The proper type and amount of alloy is made ready. (For centrifugal castings, this should be

twice the volume of the pattern.) The torch is checked, and flux and appropriate ring tongs are provided.

The casting machine is wound up. If in doubt as to the correct number of turns (at least four), too much pressure is better than not enough. The melting crucible is placed in the casting machine, and the crucible platform is removed sufficiently from the cradle to facilitate placement of the ring. Be sure that the proper size cradle for the casting ring involved is in place.

Figure 46 The torch is lit and the melting crucible preheated. (If desired, and if room in the burnout furnace permits, preheating of the melting crucible can be accomplished by placing the crucible in the furnace with the ring during the burnout procedure.)

When the flame is properly adjusted, the alloy may be placed in the melting crucible. The reducing portion of the flame is applied to the alloy to begin the melt. If old alloy is being used or oxidation is caused by inadequate flame control, flux may be applied conservatively *before* the ring is placed in the casting machine. Melting is continued until the alloy just begins to slump into a molten pool.

Figure 47 With the proper portion of the flame fixed on the melting alloy, the ring is promptly removed from the furnace and positioned in the casting machine. It is probably good procedure to tap the ring lightly against the bench top before placement into the machine, to remove any loose particles of debris that may be present in the sprue channel. If provision was made to orient the pattern in the ring to

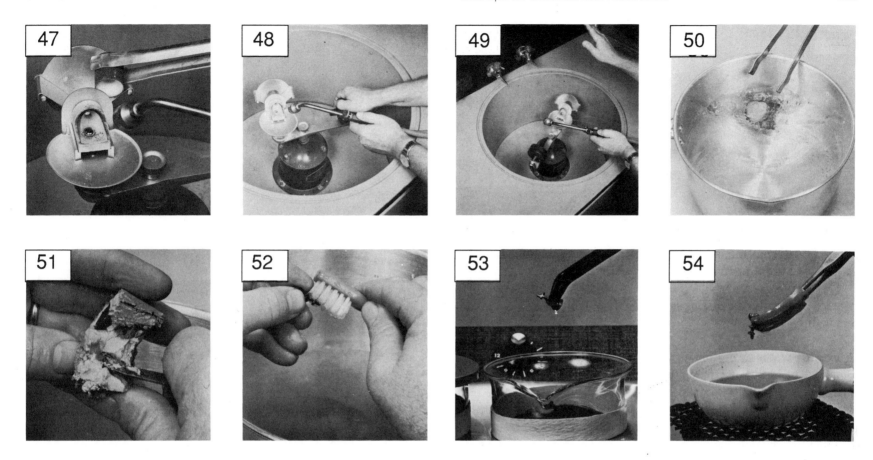

facilitate the casting, the ring is checked to assure it is properly positioned in the cradle.

Figure 48   By now the melting alloy should have slumped completely into a molten pool. To be ready to cast, one should now grasp the weighted arm of the casting machine and release the lock pin while continuing to heat the alloy. Readiness of the molten alloy for the cast may be determined by observing the color and activity of the melt. When the molten alloy becomes a bright, shiny pool that moves in keeping with slight movement of the torch flame, it should be immediately cast by releasing the weighted arm.

Figure 49   The flame must not be lifted away from the melt before the casting machine is released. Conversely, the torch must be adequately removed from the path of travel of the casting machine to avoid contact

when the machine is released. The casting machine is allowed to run down completely.

Figure 50   The ring is removed and quenched unless prolonged slow cooling is desired to heat treat the alloy. (See manufacturer's directions.)

Figure 51   Once quenched, the investment block is removed from the ring and the casting is dug out, carefully avoiding damage to the margins.

Figure 52   Gross amounts of adherent investment are scraped away, and the casting is scrubbed under running water with an appropriate brush.

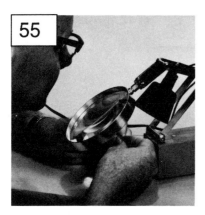
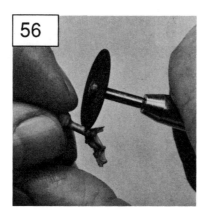
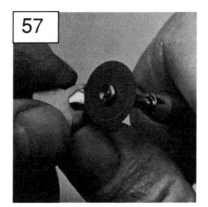
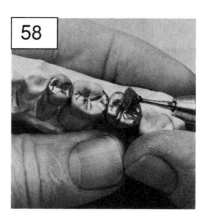

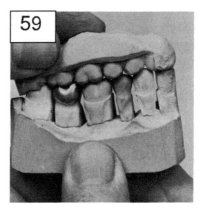
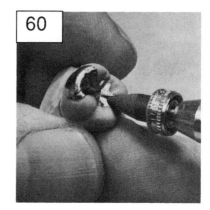

Figure 53   If available, an ultrasonic cleaner with appropriate solution may be used to further clean the casting of investment.

Figure 54   Finally, the casting is pickled thoroughly in an appropriate acid bath.

Figure 55   When the casting is thoroughly clean, it should be carefully examined using all the magnification available. Blebs or fins that would interfere with its accurate seating on the die must be removed. If there are discrepancies involving the margin that might alter the accuracy of the die, one must decide whether to take the risk of seating the casting or to develop another pattern before the casting is seated on the die. For this reason it is most desirable to have a second die on which the casting may be verified before seating it on the master die. Many technicians routinely pour a second die (and perhaps working cast) before beginning development of a restoration.

Figure 56   Once the casting is seated on the die and determined adequate, the sprue may be sectioned and the area of attachment contoured. This should not be done on the die, as the vibration might cause chipping and distortion of the stone.

Figure 57   Proximal contacts are checked and carefully adjusted, one at a time, to permit accurate reseating of the die and casting in the working cast. A disclosing solution or pencil marks may be used on adjacent tooth surfaces to identify the exact point of contact.

Figure 58   Once the die and casting are fully seated, occlusion must be

carefully checked and adjusted if necessary. Again, disclosing solution or pencil marks may be used on adjacent tooth surfaces to identify the exact point of contact.

Figure 59   Whatever the type of occlusal record provided, it should permit the accurate location of centric contacts. This is the limit of accurate occlusal contacts that can be identified by centric occlusion cores, anatomic cores, and anatomic opposing casts related on a simple hinge articulator. Eccentric contacts can be evaluated with functional cores or with anatomic casts that are related by properly adjusted semi- or fully adjustable articulators. Such limitations must be mutually understood by the technician and the dentist.

Figure 60   Once occlusal contacts have been located and adjusted, anatomy can be refined and the casting surfaced as necessary in prepa-

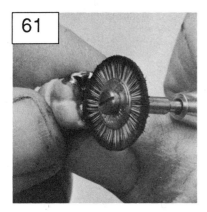
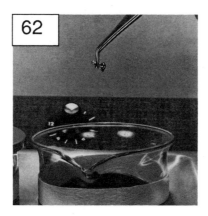
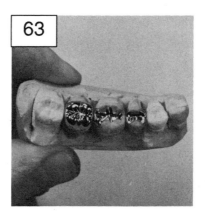

ration for polishing. Axial contours are rechecked; also absolute smoothness of tissue-contacting surfaces must be assured.

Figures 61 and 62 Polishing should be accomplished by standard procedure with care to avoid alteration of occlusal and proximal contacts and marginal contours. Removal of polishing compounds—especially rouge—is greatly facilitated by cleaning the casting and dies in appropriate solutions in an ultrasonic cleaner.

Figure 63 The polished and cleaned casting should be properly packaged for return to the dentist.

One final consideration should be made. It is well recognized that inadequate communication between dentist and technician can create much unnecessary trouble. This is a two-way problem. It is entirely appropriate and necessary that the technician relay to the dentist any information that is pertinent to the peculiarities of a restoration. This responsibility is no less significant than the dentist's responsibility to provide adequate information and instructions in the work authorization.

REVIEW QUESTIONS

1. Describe the care to be observed when preparing a root-form extension for a band impression.
2. What precautions are necessary with the die stone when making a die?
3. If there is a question regarding the accuracy of the die, what action should the technician take?
4. In developing a wax pattern, the correct position of which occlusal contacts should be determined first?
5. Once the axial surfaces are grossly developed, what is the next step in pattern development?
6. In the final contouring of a wax pattern, which portion of the die is used to establish the correct contour of the margin cavosurface angle?
7. When attaching a sprue to a wax pattern, to what area of the pattern should it be attached? What areas should be avoided on a full cast crown pattern?

SECTION 18

Resin-faced Crowns

The resin-faced (resin veneer) crown is an esthetic modification of the full gold crown. Hence, except for the development of the resin window, the technique for developing a resin-faced crown is essentially the same as that for a full gold crown. In this section, only the modifications required to produce the resin veneer are presented.

WORK AUTHORIZATION

Figure 1 An explicit work authorization should accompany the materials sent to the laboratory by the dentist. In addition to the usual functional and technical directions, the work authorization for a faced crown must also provide specific information regarding shade of the resin. Identification of the desired shade is accomplished with an appropriate shade guide. The shade tab that is to be matched may be included with the work authorization, as there is often some variation between tabs of the same shade (even though they are supposed to be identical). More than one tab may be required to match a single tooth. Frequently the gingival shade of one tab and the incisal shade of another must be combined to match the tooth in question.

Just as important as which colors are involved is the distribution of these colors—specifically, how much of the tooth is gingival shade, how much is incisal shade, and how much blend of the two is present. Unless the distribution of shades in the tooth is the same as in the selected shade tab, a diagram of the tooth showing the areas or zones of various shades should be included on the work authorization. Stains simulating exposed root surfaces, hypoplastic areas, anterior fillings, and other defects should also be denoted on the diagram.

It is inappropriate to use a porcelain shade guide for resin shades, or vice versa. Most resins are supplied by the manufacturer as premixed or preblended shades that match one of the more popular shade guides. It is most convenient if the dentist matches or selects the shade desired, using the shade guide to which the resin to be used is matched. However, conversion formulae and additives or modifiers are available with most materials, so that preblended shades can be altered.

Another major esthetic consideration is form. Diagrams are useful, but the most simple and effective mechanism for indicating form is a preoperative cast of the tooth in question or its corresponding member in the arch. Gross contours as well as minute surface characteristics are easily recorded in an alginate or rubber impression and are distinctly evident in the subsequent cast. Preoperative casts are easily modified by the addition of wax to show desired changes in contour.

The work authorization for a resin-faced crown should also specify the extent of the window occlusally or incisally. (The variations that are possible are shown later in **Figures 8, 9, and 10**.)

PATTERN CONSTRUCTION

Figures 2 and 3 The working cast and its opposing occlusal model are related as described in previous sections depending on the type of casts provided. The wax pattern is developed to full contour and occlusion in the same manner as done for a full cast crown.

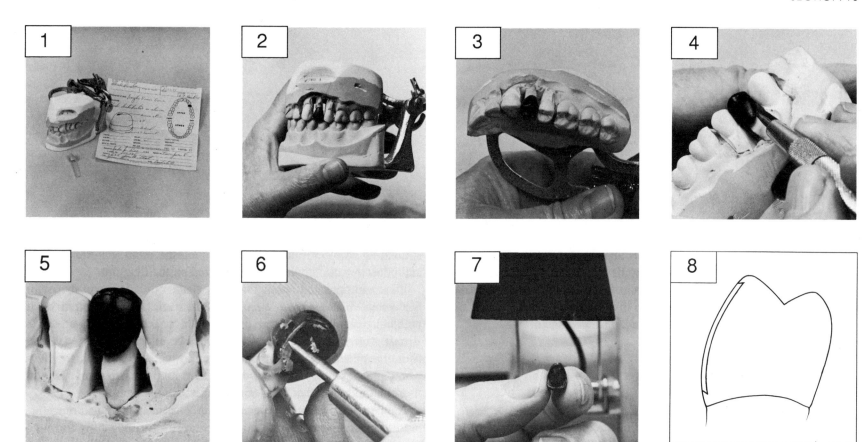

WINDOW DEVELOPMENT

Figures 4 through 7 When the pattern is complete, a window is carved in the facial surface. The window should extend into the proximal embrasures far enough to prevent any display of alloy, but without interfering with the proximal contact area, which *must be maintained in alloy*. Gingival extension should also be sufficient to prevent or minimize display of alloy, depending upon the esthetic demands of the restoration. The only safe rule is to keep the gingival collar of alloy as narrow as possible, as dies do not indicate the exact tissue level.

Figure 8 The occlusal or incisal extension of the window poses a problem. Ideally, alloy of sufficient thickness to resist occlusal wear should be present throughout the full range of occlusal contact. This usually means 1.0 to 1.5 millimeters in the posterior teeth and 0.6 to

1.0 millimeter in the anterior region. This configuration results in a display of alloy at the occlusal or incisal edge and is often forfeited in favor of esthetics. The window designs shown in the next two illustrations are more acceptable esthetically but less acceptable functionally.

Figure 9 The window may be extended to the center of the incisal or occlusofacial edge. Resin materials wear rapidly when in occlusal contact, and unprotected edges as shown here and in **Figure 10** are the object of frequent repair. If at all possible, gold coverage should be retained over the entire occlusal surface; if this is not feasible, gold coverage should be carried as close to the termination of occlusal contact as possible.

Figure 10 The window may be extended to include all of the incisal or occlusofacial edge. Because of the poor wear resistance of resin materi-

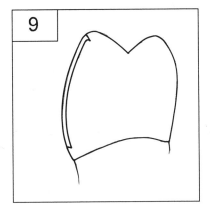
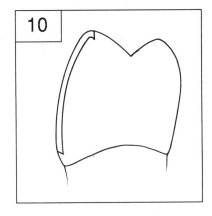
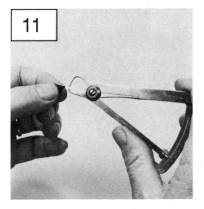
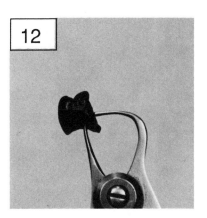

als, this is normally a very poor design for durability, though obviously the most desirable esthetically.

Positive occlusal relationship records must be provided and the working cast accurately mounted on a suitable instrument in order to be precise in establishing the final occlusal contour. Inaccurate occlusal relationships may jeopardize durability of the crown if an effort has been made to be conservative with the amount of alloy displayed on the occlusofacial or incisal edge of the crown. For example, imagine a maxillary first premolar crown developed on a simple hinge articulator with an opposing cast related in centric occlusion. The window has been carefully developed so as to leave 1 millimeter of occlusofacial alloy. The resin veneer is processed and the crown forwarded to the dentist. On trial insertion the crown is found to be premature in function. Correction requires about 0.75 millimeter reduction of the lingual incline of the facial cusp. With the resin veneer in place, it may be quite difficult to visualize the thickness of alloy that remains. The crown is cemented, only to find after very short service that the thin alloy cusp has worn through or deformed, causing failure of the veneer.

Such failures may be avoided in two ways. First, such restorations should be constructed only on articulators that reasonably accurately reproduce both centric *and* eccentric relationships. Secondly, a trial insertion of the alloy framework (especially for extensive bridges or splints) should be completed before processing the resin veneer. When this is to be done, the wax-up and resultant alloy forming the occlusal aspect of the window are purposely left too thick. Occlusal corrections are completed during trial insertion. The window side of the occlusal alloy can now be expanded to form the exact contour and dimension

of faciooclusal alloy desired, with assurance that only very minute changes might be required during final occlusal adjustment.

Figures 11 and 12   The wax pattern between the window and die must be a minimum of 0.4 millimeter thick to ensure a sound casting. When minimum thickness is desired, the window may be carved completely through to the die and the pattern for the backing of the window area formed by inserting 28-gauge wax. The use of sheet wax ensures uniform, minimum dimension. A solid casting devoid of any holes *must* be obtained in order to protect the prepared tooth.

RETENTION FOR RESIN

One cardinal fact must be kept in mind regarding the retention of resin veneers: there is no bonding or adhesion of resin to the casting, and all retention is purely mechanical. The acrylic resin that will form the facing of the crown will be packed into the window while in a doughy state. Subsequent curing will harden the resin to form the facing. Provision for mechanical retention of the resin facing must be incorporated into the wax pattern.

Several methods of providing such retention have been developed. Two or more of these methods are usually used in combination to provide sufficient retention for the resin veneer. The choice of method is left to the discretion of the dental laboratory technician and is made on the basis of the design requirements of the particular situation. The major methods for providing retention are as follows:

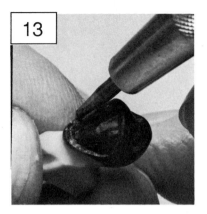

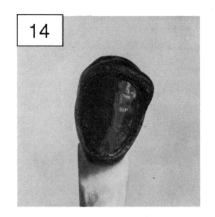

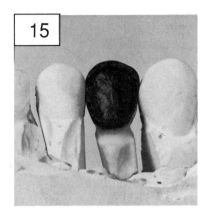

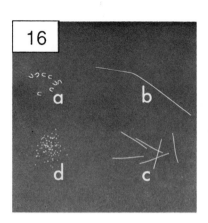

1. *Retentive loops*. Patterns for small wire loops can be developed within the window of the crown pattern using preformed wax wire, or plastic or nylon bristles. When cast, these become gold wires about which the resin can be processed. Loops can also be made by placing 27- or 29-gauge gold wire (Zephyr wire) forms in the wax pattern and casting to them.

2. *Plastic beads*. Very small (0.4 to 0.8 millimeter) plastic beads are manufactured for developing retention for resin veneers. An adhesive is applied to the wax window backing. The beads are sprinkled over the surface and held in place by the adhesive. When cast, the resulting alloy spheres offer a definite circumferential undercut. The total retentive effect is, of course, dependent on the number and distribution of the beads.

3. *Ridge locks*. A retentive lock can be developed by placing the convex surface of a suitably sized (14- to 16-gauge) half-round wax shape against the window backing about 0.5 to 1.0 millimeter within the boundary of the window. The resultant casting thus presents a bilaterally undercut ridge of alloy about the periphery of the window.

4. *Pickups*. Pickups are made by cutting *lightly* into the window backing at an angle with a very sharp instrument (Bard-Parker blade), leaving an attached, elevated spur of wax. By cutting first at one angle and then another, these spurs can be made to oppose one another and result in even greater mechanical locking. Similar roughness can be created by rolling a round bur across the backing surface by hand. Obviously these cuts will weaken the casting somewhat. They must not perforate the pattern if integrity of the casting is to be maintained for adequate protection of the tooth. Pickups are the least effective of the retentive mechanisms.

5. *Undercut excavations (grooves, ditches, pits)*. Various shapes and sizes of ditches and pits can be developed for retention where there is adequate thickness of wax (especially pontics). In particular, however, a groove or ditch in the walls about the entire circumference of the window is important. Such a continuous lock is imperative if the thinner margins of the veneer are to be kept from warping away from the casting. This is referred to both as a *peripheral undercut* or a *bezel lock*. It should be a standard retentive feature for *every* resin veneer unit.

Which type of retention should be used? It is doubtful that any one type affords the best retentive pattern for any given case. Most experienced technicians use a combination of retentive forms to obtain optimum mechanical locking of the resin. The most successful combinations involve a groove in the peripheral walls of the window, with loops, ridges, or beads on the backing surface. Such a retentive combination is indicated not only by the experience of many accomplished technicians, but also by the physical properties of the combination of materials involved.

There is no adhesion or chemical bonding between alloy and resin. The disparity in thermal coefficients of expansion of the two materials is significant enough to cause seepage or percolation of oral fluids between them due to disproportionate expansion and contraction. To help offset this, mechanical locking should be developed about the entire edge of the veneer as close to the margin as possible. This accounts for the significance of the bezel lock. In addition, retention in the central region of the veneer should be adequate to prevent warpage or pulling away of the resin from the backing. Wire loops, beads, and the ridge lock provide the most positive retention here.

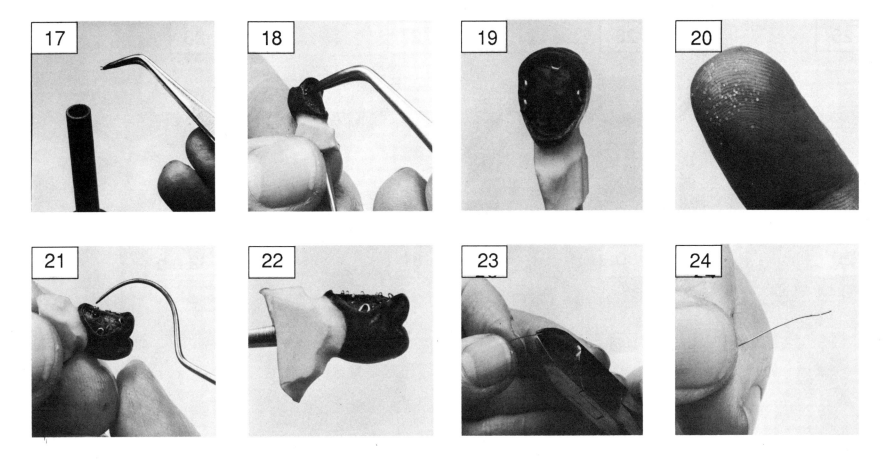

Figures 13 through 15 The peripheral undercut or bezel lock should extend completely around the excavation for the veneer and may be accentuated to form grooves on the proximal walls of the window. Space for such locking is minimal about the gingival margin. However, it is imperative that adequate retention be provided here, so that percolation and warpage will be minimized to prevent soft tissue irritation.

Figure 16 The materials for different methods of retention of the resin veneer: (a) Zephyr wire in preformed loops, (b) Zephyr wire as straight 27- or 29-gauge wire, (c) nylon bristles (cut from a toothbrush), and (d) spherical plastic beads.

Figures 17 through 19 Zephyr wire loops are first warmed in a flame and then placed about the borders of the window. These loops must not be too large or close to the surface, or they will show through the resin.

Figures 20 through 22 Small plastic beads are placed using either the adhesive supplied with the beads, or the tacky liquid used with preformed removable partial denture patterns. The beads are sprinkled over the surface and are held in place by the adhesive. They may be distributed evenly with an explorer. When cast, the resulting gold spheres offer a definite circumferential undercut. This undercut can be enhanced and the beads made more remote from the veneer surface by grinding down the cast beads to a half-spherical form.

Figures 23 through 25 Straight Zephyr wire may also be used for developing retention. The wire is first nicked with a pair of cutting pliers and then removed with a pair of tweezers.

Figures 26 and 27 The pieces of Zephyr wire are placed about the edge of the window such that they bridge across the angle formed by the

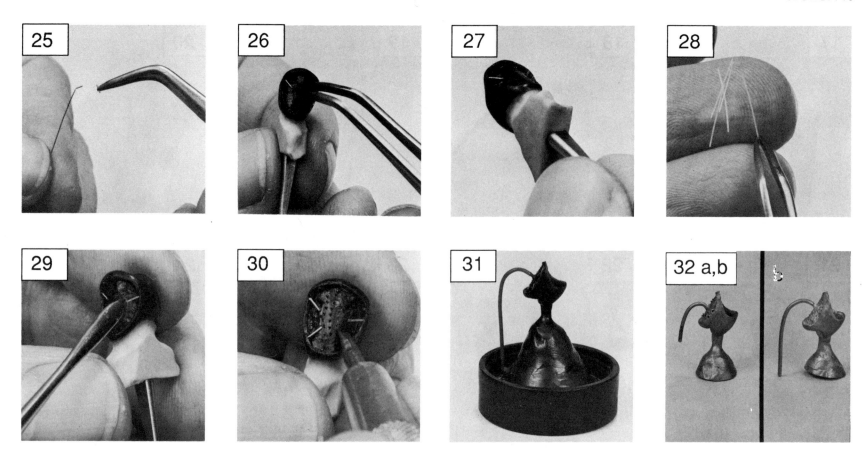

flange and backing of the window. As many pieces may be used as are appropriate. The wire is attached to the wax pattern by touching it lightly with a warm instrument.

Figures 28 and 29   Nylon bristles may be used in the same way as Zephyr wire. They are attached by placing a small amount of wax at each end of the bristle.

Figure 30   Additional retention may be provided by making pickups. These are made by cutting lightly at an angle into the wax window backing with a very sharp instrument. These cuts must not perforate the pattern. Integrity of the casting must be maintained to protect the tooth.

Additional forms of retention (ditches, pits, etc.) that may be appropriate to the pontic resin veneer are illustrated in Section 23.

Figures 31 and 32   The techniques for investing, wax elimination, casting, and finishing are identical to those utilized in the full gold crown (see Section 17). A vent sprue for the thin backing may be indicated to help prevent miscasts by removing gases from the thin facing area.

Two castings have been made for this preparation, to demonstrate the different forms of retention evidenced earlier in the wax patterns.

Figure 33   The casting is inspected carefully to make sure that there are no voids in the crown and to accentuate retentive grooves by machining if necessary. Any holes in the facing portion must be repaired by soldering before the veneer is placed. All margins about the window should be shaped so as to permit a butt joint between alloy and resin. Feathered edges of resin must be avoided.

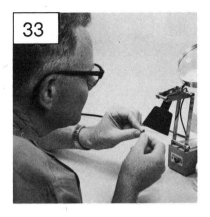

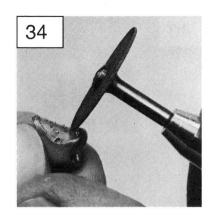

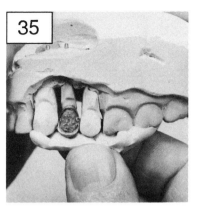

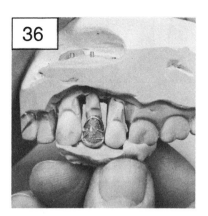

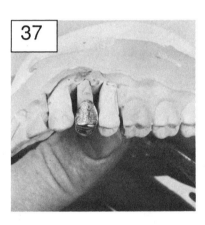

Figure 37   The crown must be completely polished before proceeding with development of the veneer.

MATERIALS FOR RESIN VENEERS

Three types of resin materials have been widely used for veneers in recent years: acrylic, vinyl, and epoxy resins. Although the manufacturers' early claims for epoxy resins were phenomenal, clinical usage soon revealed problems of toxicity and staining. These were confirmed by laboratory tests, which disclosed that the physical properties were actually inferior to those of the acrylic and vinyl resins.

The vinyl resins seemed to have superior physical properties and were the material of choice for a while. Processing requires special equipment, and the matching of shades can be a problem.

Acrylic (polymethyl methacrylate) resins have thus remained the most widely used materials for making resin veneers, although their physical properties are somewhat less desirable than those of the vinyl resins. Most resin veneers are processed as illustrated in this section. Another method of making resin veneers is to utilize a stock acrylic denture tooth as a facing and attach it to the casting with processed acrylic. An example of this technique is presented in Section 24.

In recent years, a technique has been developed for placing acrylic resin veneers utilizing special equipment with dry heat. This porcelain-like buildup-and-bake technique produces a facing with fairly good physical properties and also saves time.

Figure 34   If retentive beads have been employed, they can be ground flat on their exposed surfaces using a disc or stone. Such grinding tends to "brad" the top of the bead, thus increasing its retentiveness and making it more remote from the surface of the veneer.

Figures 35 and 36   With accuracy of fit on the die assured, the casting is adjusted as necessary for proximal and occlusal contact. In this case, adjustment for occlusion is made using both the opposing anatomic cast and a functional core.

Note the different retentive features in the two castings. In **Figure 35** a combination of Zephyr wire loops and plastic beads was used. **Figure 36** shows a nylon bristle and pickup combination. A bezel lock is of course evident in both castings.

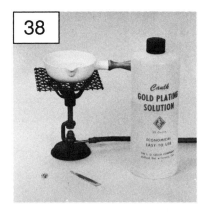

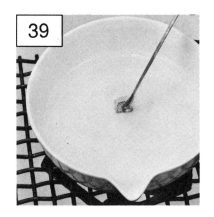

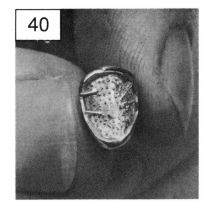

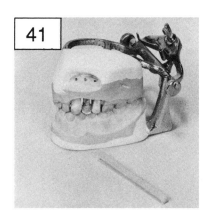

TECHNIQUE FOR PROCESSED RESIN VENEERS

Figure 38   Before waxing the veneer, it is often desirable that the window area be flash-plated with pure gold to provide the best background color and the most noble surface to prevent subsequent oxidation and discoloration of the casting. Flash plating is easily accomplished with a commercial gold-plating solution according to the following technique.

Figure 39   A quantity of gold-plating solution sufficient to cover the casting is placed in a porcelain or heat-resistant glass vessel. The solution is heated until it begins to steam. The alloy to be plated is completely submerged in the steaming solution. A strip of zinc metal supplied with the solution is brightened by scraping or sanding. The zinc strip is held in contact with the surface to be plated and is moved slowly across the casting to assure even coverage of the gold plate. The plating process requires 1 to 2 minutes. Because these solutions contain cyanide, it is essential that they be used in well-ventilated spaces, preferably under a ventilating hood.

Figure 40   The appliance is removed and thoroughly washed in tap water. The window should present a uniform bright gold surface.

Waxing and Flasking for Resin Veneers

Figure 41   After plating, veneer contour is carefully established in wax. Ivory wax is used to prevent the formation of any colored wax residue when the wax-up is eliminated during the boil-out phase of the technique.

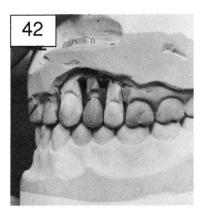

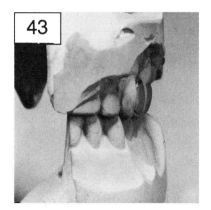

Figures 42 and 43   Care should be taken during waxing of the veneer to develop the exact contour and anatomy desired in the completed crown.

Figure 44   The inside of the crown is coated with die lubricant. A small mix of stone is used to fill the inside or core of the crown. Vibration may be used if necessary. The core must be completely filled, as lack of support, especially under the veneer window, may result in distortion of the casting when packing the facing.

Figure 45   A dowel pin or brass screw may be inserted into the stone filling the core. This will facilitate the removal of the core after processing.

Figure 46   The crown with its core is now ready to be flasked. Note the convenient handle produced by the brass screw.

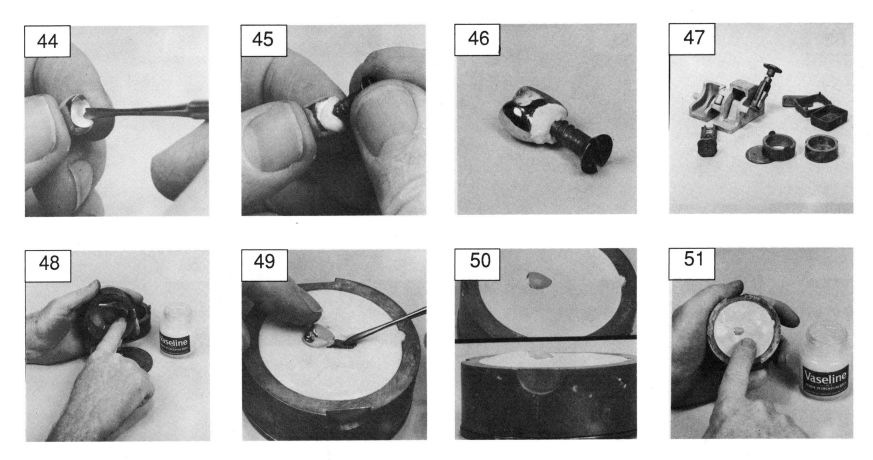

Figure 47 Many types of flasks have been developed for processing resin veneers. A denture flask may be used for single crowns or small bridges, although it is large and awkward. The smaller flat flask is best used to accommodate single crowns or small bridges. Large curved flasks may be used to process veneers on extensive bridges or splints.

Figure 48 The flask to be used is lightly coated with petroleum jelly.

Figure 49 Any exposed portion of the stone used to fill the core of the crown is painted with plaster separator. The bottom half of the flask is filled with plaster or stone, and the crown with its stone core is embedded in the gypsum with only the waxed veneer exposed. Many technicians use a mixture of plaster and stone in the flask to obtain a light buff color, which aids in matching shades during the packing process. Either quick-set or regular plaster may be used, depending upon the working time required by the individual technician.

Figure 50 The gypsum is smoothed and allowed to set. It is often easier to smooth and contour the plaster surface after initial set but before the final set has occurred. Note that the entire surface of the veneer is exposed in addition to a slight margin of alloy surrounding the veneer. The gypsum has been smoothed so that no undercuts are present.

Figure 51 A plaster separator is applied to the surface of the gypsum in the base of the flask. The surface of the wax pattern for the veneer must be left untouched.

Figures 52 and 53 The top half of the flask is poured in stone. The lid is pressed into place, and the entire flask may be placed in a press to assure metal-to-metal contact of the flask halves. The stone is allowed to set.

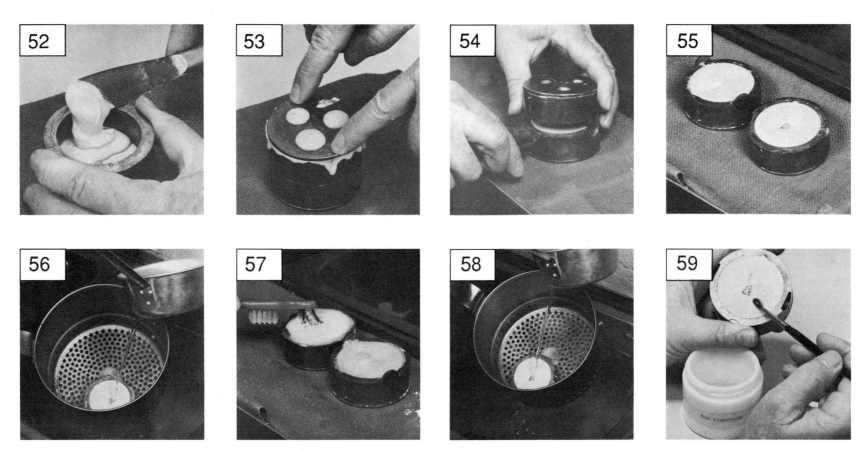

Figures 54 and 55 If multiunit wax veneers are involved, it may be best to place the flask in hot water for about 5 minutes before opening. The flask halves are separated to permit removal of the veneer wax pattern.

Figures 56 through 58 The wax is completely removed with boiling water. The veneer area is scrubbed with a detergent and is again flushed with clean boiling water.

Figure 59 The stone surfaces are checked for significant bubbles or sharp edges that might break during the packing process. These are conservatively removed. The surfaces of the gypsum mold are painted with tinfoil substitute. *Do not permit any tinfoil substitute to contact the crown.*

Packing and Processing Acrylic Resin Veneers

There are many brands of resins suitable for crown and bridge veneers. The manufacturer of each cites the merits of the particular product. The techniques vary somewhat, although they are similar in most respects. The technique illustrated here shows the basic procedures necessary to process an adequate acrylic facing.

Figure 60 The first step in packing is the application of an opaque material to mask the alloy. The opaque used here is an autopolymerizing resin that combines chemically with the veneering resin that will be applied. It is supplied as a liquid and powder in various shades, the selection of which is determined by the desired shade of the finished restoration. Different shades of opaque are used for the body and incisal portions of the veneer. In this example, appropriate quantities of

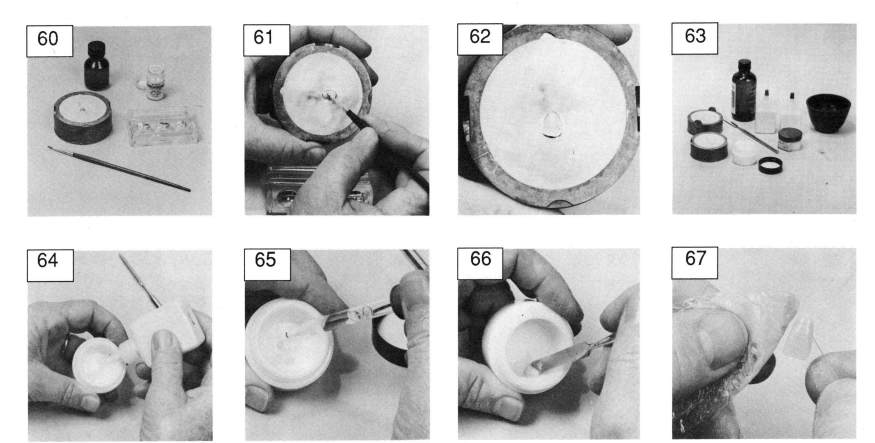

powdered body opaque and incisal opaque are placed in glass mixing dishes.

Figure 61   Liquid is added to the body opaque powder and mixed with a brush or small spatula to produce a thin, creamy consistency that can be easily painted on the veneer surface. Depending on the distribution of body and incisal shades desired in the final veneer, the body opaque is extended from the gingival to the middle or incisal third of the window. This coat of opaque should be only thick enough to mask the alloy completely and should terminate incisally in a thin, irregular edge.

Figure 62   The incisal opaque is now mixed and painted from the incisal to overlap the body material, producing a blended zone. These applications must be made quickly, as the opaque cures quite rapidly (2

to 3 minutes). The mixing vessel should be kept cool to prevent rapid polymerization of the mix. Any opaque that extends beyond the margin of the veneer should be trimmed with a sharp instrument.

Figure 63   The proper shades of body and incisal veneer resin are selected, using the work authorization and/or shade tab provided by the dentist. The powder bottles are rotated before opening to assure even distribution of the pigments.

Figures 64 through 66   Approximately ½ teaspoon of gingival shade powder is placed in a mixing jar and monomer is added, one drop at a time, until the powder is completely wetted—then stirred only enough to assure wetting of the powder.

Figure 67   The shade may be checked by wrapping a portion of the

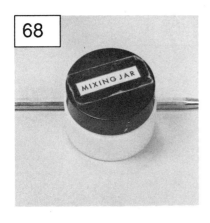

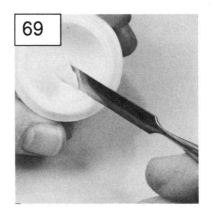

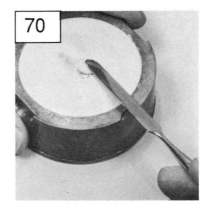

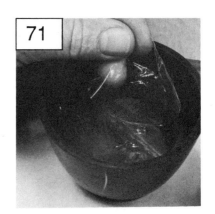

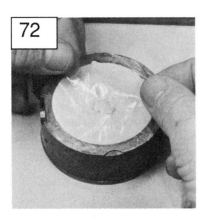

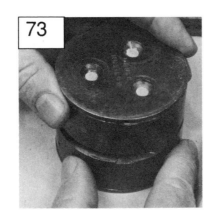

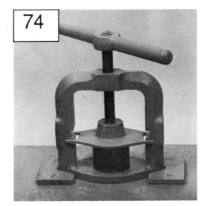

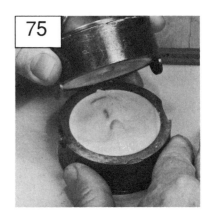

mix in cellophane and comparing it with the shade guide. If alteration is desired, it can be accomplished by mixing in a powder of another shade or modifier if available.

Figure 68   The jar is covered while the mix ages, to prevent evaporation of the monomer.

Figure 69   When the mix leaves the sticky stage, it is ready to pack. It should be doughy enough to be picked up cleanly with a spatula and carried into place.

Figure 70   A slight excess of material is carried to the flask and placed in the window.

Figures 71 and 72   Wet cellophane is used to cover the lower half of the flask.

Figures 73 and 74   The flask is closed slowly with hand pressure and is then placed in a press. The press is closed slowly, with minimum pressure. Fingertip pressure on the ends of the handles is sufficient to effect proper closure.

Figures 75 and 76   The flask is opened and the cellophane removed.

Figure 77   Excess resin surrounding the crown is removed with a sharp knife.

Figure 78   A scalpel is used to remove the excess extending over the edge of the window.

Figure 79   A scalpel blade or other suitable sharp instrument is used to trim some of the body material from the incisal portion of the veneer. The shape and amount of this excavation depends on the amount of

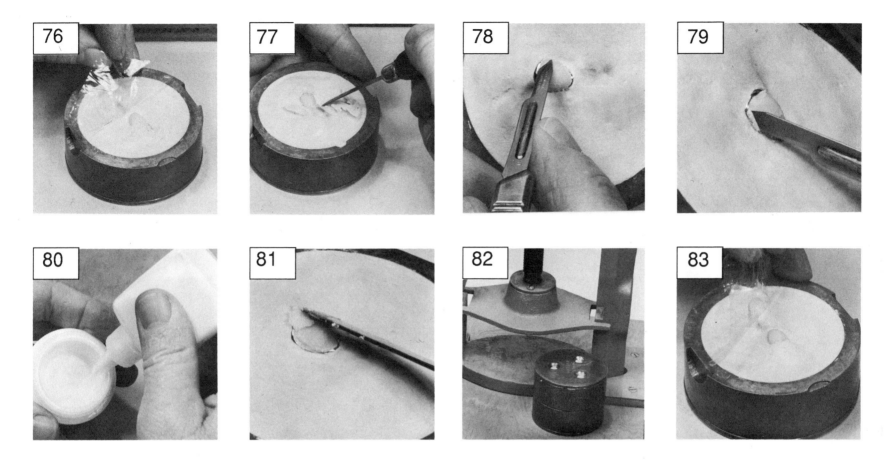

material needed to produce the incisal shade dictated by the work authorization.

Figure 80   The incisal powder and liquid are mixed to wet-sand consistency.

Figure 81   A sufficient amount is immediately placed in the incisal void, overlapping the body material to the desired degree. The lower half of the flask is covered again with wet cellophane. The upper half of the flask is placed in position and allowed to settle under its own weight as the incisal material gels. When gellation proceeds to the point that the cellophane can be pulled away cleanly, further blending can be accomplished. This may be done by working the doughy mix with a spatula through the cellophane. The same action may be obtained by rocking the upper half of the flask toward the direction of flow desired

as the flask is progressively seated. The incisal material is softest at this point, and advantage can be taken of that greater "flowability" when manipulating to obtain proper distribution of the two shades of material.

Figure 82   When distribution is correct, the flask is closed completely in a bench press, allowing a minute or two for the material to flow.

Figure 83   The flask is again opened and the cellophane removed.

Figure 84   Excess resin is removed with suitable instruments. The flask should be reassembled with wet cellophane and trial closure repeated until no more flash is produced.

Figure 85   Stains may be applied as desired at this point, or after

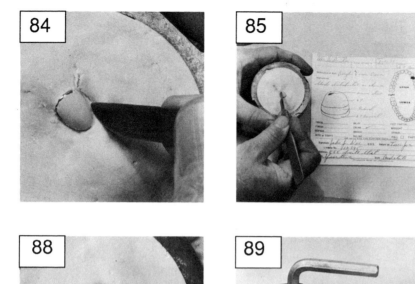

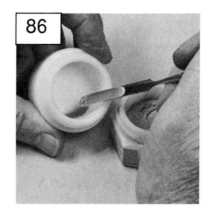

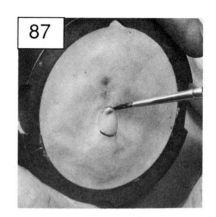

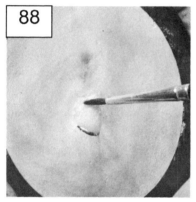

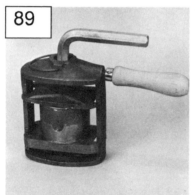

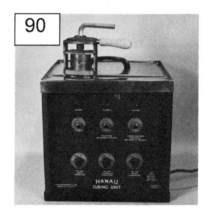

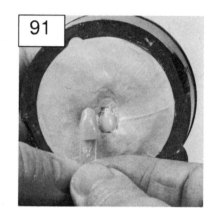

curing. Placement of stains before curing is preferred if intensity and shade can be properly determined. The desired stains are indicated on the dentist's work authorization.

If stains are to be placed, the resin material should bench cure until it may be cut cleanly with a sharp instrument. This stage may be hastened by warming the upper half of the flask in hot water during the trial packing procedure. The desired outline of the area to be stained is cut.

Figure 86   The stain shades are mixed following the manufacturer's directions. A thin mix is usually appropriate.

Figure 87   A brush or fine instrument is used to flow the stain into the desired areas.

Figure 88   The stained areas may be covered with a clear powder, as recommended by some manufacturers. A trial pack before curing is advisable.

Experience is the only real means of learning the art of blending and staining resins for shade duplication. Even experienced technicians have difficulty when batches of materials are changed or a new brand is introduced.

Characterization of form may also be accomplished at this point, although this should have been incorporated in the wax-up procedure. Indentations can be made with suitable instruments. A subtle waviness can often be created by tightly wrinkling the cellophane to be used during final closure and cure. Minute cross-striations often are desired and may be obtained by slightly scratching the appropriate surface of the stone in the upper flask half.

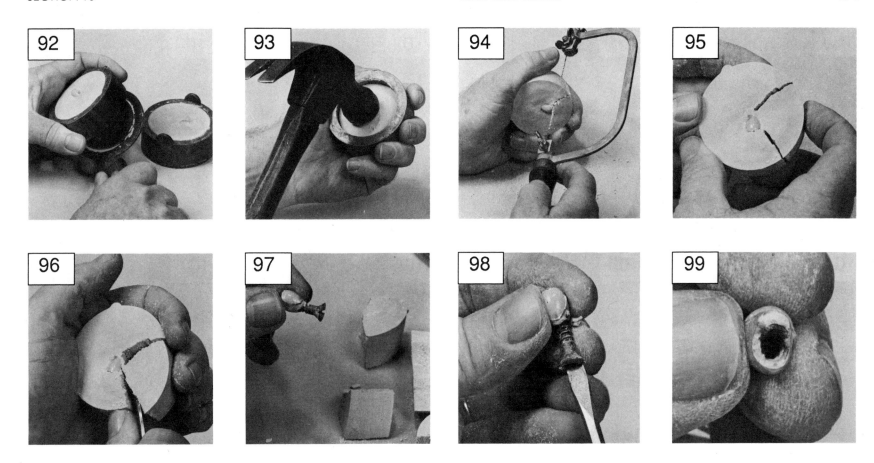

Figure 89 When all of the packing, staining, and characterization is completed, the flask should be closed and placed in a press. The flask and press should be left on the bench at room temperature for 30 minutes before curing.

Figure 90 The flask and press are submerged in 160° F water for 1 hour and then placed in boiling water for 30 minutes. A two- or three-stage curing unit is a good method for accomplishing this. An alternate curing method requires submersion in 160° F water for 9 hours. After curing, the flask is cooled slowly to room temperature.

Figure 91 The flask is opened and the shade of the cured veneer is checked with the selected shade tab. If the cured shade is incorrect, the facing may be removed by heating it with a Hanau torch and peeling it from the crown. This permits the packing procedure to be repeated without having to wax and invest another pattern for the veneer.

Figure 92 When the shade is deemed correct, the base is removed from the flask.

Figure 93 The flask and gypsum may be separated by tapping lightly with a hammer.

Figure 94 The crown is most readily recovered by using a plaster saw to place cuts that isolate a wedge of gypsum.

Figure 95 The saw cuts should extend until they approach, but do not touch, the crown.

Figure 96 A knife is used to fracture the residual stone.

Figure 97 Additional saw cuts are made and sections fractured until the crown and its core are recovered.

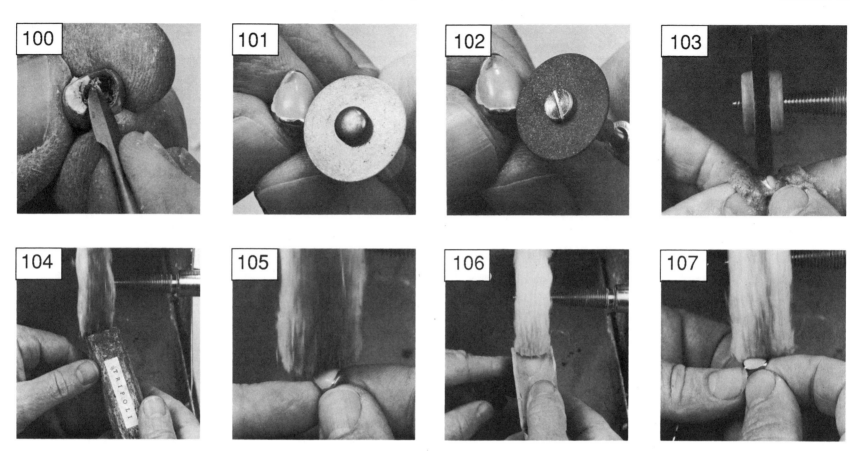

Figure 98 If a dowel or brass screw was used, it is removed. The screw used for these illustrations is being removed with a screw driver.

Figures 99 and 100 The hole left by the screw facilitates removing the stone core. If internal roughness is such that the stone core cannot be removed in one piece, the stone is carefully chipped away with suitable instruments.

Figures 101 and 102 Little excess resin should be left if trial packing was done properly. Excess may be removed with suitable discs and rubber abrasive wheels. Only light finishing of the veneer surface should be necessary if the wax-up was correctly done.

Figure 103 Wet pumice may be used to smooth the alloy and rough edge of the veneer if needed.

Figures 104 and 105 Tripoli may be used to polish the veneer and the surrounding alloy. Avoid application of too much pressure of polishing wheels on the resin facing.

Figures 106 and 107 A high-shine material is applied with a clean buff wheel to impart a high gloss to the resin veneer.

Figure 108 Rouge on a chamois or minim felt wheel is used to give a final luster to the alloy portion of the crown. Avoid contact with the resin.

Figure 109 The crown is checked against the indicated shade tab.

Figure 110 Before delivery to the dentist, the crown should be cleaned with detergent by scrubbing with a toothbrush or by placing it

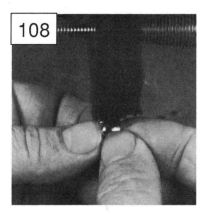 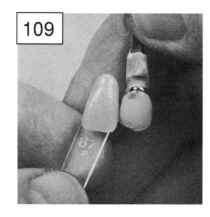 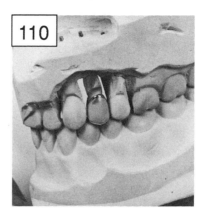

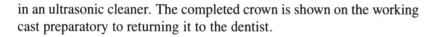

in an ultrasonic cleaner. The completed crown is shown on the working cast preparatory to returning it to the dentist.

All resin material should be kept moist from the time of finishing until delivery to the patient. This can be easily accomplished by wrapping the restoration in wet cotton and placing it in a closed, relatively airtight container for delivery or sealing it in a plastic bag with a small quantity of water.

REVIEW QUESTIONS

1. In addition to the usual functional and technical directions, what other specific information must the work authorization for a resin-faced crown provide?
2. Discuss the important considerations involved in the esthetics of a resin-faced crown.
3. Discuss the methods for the retention of a resin veneer in the casting.
4. Which type of retention should be a standard feature for every resin veneer unit?
5. Compare and contrast the types of resin materials that have been used for veneers.

SECTION 19

Post/Core Foundations

As mentioned in the brief description of types of fixed restorations in Section 2, the indications and use of cast restorations for endodontically treated teeth have changed markedly since the 1950s as a result of advancements and greater acceptance of endodontic treatment. Because of the desire of the profession and the public to preserve teeth, literally thousands of teeth that were once forfeited due to pulpal involvement are now being salvaged by adequate root canal therapy. These teeth require special considerations for proper restoration.

RETENTION AND RESISTANCE FORM

Most teeth that are endodontically treated have been extensively involved with caries and previous restoration or severe traumatic injury. This, coupled with the loss of structure associated with gaining endodontic access into the root canal(s), makes these teeth weak and more prone to fracture (**Figure 1**). Hence most endodontic teeth, especially multicusp teeth, should be restored with cast restorations of dominantly extracoronal design, that is, crowns. Even with full crown restorations, single-rooted endodontic teeth are prone to fracture transversely through the marginal or cervical region (**Figure 2**). These teeth usually require special "post" foundations in addition to the crown restoration.

Because of their much larger cross-sectional dimension molar teeth seldom fracture transversely. However, unless restored with full occlusal coverage castings, molars are very prone to vertical fractures (**Figure 3**). Thus molar endodontic teeth are usually restored with a directly placed foundation (amalgam, composite, or glass ionomer cement) followed by a cast crown (**Figure 4**).

Because of the potential for transverse fracture, single-rooted teeth are usually restored with a post/core foundation followed by a crown (**Figure 5a, b, c**). This is especially important for single-rooted multicusp teeth (premolars). Many anterior endodontic teeth that are conservatively involved (minor caries, restorations, or fractures) can be conservatively restored with composite and do not require a post/core foundation. However, those that require restoration with a crown usually do require a post/core foundation.

POST/CORE FOUNDATIONS

Post/core foundations involve a metal post that extends well into the root canal and a core portion that blankets the occluding surface(s) and replaces any missing portion of an ideal "stump" (preparation) form. Accordingly the core in conjunction with prepared remaining tooth structure creates an ideal preparation form that provides retention for the crown. The incorporated metal post, when properly extended into the root, provides retention for the core. It also dissipates stress from biting forces on the crown throughout as much of the root and bone support area as possible. It is this distribution of stress that provides the *resistance form* to prevent transverse fracture of the tooth. Thus the metal post should serve as a reinforcing or stress-distributing rod for the tooth and may also provide retention for the crown via a core.

The original post crowns (the Richmond crown and Davis crown)

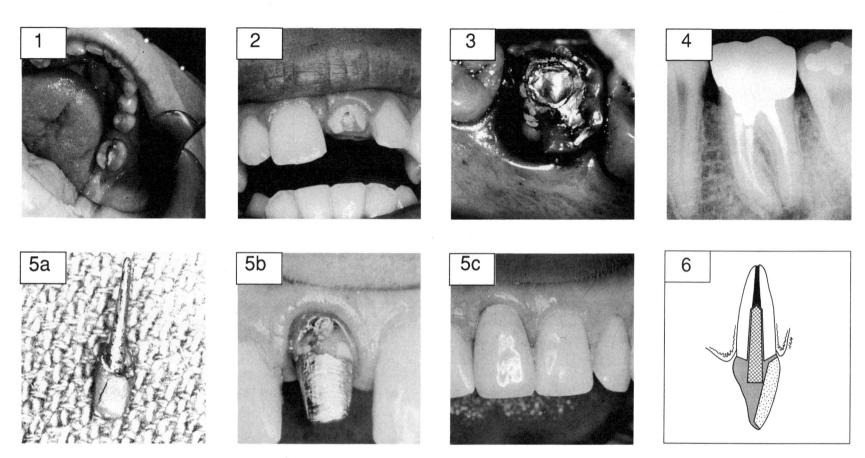

incorporated a post primarily for the purpose of retention. Teeth to receive such crowns were prepared flush with the crest of gingiva, and a crown incorporating a post as an integral part of its structure was held in place by cementing the post into the root canal (**Figure 6**).

The modern concept of the use of posts includes not only their retentive potential but also the resistance form (prevention of fracture) that they provide. No longer are teeth arbitrarily reduced to gingival level when a post crown is to be involved. Instead, a conventional crown preparation is executed to provide a stump form which preserves the maximum amount of sound tooth structure. Admittedly in many cases very little, if any, stump form remains. In these cases the post certainly provides the primary, if not sole, retention for the restoration. But the preparation must include a beveled gingival margin on sound tooth structure about which the crown will fit. This "hoop around the

barrel" serves to tie the tooth together and thus resist the tendency of the post to split the root (**Figure 7**).

Integral and Separated Post Crowns

The original post crown was a one-piece restoration; that is, the crown and post were an integral unit. Modern post crowns are generally made in two pieces (**Figure 8**). This approach offers many potential advantages. If the post and crown are developed as separate units, the path of draw for the crown is not dictated by the root canal. Many problems, notably perforation or fracture of the root wall, have occurred due to efforts to change the orientation of the root canal in relation to path of draw of the prepared stump (**Figure 9a, b**). This is particularly significant in bridge situations where one of the abutments is an endodontic tooth. The path of draw necessary for a bridge is often

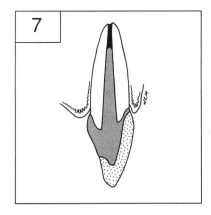

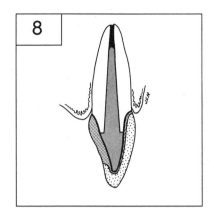

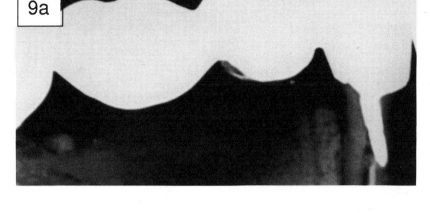

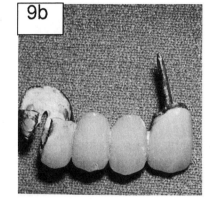

inconsistent with the orientation of the root canal in an endodontic abutment. When one-piece post crowns are used in such situations, either the abutment preparations must be modified to parallel the path of draw of the involved root canal, or the orientation of the prepared root canal must be changed to parallel the prepared stump. This challenge is most effectively resolved by using the two-piece post crown. Obviously, under these circumstances the orientation of the post need not be consistent with path of draw for the bridge.

Another significant advantage of two-piece construction occurs in situations where a post crown needs to be remade. Properly designed and cemented, a post is difficult if not impossible to remove from the root canal of a tooth. Attempts to extricate such posts by pulling them from the canal result in subjection of the tooth to marked stress, which may easily fracture the root. Consequently, removal of a post is a most undesirable procedure. The alternative procedure for removing a post crown when one-piece construction has been employed is to grind away the crown, leaving the post and appropriate stump portion of the crown on the tooth. Obviously, this too is a tedious and time-consuming task. However, when the crown and post have been made separately, the crown may be removed in a conventional manner without disturbing the post (**Figure 10a, b**).

The third major advantage of two-piece construction is the facility provided during trial insertion and cementation of the restoration. When seating a one-piece post and crown, it is extremely difficult to determine whether resistance is being provided by the post seating in the root canal or by the crown seating on the stump. As a consequence, many roots have been fractured by forceful seating of one-piece post crowns (**Figure 11a, b**). Obviously a separate post can be placed without

this jeopardy, as there is no confusion as to the source of the tactile sensation of resistance. The crown can subsequently be placed with the same tactile sensibility.

Modern techniques permit the construction of post/core foundations by either of two basic methods: the use of prefabricated posts, or the development of a customized anatomic post.

PREFABRICATED POSTS

Several problems are associated with the use of prefabricated posts. The most serious is that almost all are parallel-sided, which requires that naturally tapered root canals be arbitrarily enlarged to receive them. The alternative is to use a post so small that it fits the canal quite

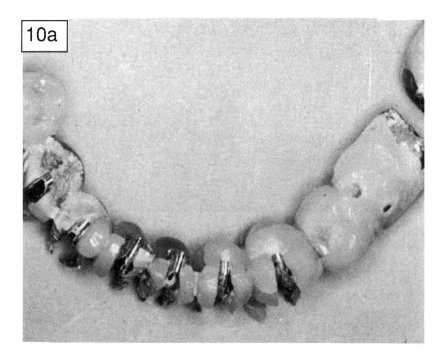

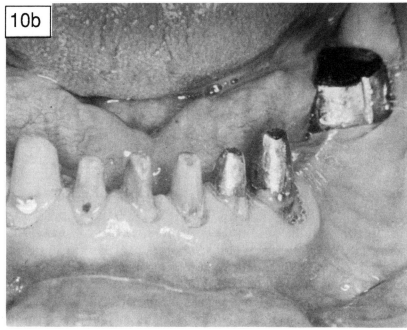

poorly in the occlusal region. Significant enlargement of the canal weakens the root and may also lead to perforation of the root. This problem is apt to arise because most prefabricated posts come with a twist drill of matching size. The canal is thus "prepared" by sinking a twist drill to the desired depth rather than by excavating gutta percha and shaping the anatomic canal space (**Figure 12**). Nonetheless prefabricated posts are quite popular because they provide a ready-made technique, require less time, and are sometimes less expensive.

Dentists use a variety of techniques to accomplish post/core foundations. Probably the most common one involves some form of prefabricated post that is cemented into the root canal, followed by a core that is developed directly with either amalgam or composite material. Although these techniques offer advantages relative to speed and cost, they inherently entail some compromise in adaptation of the post, form of the core, or structural integrity.

Another approach that uses prefabricated posts is a direct-indirect technique. The dentist may adapt a prefabricated post and then add to it a pattern for the core form using either wax or some resin material (usually Duralay). The post with attached core pattern is then invested, and the core is cast to the post. There are a number of disadvantages to

this technique as well. In addition to problems that pertain to use of prefabricated posts, the result of this approach is a casting composed of dissimilar metals. The crown that is ultimately placed is often made of yet another alloy. The result is a bi- or trimetallic system that is very undesirable from a electromotive or corrosion-resistance standpoint. When dissimilar and especially nonnoble alloys have been employed for a post foundation, roots may fracture due to the tensile stress caused by buildup of corrosion.

ANATOMIC POSTS

Because of the problems associated with the use of prefabricated posts many dentists still prefer to take the time, trouble, and expense to develop custom-fitted anatomic posts. They feel strongly that the anatomic form and dimension of the root canal should not be significantly altered, because this directly weakens the tooth. Accordingly they "prepare" the canal to receive a post by excavating sufficient gutta percha and only lightly smoothing the walls to eliminate minor under-

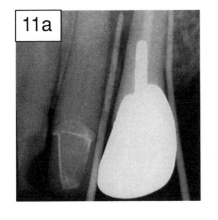

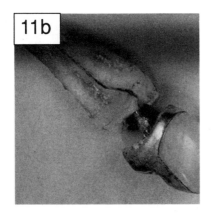

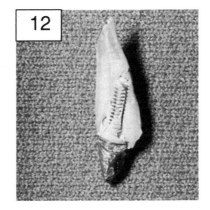

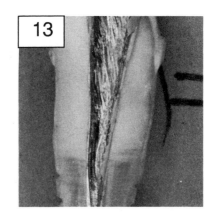

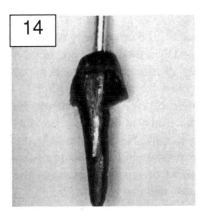

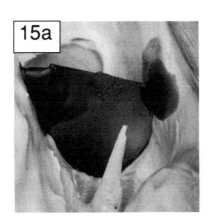

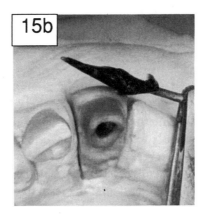

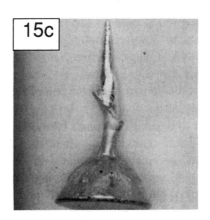

cuts. Any major undercuts are blocked out with appropriate base material. The post is developed by generating a pattern that fits the canal and provides appropriate core form. This pattern is cast with appropriate alloy—the same noble alloy that will be used for the crown restoration. Such posts are categorically known as anatomic posts because they are custom-made to fit the anatomic form of the canal (**Figure 13**).

There are two basic approaches for development of anatomic post/core foundations—a direct technique, and an indirect technique. The pattern for the post/core can be developed directly in the mouth (**Figure 14**), or an impression can be made of the prepared tooth and the pattern developed indirectly in the laboratory (**Figure 15a, b, c**).

Direct Patterns

In the past direct patterns were made with wax. Because it is quite awkward to use molten wax intraorally, these patterns were commonly formed by condensing soft sprue wax into the canal and then seating a heated metal pin or wire into the wax. This formed the pattern for the post. Molten wax was then carried to place to form the core about the occlusally exposed end of the wire (see **Figure 14**). The pattern was carved and then forwarded to the laboratory for casting. This same technique works quite well for the development of indirect patterns and is discussed further under that heading. One essential point regarding this approach must be recognized and remembered: *The metal pin must be removed prior to casting!* This is done by using the occlusally exposed end of the metal pin as the sprue (its diameter can be enlarged by addition of wax) and investing the pattern. Then, either before the investment has been placed in the burnout furnace or after it has been there long enough to soften the wax thoroughly, the pin is extracted from the investment. If this step is forgotten, the pin can still be removed after burnout—just before casting. **Figure 16** shows a crown

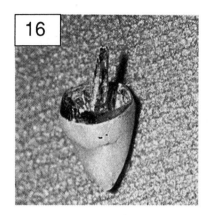
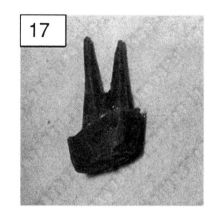
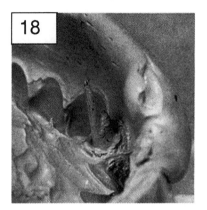
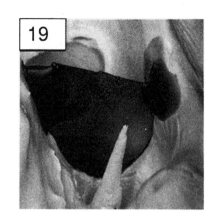

that failed because the metal pin (made from a segment of paper clip) was not removed before casting. In time (eight years) it corroded (note voids in post), causing fracture of the tooth root.

Currently the most favorable approach to development of direct post/core patterns is the use of Duralay pattern resin. By one of several means the dentist can form the resin pattern directly on the tooth, shape it to desired form, and forward it to the laboratory for casting (**Figure 17**). If made entirely of resin, such patterns can be sprued, invested, and completely eliminated in burnout. However, some dentists use a metal wire or pin in forming direct resin patterns. In these cases the metal pin must be removed *after* burnout, or at least after the resin has fully softened in the burnout furnace.

Indirect Patterns

For any of several reasons the dentist may choose to make an impression of the preparation and have the post/core pattern developed indirectly. This approach is clearly indicated when there are undercuts in the prepared canal (**Figure 18**). Some dentists routinely prefer this approach because it requires less chair time than formation of a direct pattern, or because they are not comfortable with direct pattern techniques. Some presume that even more chair time may be saved by completing marginal preparation of the tooth and having the post/core and the crown made on the same die. This approach sounds quite favorable, but it can be very problematic, for two major reasons. In many cases (primarily maxillary anterior) it can be difficult to establish ideal core form unless casts are accurately related in an adjustable articulator, permitting evaluation of full-range occlusion. Secondly, it

can be tedious to fit both a post/core and crown to a tooth. If for any reason the post/core is not precisely seated, the crown will not fit. A safer procedure is to seat the post/core and then finalize the preparation of the tooth/core complex for proper form, dimension, and occlusal clearance, followed by a separate impression for the crown.

Impressions for posts must be handled carefully. They should be poured promptly, as the extension of material that duplicates the prepared canal may distort under its own weight. For this reason many dentists prefer to incorporate a metal or plastic pin in the post impression. Even so, any force during shipment or storage that loads the extension of material duplicating the canal will cause distortion.

Another problem is the extension of post impression above the flanges of the tray. In these cases the flanges of the impression may be made higher by the placement of rope wax. *A closed system must be established* that provides for at least 3 to 4 millimeters of die stone above the end of the post impression (**Figure 19**). For stripped impressions, wider than normal matrix material or edgewise placement of material may be necessary. Care must also be exercised in placement of dowel pins. It will often be necessary to place the dowel facially or lingually in the die base in order to avoid the area of the post. Thus it might well be appropriate to mark the separating strip (**Figure 20a, b**).

In many cases it may not be necessary to make the die for a post/core removable. If margins for the core form are quite supragingival, the pattern can probably be readily developed from a solid-pour model. Even so, *a closed system* must be established for the pour such that the fluid stone mix can reach equilibrium about the post impression.

There are three challenging aspects to the development of an indirect pattern for a post/core foundation. The first challenge is to ensure that

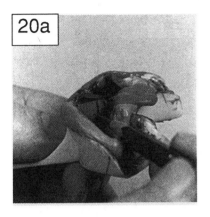
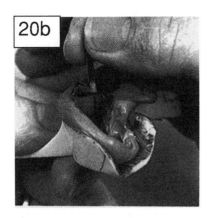
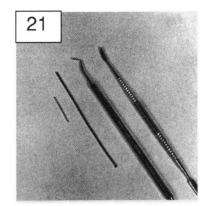
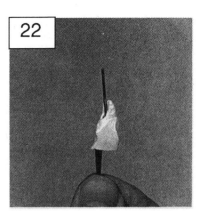

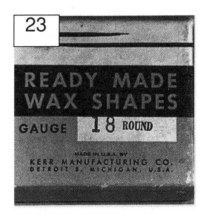
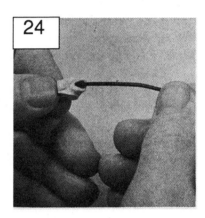

wax is accurately adapted to the full extent of the post space. The second is recovery of the pattern, especially if it is long and/or roughness and undercuts are present in the canal walls. Determining and establishing proper dimension and contour of the core often presents a third challenge.

Post/core patterns may be developed in many ways. The following has proven to be a very simple, dependable technique.

Figure 21 The die is thoroughly lubricated. If lubricant cannot be placed via brush all the way to the apex of the space, the space should be filled with lubricant, which can be gently pumped into place with a toothpick or probe (one must be careful not to scar the die). While lubricant is soaking into the die, the armamentarium for development of the pattern can be assembled:

—a segment of paper clip or arch wire long enough to seat to the base of the post space and extend out of the die to form a sprue
—a length of small diameter sprue wax (18-gauge preformed "wax wire," the same as used for open vents in spruing, is best)
—a long, small-diameter plugger or probe
—waxing instruments
—lab tweezers
—Bunsen burner

Figure 22 The wire is cut to proper length to seat fully into the die and extend far enough to form a sprue. It must be definitely smaller in diameter than the post space. One end may have to be tapered (by

rotating it against a revolving Carborundum disc) so that it will seat freely into the die. Its surface should be notched or scarified to enhance retention of the wax.

Figure 23 A length of wax that can be inserted to the end of the post space must be fashioned. This is most easily done by using 18-gauge "wax wire." The middle portion of a length of wax wire is lightly warmed and slowly pulled apart. This forms a finely tapered length of wax that can be inserted to the base of the post space. If preformed wax is not available, a long taper may be formed from sprue wax, beeswax, or other nonbrittle wax.

Figure 24 Excess lubricant is blown from the die, and the wax taper is seated to the base of the post space.

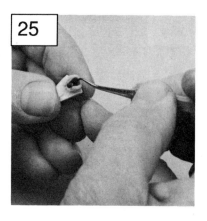
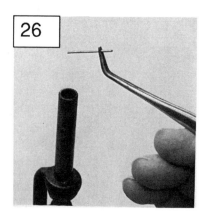
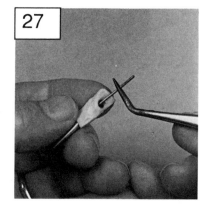
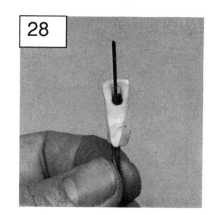

Figure 25   With a small plugger or probe the wax is compacted down into the post space (be very careful not to scrape the die). The post space should be stuffed completely full of wax.

Figure 26   The prepared metal wire is gripped with lab tweezers, and the tapered end is held over a Bunsen flame until hot.

Figure 27   By touching the wire repeatedly to the wax, one can determine when the wire has cooled just enough to not smoke the wax.

Figure 28   The wire is seated to the base of the post space, and wire and wax are allowed to cool completely. Because of surface tension the molten wax will shrink into the post hole as it cools, leaving it well adapted.

Figure 29   The post pattern is removed to verify withdrawal and accuracy of adaptation. If undercuts were present in the die, the soft wax pattern will drag as it is removed. Careful visual inspection will reveal where the wax has been scuffed and pulled by the undercut. This displaced wax can be removed with a sharp carving instrument. The pattern is then reseated and the removal, inspection, and relief procedure is repeated until all excess is removed and the pattern will fully reseat in the die.

Occasionally voids will be present. If small, they are meaningless. If large enough to affect the strength or adaptation of the post, they should be corrected. This can often be done by adding wax in the voided area,

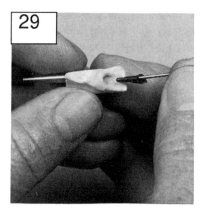
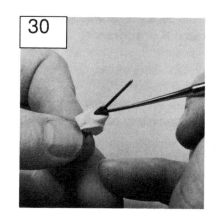

being very careful to keep the addition slightly deficient. The pattern must be reseated immediately to correct any distortion. If the pattern does not fully reseat, or if significant or numerous voids were present, it is best simply to strip the wax from the pin and repeat the pattern process.

Figure 30   Once the post pattern is complete, it is carefully reseated (be certain that it is fully seated) and inlay wax is added as needed to form the core. Proper core form should *always* cover the entire occludable portion of the tooth (occlusal surface of posteriors, incisal edge of mandibular anteriors, lingual and incisal surface of maxillary anteriors). The tooth should have been adequately prepared to permit this. In addition to blanketing the occluding surfaces, the core should replace any missing portion of an ideal stump form (preparation form),

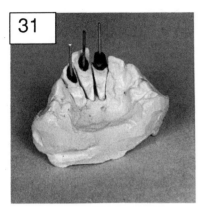

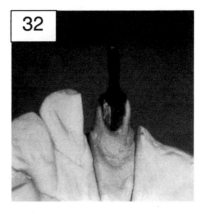

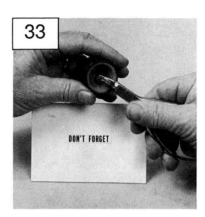

thus ensuring adequate retention form for the crown. However, the core must not be so large as to invade adequate "crown space" either occlusally or axially.

Proper core form is the third challenge that was identified in developing adequate post/core foundations and is just as important as an adequate post. If the core form is too small or tapered, it will not provide adequate retention form for the crown. If too large or improperly contoured, it will interfere with normal crown space and present the dentist with the difficult and time-consuming task of cutting it back to proper form.

Just as when carving an onlay or crown, core contour is determined primarily by relationship to adjacent and opposing teeth. But two factors make this more difficult for a core. First, opposing models are usually not provided. If they are, their use precludes extending the metal wire or pin to be used as a sprue. However, this obstacle can be readily overcome by shortening the pin sufficiently to clear occlusion and then, when the pattern is complete, placing a hollow plastic sprue pin over the exposed end of the reduced pin. (As will be discussed later, the metal pin must be removed from the investment mold prior to making the casting. Pins that are cut off must be removed after burnout by gently tapping the inverted investment ring.) The second problem is that technicians are not initially skilled in determining ideal preparation form. With study and experience this can be learned, however, just like all other aspects of contour.

Figure 31   Core patterns may range from a simple blanket covering the

occluding surfaces to almost the entire stump form for the crown. Unless an opposing model is used to help establish the occlusal dimension of the core, the metal pin should be left long enough to serve as a sprue.

Figure 32   The diameter needed for an adequate sprue can be obtained either by adding wax to the exposed pin or by placing a hollow plastic sprue over the pin. The pattern should be invested as for a full crown. The type of investment depends on the alloy to be used for the casting. Patterns for conventional gold alloy castings can be embedded in hygroscopic investment. Dentists who wish to use the same alloy for both the post/core and crown will often require castings made with one of the several ceramic alloys. These require the use of phosphate-bound investments, which are not covered in this manual.

Figure 33   Burnout of the pattern will depend on the type of investment used.

Do not forget to remove the metal pin before casting!!

When the casting is recovered, it must be thoroughly cleaned. Conventional gold alloys should be carefully pickled in clean solution. Other alloys should be prepared according to manufacturers' directions. The casting should be thoroughly inspected under magnification, and blebs and other irregularities should be completely removed. If available, an air-abrasive unit (using aluminum oxide) is best for final cleaning and finishing.

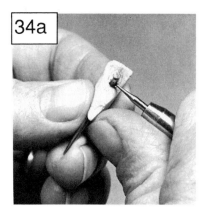
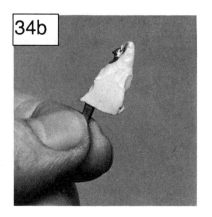
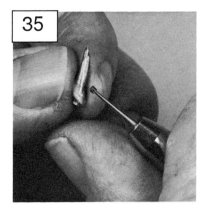
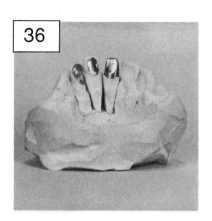

When clean, the post is placed in the die but *not* forced into place. Posts very often bind. The point(s) of interference must be discovered and relieved. These areas can usually be determined by observing abraded stone particles on the surface of the casting or die. It is not critical that the post fit tightly—in fact this is undesirable, as it would create tensile stress in the tooth root. The fit should be stable but passive. Likewise marginal discrepancies are not critical, as all margins should be completely covered by the subsequent crown.

Figure 34   On a simple post (one having no blanket or core form), it is appropriate to form a "button" handle when removing the sprue. This can be accomplished by leaving 1.5 to 2.0 millimeters of the sprue and creating a groove around this sprue stump with either a small round bur or a separating disc. The button will facilitate removal of the post during try-in procedures and then can be removed prior to or just after cementation.

Figure 35   The dentist may wish to have the post vented, to facilitate escape of cement for relief of hydraulic pressure during cementation.

This is easily done by cutting a small groove from the apex of the post to and through the margin of the core form, using either the corner of a bur or a sharp-edged disc. Any metal that is "picked up" during the procedure must be ground away to prevent binding of the post.

Figure 36   The post/core foundation should now be ready for trial insertion by the dentist.

REVIEW QUESTIONS

1. Describe the advantages of two-piece construction of a post and crown.
2. Discuss the advantages and disadvantages of prefabricated and anatomic posts.
3. How are retention form and resistance form provided for in post/core foundations?

SECTION 20

All-metal Bridges

The simplest fixed partial prosthesis is the all-metal bridge, the most popular form of which is commonly called the *hygienic bridge*. The term *hygienic* relates to the contour of the pontic, which is, in essence, a bar of metal that spans the edentulous space. This bar duplicates only the occlusal one-fourth to one-third of the missing tooth. As a result, a space of approximately 2 millimeters is left between the gingival surface of the bar and the crest of the residual ridge (**Figure 1**). This space permits the patient free access to clean the gingival surface of the pontic and the approximating surfaces of the retainers; hence the name "hygienic."

Without question, this form of pontic is the most compatible with the soft tissue, not only because it permits the patient to cleanse the area freely, but primarily because it does not contact tissue and hence cannot irritate it. However, as the all-metal pontic is not esthetic, these bridges are confined almost exclusively to the posterior segments of the mouth. They are the most common type of bridge used in the lower posterior quadrants and also are occasionally used in the maxillary posterior quadrants.

HYGIENIC BRIDGE CONSTRUCTION

The following pages describe the construction of an all-metal hygienic bridge for a dentoform. In this example the working cast was developed from a coping transfer impression—a procedure normally used only for some large multiabutment bridge cases. It is used here to permit review of the technique and to exemplify the resultant working cast.

Retainer Development

Figure 2 When a working cast is to be developed by means of incorporating individually derived dies of the abutments, the dentist must provide a transfer impression into which the dies can be seated. As described in Section 8, the most accurate of such impressions involves either resin or cast metal copings. This example involves cast copings.

Figure 3 If a coping is not absolutely stable in the impression, it should be removed and the relationship of coping and impression carefully evaluated. If a stable relationship cannot be achieved, the transfer impression must be retaken.

Figure 4 If the root portion of the dies has not been tapered to facilitate removal from the working cast, this must now be accomplished. Each die must be accurately seated in its coping. For copings that are readily removable from the impression, it may be desirable to seat the die into the coping and then seat the joined coping and die into the impression.

Figure 5 Once accurately seated, the coping and die must be secured in position. Sticky wax is commonly used. In addition to luting the coping/die unit to the impression, the wax must also block out all undercuts in the exposed surface of the die. Many use molten rope or boxing wax in these areas; baseplate wax may be more convenient,

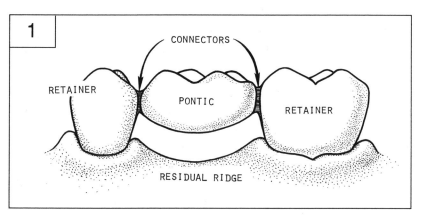

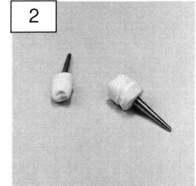

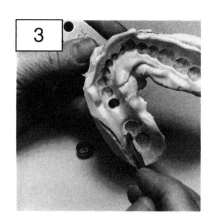

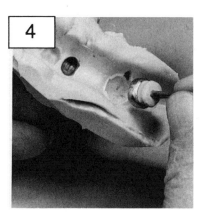

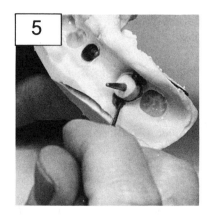

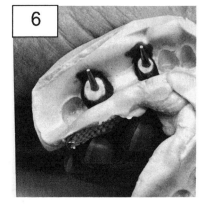

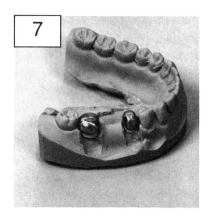

however, because it can be more readily removed from the die after recovery of the model.

Figure 6 After sufficient wax is flowed into place to eliminate all undercuts, it is good technique to extend wax over to the surface of the impression on a level even with the base of the die on the facial surface. This extension of wax will expose the junction between the base of the die and the cast when poured, thus permitting visual inspection for complete seating of the dies. Note that no wax is allowed to flow onto the base portion of the dies, because this surface must provide a positive index with the cast to ensure accurate, stable seating of the die. Gypsum separator is applied to all exposed die surfaces. The cast is poured with a good mix of dental stone, using a minimum of vibration to avoid displacement of the dies and/or copings.

When the base pour of stone has set, the cast may be separated from the impression. Depending upon the number of dies and how fragile they are, the cast may be pulled directly from the impression; or the tray may be separated from the impression and then the impression material carefully removed from the working cast and copings. Any trimming of the cast on a model trimmer must be accomplished before the copings or dies are removed. The dies should be readily removable by tapping or applying pressure on the exposed ends of the dowel pins.

Figure 7 Once the dies are removed, all wax adherent to the die surface or to the die seat area of the working cast is thoroughly removed to eliminate the possibility of its lodging in the dowel pin hole and preventing accurate reseating of the die. Note that the junction between base of die and cast is readily evident as a result of having extended wax in this area prior to pouring the impression.

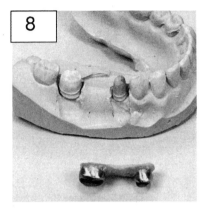

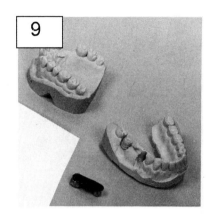

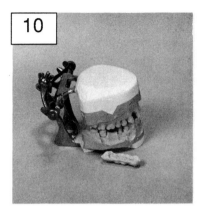

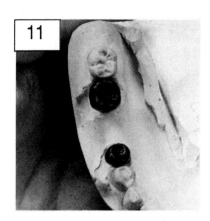

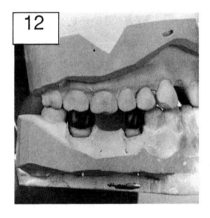

Careful inspection for, and removal of, any blebs on occlusal surfaces of teeth included in the cast completes development of the working cast.

Figure 8 Because the interrelationship of copings may be somewhat unstable when embedded in elastic impression materials, many dentists choose to index the relation of the copings by locking them together in a matrix of Duralay resin (see Section 8). When this approach is used, resin can also be carefully added at appropriate places to index the centric occlusal relationship. Accordingly the dentist may advise that the resin/coping index be recovered from the impression so that it can be seated on the dies to facilitate accurate mounting of the working cast. This technique is especially appropriate when the terminal posterior teeth are involved and in large bridges where most or all of the remaining teeth are involved.

Figure 9 In similar fashion the dentist may choose to use the resin/coping index to form a functional occlusal registration. When this is done, the index can be used both to facilitate mounting the casts in centric and to form a functional core. This approach is exampled here.

Figure 10 With the working cast and its opposing anatomic cast accurately mounted on a simple, rigid articulator, and with the functional core, all necessary occlusal records are at hand to permit proper development of occlusion for the bridge.

Figure 11 Wax patterns for the retainers are developed in the conventional manner. Many points are considered when establishing contour of the retainers. The occlusal surface must be established first. When the functional core is available, it is used to establish gross occlusal contour. It is difficult to establish the entire occlusal surface with the functional core at one time: a buildup approach, involving one cusp at a time, should be employed. The functional core can then be applied to mold each segment of the occlusal table.

Figure 12 When the occlusal table of a given pattern has been formed by the functional core, it is then related to the opposing anatomic cast for verification of centric holding contacts and further evaluation of other occlusal relationships, such as marginal ridge compatibility and occlusal embrasure form, location of grooveways, and amount of horizontal overlap. As mentioned in Section 9, the functional core is an index of maximum noninterfering contour. Appropriate restrictions of this maximum contour must be determined in conjunction with an anatomic opposing cast.

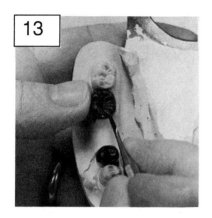
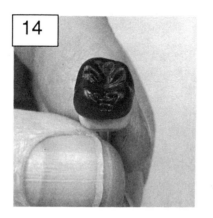
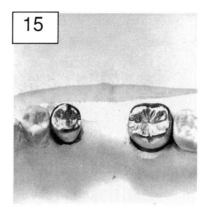
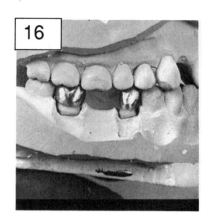

Pontic Development

Three possibilities exist for developing the complete assembly of an all-metal bridge. Each retainer can be waxed and cast, the pontic then waxed and cast, and then the bridge united by two solder joints. The second method is to wax and cast one retainer, usually the anterior; the other retainer and pontic section can then be waxed and cast together, and the bridge united by a single solder joint. The third method is to wax all components individually, unite them, and cast the assembly in one piece. For the novice, it is recommended that the first procedure be followed, as illustrated here.

Figure 13   When a soldered joint is anticipated in the construction of a bridge, a boxed soldering rest is developed in the retainers. Such rests are simply box-like excavations in the occlusoaxial aspect of the pattern next to the proposed pontic. To be effective, these excavations must be 2 to 3 millimeters wide faciolingually and 1 to 2 millimeters deep occlusogingivally.

Figure 14   They can be in the form of a simple box that is approximately 1.0 to 1.5 millimeters deep into the axial surface, or a compound box that has this depth into the axial surface and in addition extends onto the occlusal surface for an additional 1.0 to 1.5 millimeters. Because of the reduction necessary to remove the bell-shaped contour of the proximal surfaces of most posterior teeth to permit draw, sufficient bulk is generally present in this area of the wax pattern to allow an excavation of these dimensions. It is not the purpose of these soldering rests to provide precision fit for the cast pontic; hence no effort need be made to keep the opposing walls parallel or to develop

sharp angles in the box form. The pontic pattern will be waxed with a lug that fits into the boxed rest on the retainer.

Soldering rests are not mandatory for developing an adequate solder joint, but they do serve to help stabilize the pontic wax pattern during its development, and this lug-rest relationship does provide potential for a stronger solder joint. This is not due to the precision fit of the pontic in the rest, but rather to the greater total surface area that is joined by the solder.

The retainers are cast, thoroughly inspected and carefully seated on their dies. If the casting does not readily seat, one must decide whether to risk abrading the die or to remake the casting. If a second set of dies is available, the initial seating should be accomplished on these second dies (see Section 15).

Figure 15   The retainer castings are placed in the working cast and accurately related to their adjacent and opposing structures. The first check to be made when seating the crown in the working cast is proximal contact. If an excess of wax was placed on the pattern to ensure adequate contact, adjustment will have to be made to establish proper contact with the adjacent tooth. If contact is insufficient, due either to original contour of the casting or to subsequent adjustment, this will have to be corrected by soldering. It is usually appropriate to make such soldered corrections at the same time that the joints are soldered.

Figure 16   Occlusion must also be checked and adjustments made before the pontic pattern is developed. First, one must always make sure that dies and castings are completely seated. Necessary adjust-

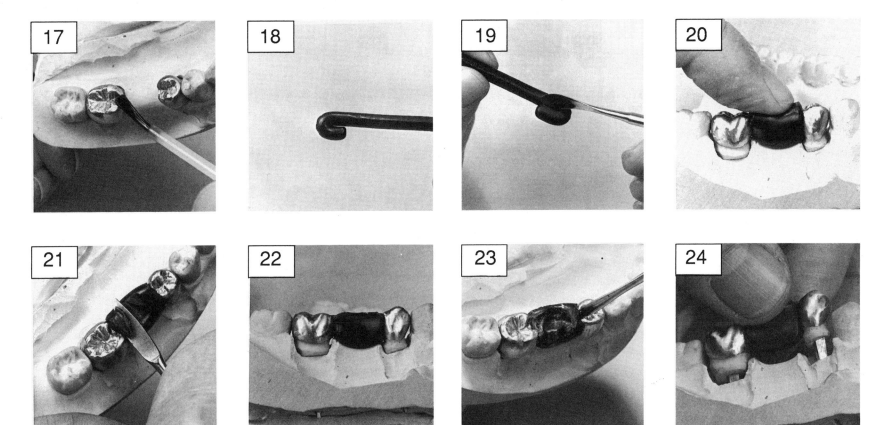

ments may be indicated by applying a dye (Merthiolate) to the core, or by using articulating ribbon with the opposing cast. Either method will indicate premature contacts, which must be selectively ground until the core and/or opposing cast is properly related to the retainers. Length of cusp slopes and position of the occlusal marginal ridge adjacent to the edentulous area are determined by their occlusal relationship. Consideration should be given to the mesiodistal space available for the pontic, especially as this might relate to position and potential for interdigitation of the cusps.

Several possibilities exist for stabilizing a bulk of wax in proper position during the carving of the pontic; the example shown here is adequate for most situations.

Figure 17   Die lubricant is applied to the soldering rests of the retainers.

Figure 18   A stick of inlay wax is softened and bent double to a length slightly in excess of that of the edentulous space.

Figure 19   The folded surfaces of the wax stick are sealed together with a hot spatula. The folded segment is sectioned from the stick.

Figure 20   This softened wax can be molded somewhat with the fingertips and is pressed into place between the retainers against the crest of the edentulous ridge.

Figure 21   Any gross excess is removed with a suitable instrument.

Figure 22   The wax mass should be firmly seated and may be sealed with a hot instrument against the edentulous ridge area of the cast for stability.

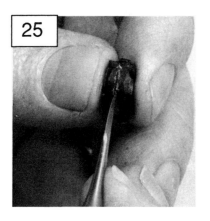
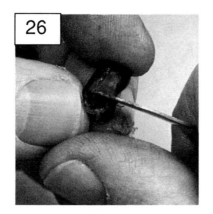
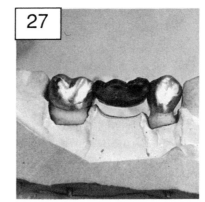
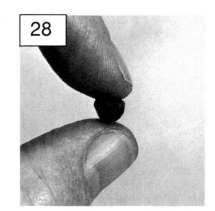

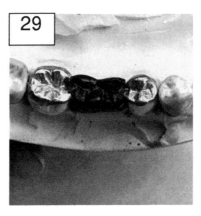
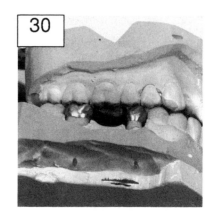

Figure 23   Wax is flowed into the soldering rest areas to help stabilize the position of the wax mass. The occlusal table is formed using the functional core and the anatomic opposing cast. Contour and anatomic detail of the occlusal surface are completed before the wax is removed from the cast. The appropriate location of contact of the centric holding cusps should always be kept in mind. It should be remembered that the functional core represents maximum nonpremature contact. Overextension and excessive steepness of cusp slopes must be corrected.

Figure 24   When the occlusal surface is completed, the pattern is removed from the working cast.

Figure 25   The crest of the residual ridge is evident in the gingival surface of the wax pattern. This area is scribed from mesial to distal with a sharp instrument to a depth of about 2 millimeters.

Figure 26   With the scribed groove serving as a depth gauge, gross excess is removed from the facial and lingual aspects of the gingival surface of the pattern to provide clearance between the pattern and crest of the residual ridge.

Figure 27   This clearance should be a minimum of 1.5 millimeters, preferably 2 millimeters, and should follow the mesiodistal outline of the crest of the edentulous ridge.

Figure 28   The facial and lingual aspects of the gingival surface of the pontic are rounded to produce a *heart-shaped* form in cross section. The linear vertex should be directly over the crest of the residual ridge.

Figures 29 through 31   The pontic pattern is returned to the working cast to verify occlusal contour and relationship and overall contour. The pattern is now ready to be sprued and invested.

Figure 32   Conventionally such patterns have been sprued in the center of the gingival surface. This technique often results in porosity in the area surrounding the sprue, due to shrinkage. A more effective method is to attach the sprue to one end of the pattern, just beneath the soldering lug. This method keeps the pattern ahead of the sprue and establishes an effective position for placement of an open vent. During casting, molten alloy will fill this large, open mold cavity progressively, from the remote end back toward the sprue—like pouring water in a bucket. As a result mold gases are backed up toward the sprue. Therefore the terminal flow point, and hence the most efficient and effective position for an open vent to be placed, is level with or below

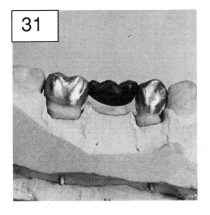

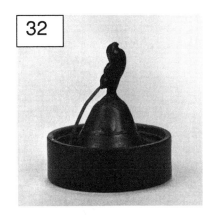

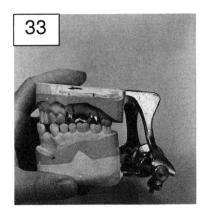

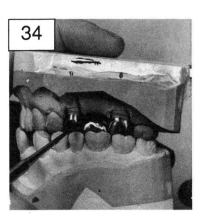

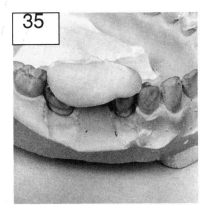

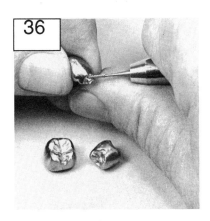

gingival surface is easier now than it will be after the bridge is united and margins of the retainers are present to restrict access to this area.

Soldering

The pontic is related to the retainers by placing it in the working cast in proper centric occlusion. For a mandibular bridge, this positioning is facilitated by inverting the articulator so that gravity will hold the pontic in position against the occlusal surfaces of the opposing teeth.

Figure 34 Once it is ascertained that the retainers and their dies are accurately seated and that the pontic is in accurate centric occlusion, this position is stabilized by the addition of sticky wax to the joint areas.

Figure 35 Transfer of the relationship between the pontic and its retainers for investment soldering is done by means of a plaster occlusal index. The quick-set plaster should index only the occlusal one-fourth of the castings.

Figure 36 The joint areas of the retainers and the pontic are carefully cleaned before the assembly is invested for soldering. This is most effectively accomplished by machining, which also provides the necessary clearance (.005 to .01 inch) for the joint area between the retainers and the pontic.

Figure 37 The plaster index should be trimmed with a sharp knife such that only a registration of the occlusal surface remains.

the supply sprue. Such a position is readily available at the soldering lug on the pattern. If shrink-spot porosity were to occur under these conditions, it would be located in the area of the solder joint and could be corrected by the solder.

The wax wire establishing the open vent channel is attached to the crucible former (sprue base) as close to the ring as is possible without conflicting with the ring or its liner. Because the dimensions of the pontic are not extremely critical, it may be invested at a convenient water/powder ratio, normally the same ratio used for full crowns. Casting and cleaning are accomplished in a conventional manner.

Figure 33 The cast pontic is surfaced and smoothed. The gingival surface of the pontic is smoothed to final form. Finishing of the

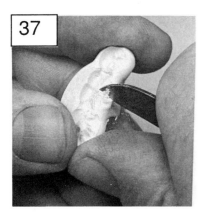
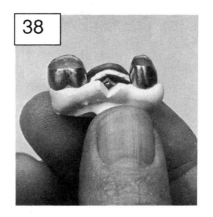
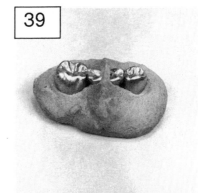
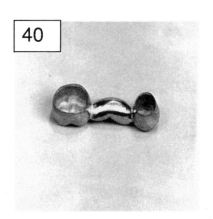

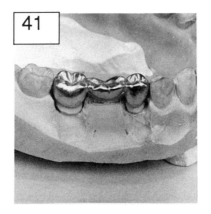
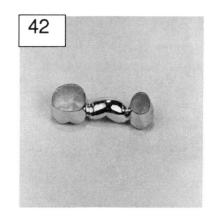

Figure 38 After careful inspection to see that no debris is present in the index or on the occlusal surfaces of the castings, the units of the bridge are assembled in the plaster index. Some provision must be made to allow the soldering investment to lock the pontic into position. This is best accomplished by carving a notch in the plaster index in the area of the occlusofacial and occlusolingual grooves of the pontic.

Because of the soldering lugs, the pontic must be positioned in the index first and should be stabilized by spot luting with sticky wax along its facial and lingual borders. A very thin film of flux is placed on the joint surfaces.

When the retainers are positioned in the index, they are held firmly in place while sticky wax is added to the joint area and allowed to cool. Additional sticky wax or utility wax is built up and extended facially and lingually to provide an airway beneath the joint in the investment. Thus the wax placed in the joint areas serves three functions: it stabilizes position of the units, seals the joint against debris and contaminants, and provides a future airway in the investment. Investing is accomplished in the conventional manner (see Section 16).

Figure 39 The rib of investment reaches across the occlusal surface of the pontic to serve as a tie-down or lock. Stabilization of the pontic position is important for three reasons. First, it prevents the pontic from being dislodged from its position by the air blast from the torch. Secondly, it maintains relationships if the investment block tips over during the soldering operation. Thirdly, it prevents effervescence of the flux from dislodging the pontic from its position during the early stages of preheating.

Wax is flushed from the assembly with boiling water or under the force of hot tap water. Flux is added to the joint areas, and the soldering operation is completed (see Section 16).

Finishing

Figure 40 After soldering, the joint areas are surfaced and contoured.

Figure 41 The bridge is carefully replaced on the working cast to verify accuracy of relationship. If the relationship is inaccurate, a decision must be made as to which joint will be desoldered. Clearance in the desoldered joint is established with burs or stones, a new index is made, and the joint resoldered.

Occlusion must also be rechecked and adjusted in the areas of the

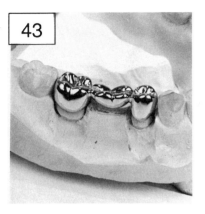
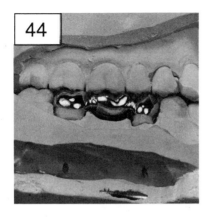
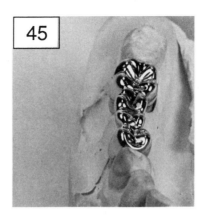

joints. The marginal ridge and occlusal embrasure between pontic and retainer must be established.

Figure 42 When contouring is complete, the bridge is ready for polishing. The finished bridge should be devoid of any scratches or irregularities. This is particularly important on the gingival surface of the pontic and about the margins of the retainers. The gingival surface of the pontic and joint areas should be smoothly rounded, with no sharp angles or grooves.

Figure 43 The bridge should be reseated on the working cast and adequacy of the proximal contact areas checked. Embrasure forms and the relationship of the vertex of the gingival surface of the pontic with the crest of the residual ridge are reexamined.

Figure 44 A final evaluation of occlusion verifies the position of centric contacts, functional and nonfunctional relationships, and overjet (horizontal overlap).

Figure 45 Heights of contour of the facial and lingual surfaces should be compatible with the adjacent teeth. Marginal ridge height and cuspal inclination should also be consistent with adjacent teeth. The alignment of facial cusps and reduction in lingual dimension (especially of the pontic) is evident in this photograph.

The beauty of a properly finished bridge provides a satisfaction of accomplishment that justifies the hours of artistic and technical effort required for its development.

REVIEW QUESTIONS

1. What is the simplest fixed partial prosthesis?
2. What are the features of a hygienic bridge?
3. Name the parts of a fixed partial prosthesis.
4. What are the three ways or possibilities for developing the complete assembly of an all-metal bridge?
5. What are the usual effective dimensions, occlusogingivally and faciolingually, of a soldering rest?
6. What is the minimum clearance between pontic pattern and the crest of the residual ridge of a hygienic bridge?

Porcelain-faced Bridges

Just as the first modern denture teeth were made of porcelain, so were the first modern facings for fixed partial dentures. Through the years, several types of facings have been developed for this purpose. Porcelain denture teeth were initially used as such facings, and on occasion are still used for that purpose. It is important to realize that for many years the porcelain denture tooth or porcelain facing was the only esthetic veneer available for fixed replacement of missing teeth. Manufactured resin facings, processed resin facings, and porcelain-fused-to-metal are now used in addition to the porcelain facings.

Most of the facings that have been developed through the years are still made today, though possibly by different manufacturers. However, use of manufactured porcelain facings has decreased markedly during recent years due to the advent and growing popularity of porcelain-fused-to-metal restorations. Other than denture teeth, the facings available for pontic construction can be grouped into two categories: *pin facings* and *slot facings*. In general, the slot facings are intended to be interchangeable; these are dealt with as a group in Section 22.

Figure 1 Pin facings are available with long and short pins, and in a variety of shades and molds, both anterior and posterior. They are used with metal coverage to protect their incisal or occlusal edges. One facing with pins, the Pin Pontic, is designed so that it might be used without metal coverage of the incisal if desired. This facing is available only in anterior molds.

As mentioned in the brief discussion of the porcelain-faced crown in Section 2, any of these facings or a porcelain denture tooth may be used for establishing a veneer for a crown. Porcelain-faced crowns are seldom used, although porcelain-faced pontics are still employed. The retainers for such bridges are usually either partial crowns or resin-faced crowns.

MAXILLARY POSTERIOR BRIDGE WITH PORCELAIN-FACED PONTICS

Figure 2 This example involves a bridge between the maxillary left canine and first molar. Modified three-quarter crowns are used as retainers on both abutments. For contrast, the facings for the premolar pontics will be developed from a denture tooth and a long-pointed pin facing.

A full arch cast with removable dies for the abutments and adjacent teeth has been developed from a tray rubber impression. Note that the residual ridge has been carefully preserved in the base pour of the cast. Such preservation requires careful placement of strips and the wax used to locate the strips, or careful placement of saw cuts.

Figure 3 Establishing occlusion for a porcelain-faced construction is extremely critical. This is because (1) The facings are contoured and positioned on the working cast in the laboratory; (2) castings are made dependent on such positioning without the possibility of trial insertion in the patient; and (3) the limited thickness of gold covering the incisal or occlusal of such facings places definite constraints on the correction of any occlusal discrepancies produced by the mounted casts. If an

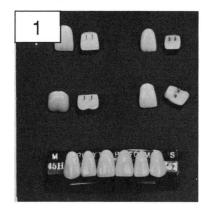
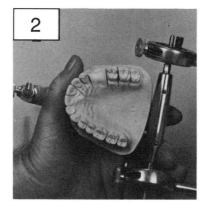
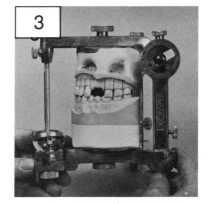
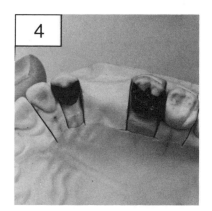

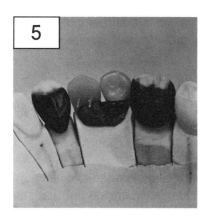
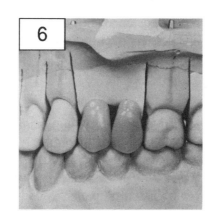
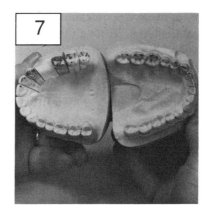
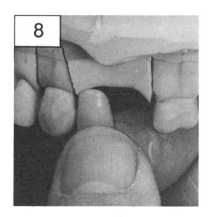

effort has been made to be esthetically conservative with the dimension of the gold coverage on the occlusal of the facings, there is little latitude for error. Consequently such bridges should be constructed on carefully adjusted semi- or fully adjustable articulators.

Retainer Development

Figure 4   Patterns for the retainers are waxed. One should remember that internal adaptation for partial crowns must be extremely accurate. Attention must be given to the position and stability of centric contacts, and to the functional contacts that are appropriate to these retainers. Canine contour is extremely important in lateral guidance and must normally provide for positive functional contact from centric all the way to terminal functional relationship.

Figure 5   Before the retainer patterns are sprued and invested for

casting, the size and position of the pontic facings is determined, as these factors may influence the desired contour of the approximating retainer surfaces.

Figure 6   Ideally the pontic facings should be wide enough to fill the edentulous space without display of alloy on the proximal of the retainers. This is especially significant in the anterior facial embrasure (between canine and premolar).

Figure 7   When the retainer patterns are complete, they should be carefully sprued and invested. Careful investing of the partial crown is imperative to assure a snug fit. (Because of their design—limited coverage and dimension—and because of the stress that could be expected to be applied to a bridge of this span, the retainers shown here were cast using a Type IV alloy.) After careful inspection, the retainers

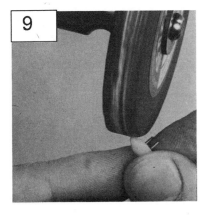
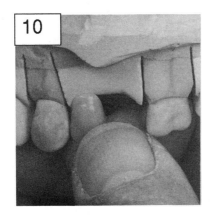
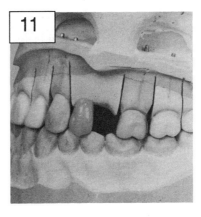
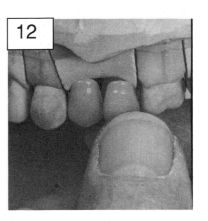

are seated on their respective dies and examined for accuracy of fit. Proximal contacts are verified as the castings are seated in the working cast. Once accurately seated, the castings must be carefully inspected and adjusted for centric and functional occlusal contact.

Positioning and Contouring Pontic Facings

Figure 8 A Trubyte long-pointed pin facing has been selected for the first premolar pontic. It will be developed with a baked porcelain gingival tip. The facing is held in approximate position against the cast to evaluate tip contour as it relates to residual ridge contour. As seen in the photograph, reduction is usually necessary to provide clearance in the area of the papilla adjacent to the abutment. The ultimate objective is to establish a uniform clearance of approximately 1 millimeter between the tip of the facing and the residual ridge to provide room for addition of the baked porcelain tip.

At the time this is being considered, a decision must also be made as to length of the facing. Usually a facing that is somewhat too long is selected. In such cases a choice must be made as to whether the gingival or occlusal end of the facing will be shortened. Several factors are important to this decision.

The most critical factor is the location of the pins in relation to the crest of the residual ridge and the opposing teeth. Sufficient clearance must be provided between the opposing teeth and the pins, and between the crest of the residual ridge and the pins, to allow for adequate coverage with gold alloy.

Another factor is the height of contour of the proximal surfaces of the facing. It is desirable to take advantage of the proximal contact heights of contour that are present on the facing. To do so, this contour must be matched to the proximal contact area of the adjacent retainer. Such matching will limit the occlusogingival position of the facing. The facial height of contour of the facing is less important but must be considered.

If other factors permit, the decision whether to grind the gingival or incisal of the facing may be based on desired shade. This choice may permit a reduction of the amount (distribution) of either the gingival or incisal shade of the facing. In the example shown here, grinding was done on the gingival.

Figure 9 The gingival end of the facing is shaped to conform with residual ridge contour either by minimum reduction, or by reduction sufficient to permit a gingival shift in the occlusogingival position of the facing. Fine-grit Carborundum or diamond stones on the bench lathe or in the handpiece may be used for contouring the facing.

Figure 10 By trial and error the gingival end of the facing is contoured to conform generally with the shape of the ridge.

Figure 11 With gross contour of the gingival end established, the facing is positioned on the working cast to evaluate other relationships. If necessary the occlusal of the facing may be reduced to facilitate positioning. Note in this photograph the desirable gingival embrasure and proximal contact form between the facing and the adjacent canine abutment.

Figure 12 A porcelain denture tooth is used for the second premolar

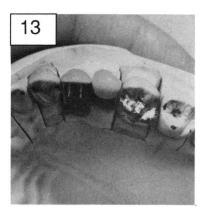

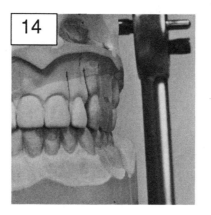

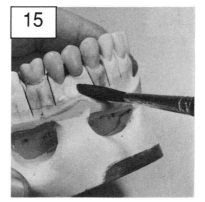

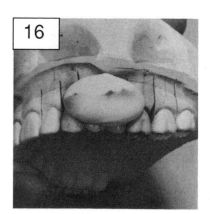

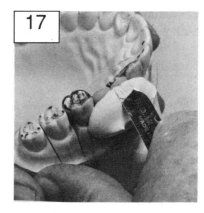

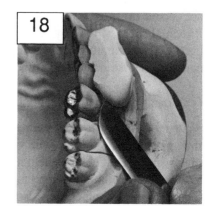

facing. This example is appropriate, as situations occur where there is not sufficient space between crest of residual ridge and opposing occlusal surfaces to permit placement of a pin facing that will allow sufficient coverage of the pins by the casting. In these cases a pinless facing is necessary. Shade selection and availability of pin facings may also favor the use of denture teeth for facings. Adjustment of the gingival contour for this facing proceeds essentially the same as for the long-pin facing, even though the gingival tip of this pontic is to be formed of gold alloy.

When length is established, proximal or occlusal reductions sufficient to permit positioning of the facing should be made if necessary.

Figures 13 and 14 The facings are carefully positioned to align their facial and proximal surfaces with the arch. Their potential occlusal relationship with their opponents must also be considered. Proper horizontal overbite should be obtained by positioning; proper vertical overbite may be obtained by subsequent reduction for occlusal clearance. Note that utility wax is placed at the linguogingival aspect of the facings to facilitate positioning.

Figure 15 Once a final accurate positioning of the facings has been obtained, a positive index must be made to record this position permanently. This is easily done by making a facial plaster index. Gypsum separator is generously applied to the exposed surfaces of the adjacent dies and land area.

Figure 16 A firm mix of quick-set plaster is puddled over the facings

and adjacent land area. The utility wax prevents plaster from extending through the embrasures. The plaster should not be allowed to extend over the incisal edge of the facings or adjacent teeth.

Figure 17 The facial index is beveled short of the incisal edges of the facings to permit visual access for evaluation of occlusal relationships. This is done with a sharp knife before the plaster completely sets, or may be accomplished later on a model trimmer.

Figures 18 and 19 When set, the plaster index is teased from the working cast. The facings may remain locked in the index because plaster extends into the embrasures. To prevent this (which may be annoying during subsequent procedures), the plaster extending into the embrasures is trimmed away with a sharp instrument. Once the final position of the facings is established, reduction for occlusal clearance

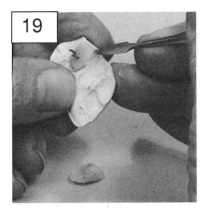

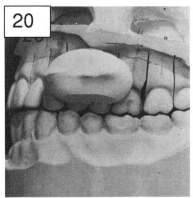

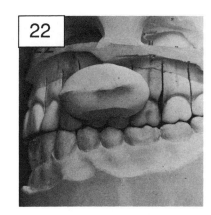

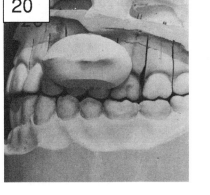

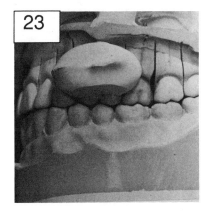

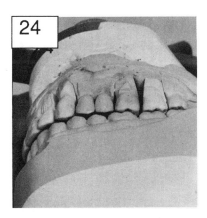

must be accomplished. This is best done with the plaster index in position to stabilize the accurate positional relationship of the facings.

Figure 20   The occlusal surface must be reduced to provide a minimum of 1 millimeter clearance between the facing and the opposing teeth (in all excursions). This space is required to provide an adequate thickness of alloy for the occlusal surface. Though not esthetic, such coverage is necessary if the facing is to be protected from occlusal forces. This illustration demonstrates adequate clearance of the distal arm of the facings, but little or no clearance exists on the mesial arm of the facings in the terminal functional relationship (end-to-end position).

Figure 21   The mesial arm of the first premolar facing is reduced to provide adequate clearance. Occlusal or incisal reductions are made at

a 45° angle to the lingual to provide maximum alloy coverage of the occlusal surface of the facing.

Figure 22   The first premolar facing has been reduced to provide uniform clearance on both mesial and distal arms as it is evaluated in centric occlusion and excursive movements. This illustration shows the uniform clearance available with the teeth related in terminal function (end-to-end) position.

Figure 23   Comparable adjustment is made for the second premolar facing. This view of the functional position of the facings with the opposing teeth shows that there will be an even distribution of alloy along the occlusofacial angle of both facings.

Figure 24   Due to the *inclined* reduction of their occlusal surfaces, there is ample clearance between the facings and opposing teeth in centric occlusion.

Final preparations must be made for developing the gingival tips of the pontics before the backings may be waxed. In the examples that follow, the second premolar pontic will be developed with an alloy tip; the first premolar pontic will be developed with a baked porcelain tip. This is being done for illustrative purposes. Under normal circumstances all pontic tips in a given bridge would probably be the same type and design.

The dentist determines the type of pontic tip and indicates it on the work authorization. A *ridge-lap tip* is developed by adapting the wax pattern and/or the porcelain directly to the unmodified residual ridge.

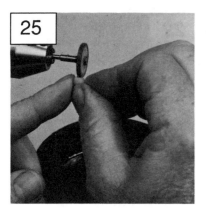 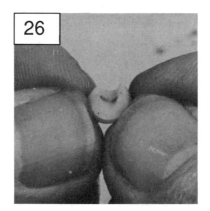 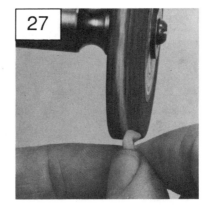 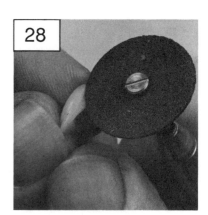

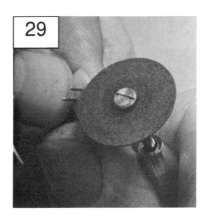 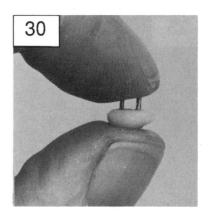

The dentist may prescribe that the ridge be smoothed to avoid incorporating any irregularities in the tip. This is accomplished by lightly scraping or sanding smooth the residual ridge area on the working cast.

The *convex pontic tip* involves slight compression of the soft tissue covering the residual ridge. This should be less than 0.5 millimeters and is developed by relieving the residual ridge on the working cast. This may be done with hand instruments (such as a knife or vulcanite scrapers) or rotary instruments (mounted stones, discs, carbide trimmers, and the like). The decision as to amount of relief, and hence the amount of compression of soft tissue that will occur when the bridge is placed in the mouth, is made by the dentist on the basis of examination of the soft tissue covering the edentulous ridge. The best way to indicate the amount of relief is for the dentist to relieve the working cast. On occasion, however, the technician may be directed to accomplish this relief. An orderly sequence for this procedure is presented here.

The desired occlusogingival length of the facing was previously determined as illustrated in **Figure 15**. The facing tip should not be allowed to extend into contact with alveolar mucosa, and areas of frenal attachment must be avoided. The desired extension of the facing tips is determined by compromise between matching the length and facial prominence of adjacent teeth and providing facial contour that blends smoothly with contour of the residual ridge.

Figure 25   Retention for the second premolar facing is developed by hollow-grinding the lingual surface of the denture tooth. Mounted stones or diamonds in a bench lathe or handpiece may be used. Frequent dipping of the facing in water provides a coolant and lubricant for the grinding procedure.

Figure 26   The facing is ground so as to provide opposing parallel internal walls.

Figures 27 and 28   In addition, external opposing walls are provided by beveling or boxing with mounted stones or discs (See **Figure 31**).

Figures 29 and 30   A Carborundum disc is used to bevel the linguoproximal angles of the pin facing. The incisal bevel (created during occlusal adjustment) should be made smooth and continuous with the proximal bevels. Care must be taken to avoid scarring the pins.

Figure 31   The bevels placed on the proximal aspects of each of the facings should be extended to coincide with the finish lines of the adjacent facing and retainer. When esthetically acceptable, it is advisable slightly to overextend the finish line or bevel on the distal of

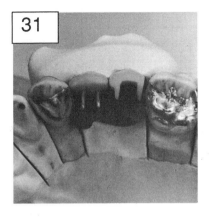

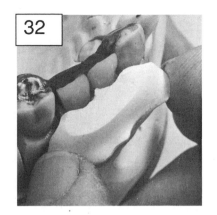

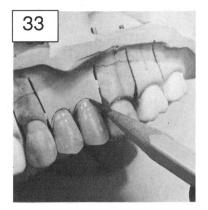

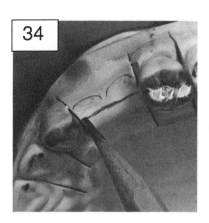

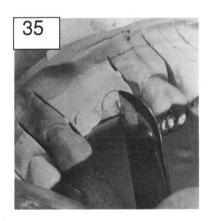

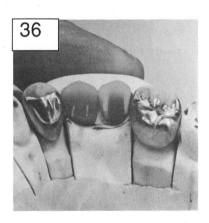

posterior pontics to provide better access to this margin and the subsequent soldered joint.

As shown in this photograph the facings are appropriately positioned and the proximal bevels properly extended.

Developing the Pontic Tips

Figure 32   To evaluate ridge relationship, the facings are carefully stabilized with utility wax and the plaster facial index is removed.

Figure 33   Correct positioning (extension) of the tips of the facings is obtained by additional contouring if necessary. Once correct, this position can be scribed directly on the cast by tracing the outline of the facings.

Figure 34   The area of contact for the convex pontic tip should extend from the location of its facial edge to the crest of the residual ridge. When a line is traced along the crest of the ridge, an outline of tissue contact to be established by the pontic tips will become evident.

Figure 35   The ridge is relieved to present a slightly concave form that will receive a convex pontic tip. (See **Section 2, Figure 37**).

Figure 36   With the ridge altered, the facings are positioned to permit evaluation of the space available for placement of the tip material.

Development of a baked porcelain tip (first premolar pontic in this example) requires a minimum clearance of 1 millimeter between the faciogingival edge of the facing and the relieved ridge for placement of porcelain. If relief of the ridge has not provided the desired clearance, the facing should be shortened so as to provide ample clearance.

Because the manipulation of porcelain is not covered in this manual, the technique for developing the baked porcelain tip is not presented here. Suffice it to say that at this point a grossly convex porcelain tip is arbitrarily established on the facing by the addition of baked porcelain.

Figure 37   The facing with the baked tip addition is illustrated. Note that the tip has purposely been made oversize, and that the lingual shelf is slightly divergent with the retentive pins, thus facilitating draw.

Figure 38   A proximal view of the facing, showing the roughly convex form of the baked tip.

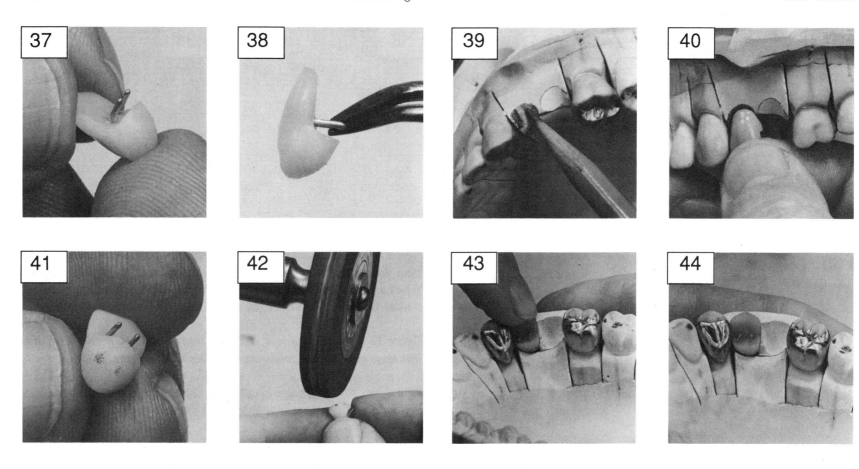

Figure 39　The ridge area on the working cast is blackened with a soft lead pencil to facilitate determination of points of contact between the facing tip and ridge.

Figure 40　Initially, the facing is grossly positioned with the fingertips and lightly rubbed against the cast to mark areas of contact.

Figure 41　Points of contact are evidenced by the transfer of the pencil carbon to the pontic tip.

Figure 42　Contour of the tip is adjusted by grinding with appropriate stones.

Figure 43　After gross corrections are accomplished, more accurate positioning of the facing is accomplished by carrying it to place with the plaster index.

Figure 44　By repeated trial, the facing tip is adjusted until it can be reseated in its correct position as indicated by the plaster facial index.

Figure 45　Final smoothing and shaping to an arbitrary convex form is accomplished using fine stones and rubber abrasive wheels. A glass-like smoothness is desired to enhance biologic acceptance by the soft tissues against which the tip will be imposed. The tip should be smoothed as much as possible before being glazed. To obtain this smoothness, abrasive rubber porcelain-polishing wheels may be used, preferably on a wet surface. A wet rag wheel and flour of pumice is another effective means of smoothing the tip surface. When smooth, the facing is returned to the porcelain furnace for glazing of the tip.

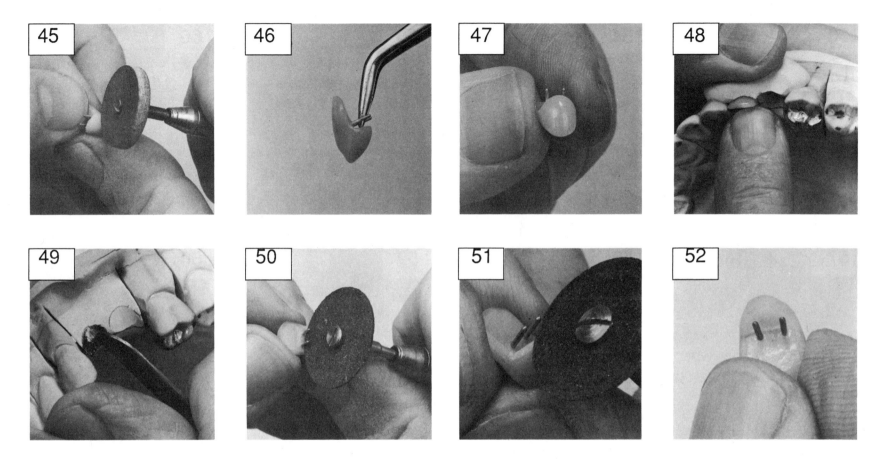

Figures 46 and 47   The glaze firing should result in a smoothly convex glass surface.

Figures 48 and 49   Once the tip is glazed, no further alterations should be made on the tissue contacting area. If any conflict is discovered upon reseating the facing against the working cast, the tip must be relieved and reglazed. Any needed correction of the incisal or proximal bevels should be made with appropriate stones or discs.

Figure 50   This leaves only the lingual shelf to be prepared before the wax pattern for the backing is developed. If the shelf surface is irregular, or not in line with the desired path of draw, it may be corrected by discing. One must avoid any scuffing of the retentive pins.

Figure 51   The cavosurface angle of the shelf must be beveled to provide a finish line for the pattern and backing. This bevel, easily made with a Carborundum disc, should be extended to blend with the proximal bevels. Here again, it is important to avoid scarring the pins.

Figure 52   If the pins are not quite parallel at this point, they should be carefully bent to provide parallelism.

Figure 53   The position of the bevels in relation to the adjacent retainer and the residual ridge should be evaluated. The junction line between the facing and backing should never be allowed to contact soft tissue.

The second premolar facing, which is to have a tip formed by gold, has been acutely beveled so as to provide a positive finish line at the faciogingival angle of the facing. Ideally, this permits gold to form the

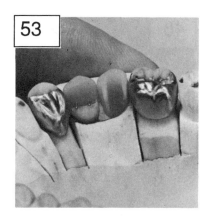
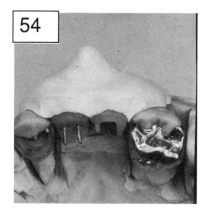
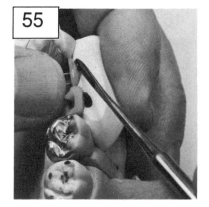
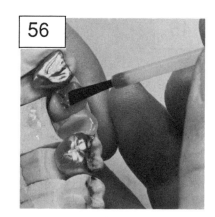

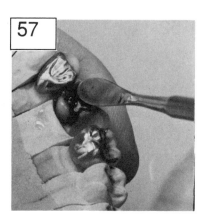
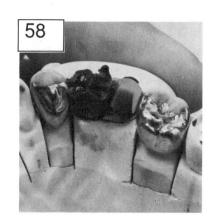
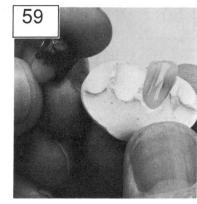
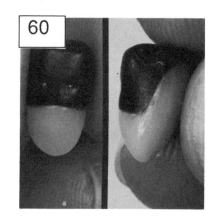

entire tissue contacting surface, even though gold is restricted in facial extension so that it is not displayed along the gingival margin of the facing.

Waxing the Pontics

Figure 54   The proximal bevel and occlusal relationship between the two facings is verified. If necessary, the facings are repositioned and a new index poured.

Figure 55   To ensure that the facing is maintained in position during waxing, it may be luted to the plaster index with sticky wax.

Figure 56   Die lubricant is applied to the facing, adjacent retainer, and adjacent surface area of the working cast.

Figure 57   Wax is added by flow-on addition with a wax spatula.

Figure 58   When the buildup of wax is sufficient, occlusal relationship is registered.

Figure 59   When the gross buildup is complete, it may be desirable to remove the facing and pattern from the index to facilitate carving.

Figure 60   This illustrates a typical problem encountered in developing a backing for the baked-tip pontic. Note that two definite dimples are required to expose the ends of the retentive pins in the pattern. Such dimples are breaks in normal contour and are undesirable. Two possibilities exist for overcoming this problem. One is to wax the pattern to full contour, leaving the pins covered with wax. This is the usual and most simple procedure. However, to facilitate seating and cementing the facing, many prefer that the pins remain exposed. Hence the second possibility is to alter the contour of the pattern and/or the porcelain tip so as to reduce the thickness of the backing in the area of the pins. This

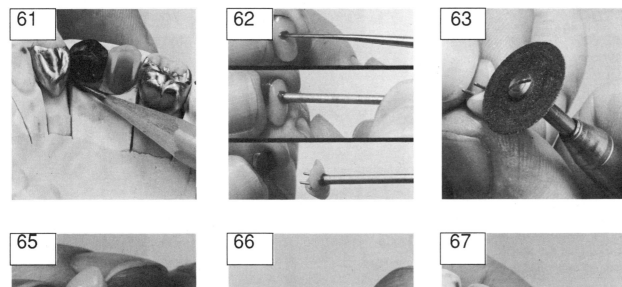

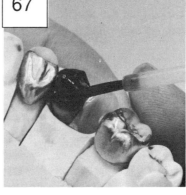

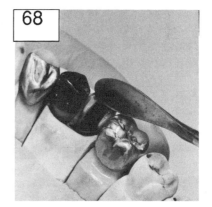

approach is preferred if consistent with the desired final contour of the pontic. The limiting factors in effecting these changes in contour are that (1) the lingual cusp tip of the pattern must be maintained in position to provide a postive centric stop, (2) the porcelain tip cannot be altered on the tissue-contacting surface without reglazing, and (3) the finish line (alloy-porcelain junction) must be kept from contacting soft tissue.

Figure 61 If it is desired to keep the ends of the pins exposed, the facing and pattern for the backing are repositioned in the working cast and evaluated. It is evident that the finish line between the tip and backing may be moved gingivalward without bringing it into contact with the edentulous ridge. Because of the taper of the porcelain tip, such a shift of the finish line will result in a reduction of the faciolingual dimension of the backing in the area of the pins.

Figure 62 The facing is separated from its backing. A steel bur or metal sprue pin inserted into a drop of hot sticky wax makes a convenient handle for the facing.

Figure 63 The bevel is extended so as to move it gingivalward.

Figure 64 Lubricant is again applied to the facing, especially in the area of the correction.

Figure 65 Wax is applied to the area of the shelf margin to reestablish contour of the pattern. Light fingertip pressure on the softened wax as it hardens ensures good adaptation.

Figure 66 The tip and backing pattern now form a smooth, continuous surface without any depressions. (Compare **Figure 60**, which shows the undesirable dimpled contour.)

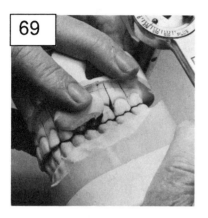

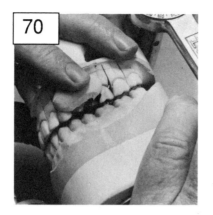

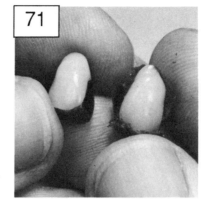

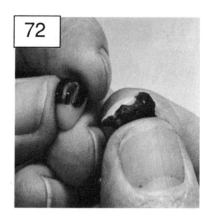

Figure 67   With all units repositioned in the working cast, and with die lubricant applied, the pattern for the backing of the second premolar facing can be initiated. Note that die lubricant is applied to the adjacent cast retainers and pontic wax patterns.

Figure 68   Wax is applied by the flow-on technique with a suitable spatula. (Gross additions of wax before the facing has been seated in the working cast make it easier to ensure adaptation, but more difficult to establish relationships with adjacent structures.)

Figure 69   Occlusion may be established by building to excess, registering occlusal relationship, and then carving back. However, the buildup technique of establishing the position of cusp tips, then waxing in cusp slopes and marginal ridges, is preferred. In either case it is important that centric contacts be positively established and accurately located.

Figure 70   Because this situation presents a segmented-group-function occlusion, contact is being established throughout the full range of functional excursion.

Figure 71   The pontics are removed to complete the margins and final contour.

Figure 72   The two pontics separate easily if the first was lubricated correctly and not touched with the hot spatula.

Figure 73   The proximal excess is removed.

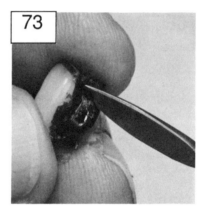

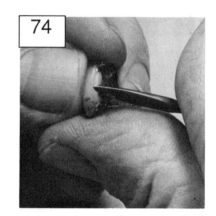

Figure 74   The wax buildup of the second premolar backing was established directly on the cast, resulting in a saddle-tip configuration. The lingual bulk of this wax is reduced to establish a convex or modified ridge-lap tip form, and the pattern is carved to margin.

Figure 75   The pontics are repositioned in the working cast for final evaluation of form and extension. If soldering rests have been developed in the retainer castings, the pontic lugs should be waxed at this time.

Figures 76 and 77   A final, careful check for adaptation of margins and surface smoothness is made for each backing pattern. Note that the occlusal margin of the pattern has been carved in line with the surface of the facing and has not been "rolled" or rounded. This rounding will be accomplished after the casting is made and should not be done in the

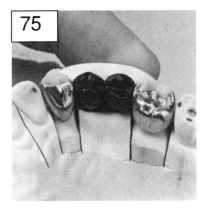
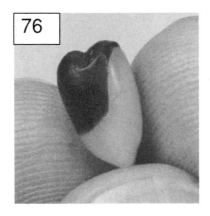
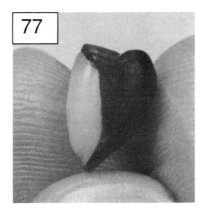
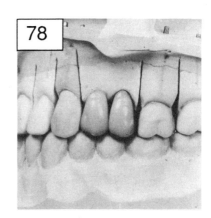

wax pattern stage, as this creates a tendency for short margins. In **Figure 77** the gingival margin has been handled in the same manner.

Figure 78   The pontics are repositioned in the working cast via the plaster facial index for final evaluation of position, marginal extension, and occlusion. If it is desired that the backings be cast in one piece, they may be luted together at this time. This is accomplished using a heated explorer tine or other suitable thin-bladed instrument to melt the adjacent backing surfaces together. This is done from a lingual and occlusal approach, being careful not to involve the margins. However, the union must closely approach the facial margins in order to prevent the formation of a crevice between the backings and to provide adequate strength in the joint. Some alteration of the lingual and occlusal marginal ridge contour will usually result and must be corrected before casting. The union must be smoothly filleted.

Investing and Casting the Pontics

Casting two or more backings in one piece creates a strong union, less probability of distortion of relationship, and elimination of a critical investment soldering procedure. However, potential marginal distortion during the luting procedure, and a more complex spruing, investing, and casting procedure are disadvantages. In addition, a one-piece casting may make it more difficult to reseat the facings in their respective backings; it also becomes almost impossible to gain access to the interposed proximal margins for polishing and finishing them to the facings. Whether the backings are cast together or individually is essentially a matter of personal preference. In this example they have

been cast individually to provide better access for photographs and to permit demonstration of the soldering procedure.

The appropriate position for attachment of the sprue is on the lingual aspect of the lingual cusp for both of these backings. The sprue must not destroy the accuracy of the centric contact. It should be attached before the backing is separated from its facing, and should be of large diameter (8 or 10 gauge).

Special consideration must be given to accurate maintenance of the pin holes in the backing for the pin facing. Two basic techniques are available. The first is to allow investment to fill the holes in the pattern. This can be done only when the pin holes pass completely through the backing and are open at both ends. Such small rods of investment extending across the mold cavity are fragile and subject to fracture under the pressure of the molten alloy as it rushes into the mold. Moreover, these investment rods may have an irregular surface, making it difficult later to seat the pins in the casting. The investment procedure for duplication of the pin holes is not recommended.

The other technique involves the placement of some rod of appropriate diameter into or through the pattern pin holes about which the casting can be made. Two types of rods are commonly used: carbon rods, and stainless steel wire. Carbon rods of .027-inch diameter should be available from the facing manufacturer, or pencil leads of proper size may be used. Stainless steel wire of 23-gauge (.026-inch) diameter is also effective. (The facing pins are .025 inch in diameter.)

Figure 79   To demonstrate both, a carbon rod and a stainless steel rod are used for this backing.

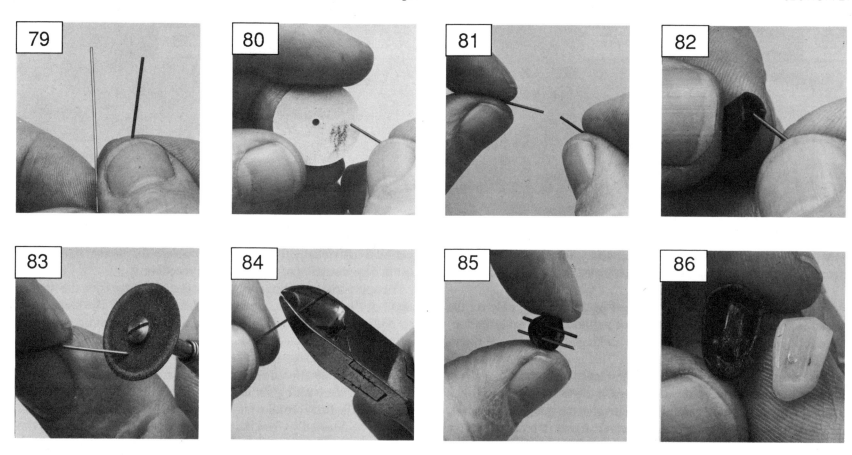

Figure 80   The carbon rod is prepared by beveling one end to a rounded point that will not drag wax from the walls of the pin hole as it is inserted into the pattern. This is done by rotating the tip of the rod against fine-grit sandpaper.

Figure 81   The rod is broken to a length that will extend completely through the pattern, leaving at least 1 to 2 millimeters exposed on either side. If blind pinholes (not extending completely through the pattern) are involved, the rods are carefully inserted to the base of the pin hole in the pattern and should be of such length to extend 3 or 4 millimeters from the face of the pattern.

Figure 82   The facing is removed from the backing (**Figure 62**). The rod is inserted in a pin hole and is gently pushed into place with a slight rotating motion.

Figure 83   The same procedure is followed with the stainless steel rod. The end to be inserted is beveled by rotating it against a slowly revolving Carborundum disc or stone.

Figure 84   The rod is cut to the appropriate length, using a disc or pliers prior to inserting into the pattern.

Figure 85   Both rods are now in position in the backing, and it is ready to be invested. The second premolar pontic facing is removed, using a sticky wax handle (**Figure 62**).

Figure 86   The pattern is carefully examined to insure that no margins have broken or deformed during removal of the facing.

The backings should be immediately invested. As with a porcelain-

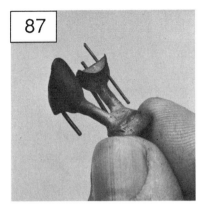

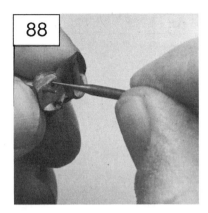

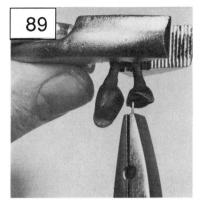

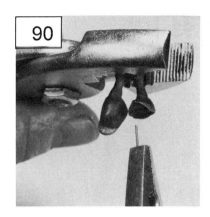

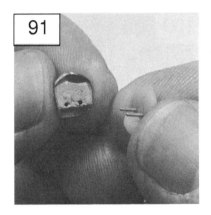

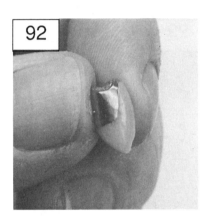

faced crown, maximum expansion is required for any casting to receive a porcelain facing. The investment technique should be pressed for slightly greater expansion than is customarily required for a full cast crown. The backings are cast of the same alloy used for the retainers.

Figure 87   After the casting has been cleaned, the stainless steel rod is still in position. The carbon rod was broken during recovery. Note the open vents that were attached just lingual to the facioocclusal edge of each pattern.

Figure 88   The part of the carbon rod that was left embedded in the casting must be removed. This is commonly done using a number ½ or number 1 round bur in a straight handpiece. This procedure is dangerous, as the head of the bur may bind and break in the backing—and be impossible to remove. If a bur is used with a handpiece, it should be

withdrawn after each millimeter of carbon is penetrated. If this is not done, debris builds up behind the bur, making its withdrawal difficult.

A safer procedure is to use the same bur by rotating it with the finger tips. Once the carbon rod is grossly removed, the bur may be used in the handpiece to hone the walls lightly.

Figure 89   The stainless steel rod requires a positive force for its removal and must be removed before the sprue is separated. The sprue may serve as a handle by which the backing can be firmly grasped with pliers. The stainless steel rod is also firmly held with a suitable pair of serrated-tip pliers.

Figure 90   A very firm pull in conjunction with a slow, steady rotation of the pin will effect its removal. Note that the pliers grasping the pin have rotated approximately one-quarter turn during removal of the pin.

Figure 91   After all debris has been removed and blebs and irregularities have been corrected, the facing can be seated to check the accuracy of the casting.

Seating Facings in Pontic Castings

Figure 92   The facing should go firmly and accurately into position. If it does not, it should again be inspected for errors in the casting. Regardless of the problem encountered in seating the facing, *do not alter the pins*. To do so may weaken them and require forfeiture of the facing. Certainly it would be much easier to redevelop the backing than

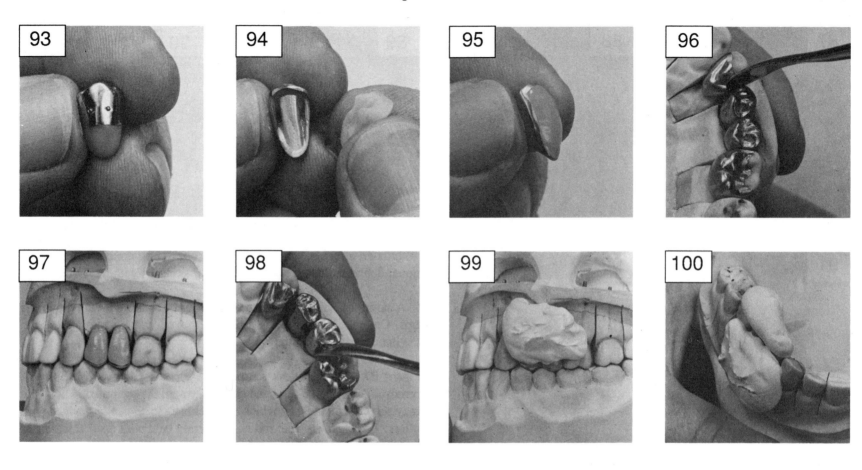

to have to make a new facing with baked tip. If, however, the backing has been developed to completely cover the pins, their pointed tips should be removed.

Figure 93 The pins should ideally extend through the cast backing. Exposed ends of the pins should not be reduced at this time.

Figure 94 The denture tooth facing, because of greater surface coverage and the angles involved, may prove more difficult to seat in its cast backing. Again, the casting should be carefully inspected and all debris and any positive defects removed before attempting to seat the facing.

Figure 95 The facing should seat completely and accurately. If it does not, and no defects are found, sharp angles either in the casting or on the facing may be lightly relieved. Do not alter the margins.

Assembly and Soldering

Figure 96 The pontic assemblies are repositioned in the working cast. This is accomplished using the previously established plaster facial index. Sticky wax is added at appropriate points to stabilize this position.

Figure 97 Relationships of the pontics should be carefully evaluated. If for any reason a change is desired, the sticky wax may be softened and the position of the pontics changed as indicated.

Figure 98 When the pontics are finally positioned, sticky wax is added in the lingual embrasures to further stabilize their position in preparation for a new index.

Figure 99 Gypsum separator is applied and a new quick-set plaster facial index is poured.

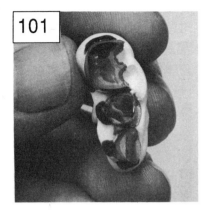

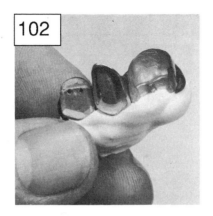

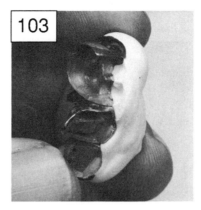

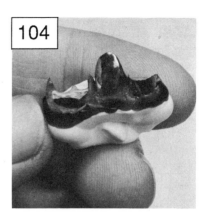

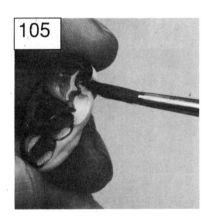

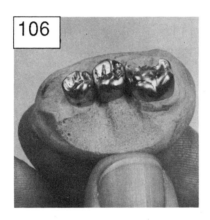

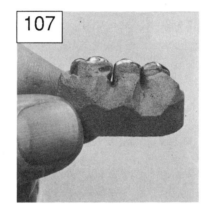

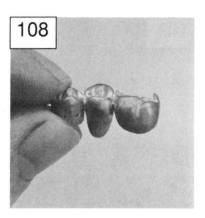

Figure 100   A quick-set plaster occlusal index is poured to facilitate transfer for investing for soldering. Note that the anterior retainer has not been included in the occlusal index. Because there must be four solder joints in this bridge, the possibility of soldering error may be minimized by joining three of the units at one time, and then establishing a new relationship index for the final joint.

Figure 101   The pontic backings and posterior retainer have been carefully positioned in the occlusal index and fixed with sticky wax.

Figure 102   Sticky wax has been added in the joints to maintain access to these areas in the investment model, and also to seal them against the possibility of inclusion of debris.

Figure 103   Note that although the joint area has been filled, no wax has been allowed to extend over the margins of the retainer or backings.

Figure 104   Additional wax has been added about the lingual of each unit to limit the investment coverage and to provide airways to the joints.

Figure 105   Gypsum separator is applied to the exposed areas of the plaster index. The index may be boxed by wrapping with sheet wax, or the investment model may be poured freehand.

Figure 106   When setting is complete (about 30 minutes), the investment cast is trimmed to provide access to the joint areas, and all wax and debris is removed by flushing with boiling water.

Figure 107   Though small, an open airway exists through each joint area.

Figure 108   When the joints have been soldered, the framework is

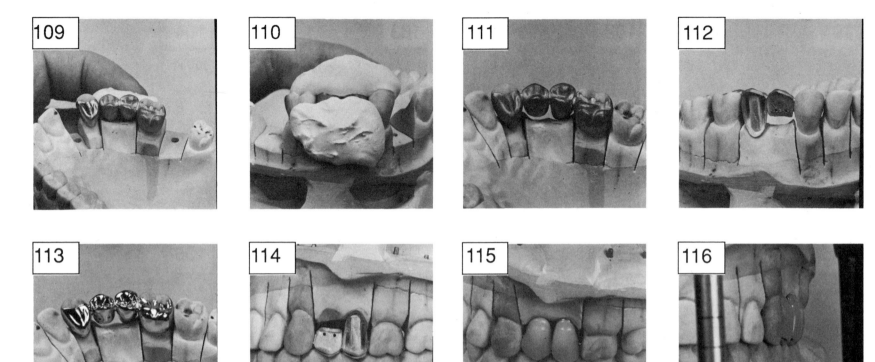

thoroughly pickled and recleaned in preparation for soldering the anterior joint.

Figure 109 The facings are repositioned to be sure that no conflict has developed as a result of the soldering procedure. All units are carefully reassembled in the working cast, using the plaster facial index for additional stability if desired. *Every precaution must be taken to ensure that the dies and retainers are accurately seated before the occlusal index is made for the final joint.*

Figure 110 An occlusal index is made, and the anterior joint is completed in conventional manner. Because this bridge has been made of Type IV alloy, it may be allowed to bench cool after this last heating procedure, to effect heat hardening of the alloy if desired (see manufacturer's directions).

Figure 111 When soldered and thoroughly cleaned, the framework assembly is reseated on the working cast to verify its accuracy.

Figure 112 Note that the dies are completely seated in the cast and the bridge is seated on the dies.

Figure 113 Any occlusal discrepancies due to the soldered joints are corrected, and the framework is polished.

Cementing the Facings and Finishing the Bridge

Figures 114 through 116 The completed framework is ready to be returned to the dentist along with the facings for trial insertion. The facings are never cemented until after trial insertion of the framework, as it would be impossible to correct any discrepancies in relationship

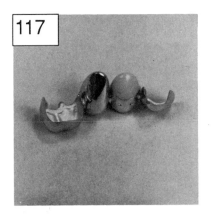 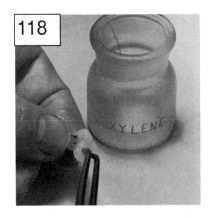 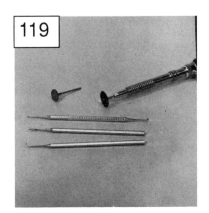 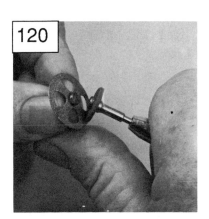

once the facings are cemented. Hence alloy about the facings has not been rounded to final form.

During trial insertion, the dentist will usually make some occlusal adjustments. Proximal contacts may also be adjusted. Open or light contacts will have to be corrected by soldering. Alloy pontic surfaces may be adjusted and repolished, but glazed porcelain pontic tips are hopefully not adjusted. A porcelain facing with a baked tip will distort enough to prevent accurate seating in the backing if it is reglazed. Any adjustment of the tip will result in forfeiture of the glazed surface. Should this occur, the tip must be carefully polished.

If an error in relationship is detected, the appropriate joint of the bridge is desoldered, a new relationship index established, and the joint resoldered. The dentist will usually desolder or section the bridge framework such that the error can be immediately evaluated, and make a new index. However, the framework may be returned to the laboratory for this procedure. (See **Section 16, Desoldering**.)

Figure 117   After all corrections have been completed and the framework is repolished, the facings can be cemented. Normally the dentist will cement the facings after trial insertion. However, on some occasions the bridge may be returned to the laboratory for cementation and final finishing.

Figure 118   To ensure maximum bond of the cement, all debris and oily substances from handling the facings and framework must be removed. This may be done by cleaning with xylene or alcohol. The

framework and facings are thoroughly dried. A good-quality zinc phosphate cement of desired shade is selected.

Figure 119   Before the cement is mixed, careful inspection of all marginal areas should be made to determine if any finishing is to be done during the cementation procedure. All instruments to be used for these finishing procedures are made ready for immediate use. The instruments required depend upon the nature of the marginal discrepancies present. In general the discrepancies may be of three types: excess porcelain contour, excess alloy contour, or an open gap between alloy and porcelain. Correction of any significant discrepancies is best made before cementing the facings. The instrumentation for correcting such discrepancies is essentially the same as that which will be needed for final correction during cementation.

The armamentarium pictured here includes a slow-speed straight handpiece with mounted Carborundum separating disc and medium-grit abrasive rubber wheel. The hand instruments are a small ball burnisher, a beaver-tail burnisher, and a sharp discoid-cleoid carver.

Figure 120   The mounted disc and rubber wheel should be trued and shaped by lathing against an abrasive surface. An old diamond instrument is excellent for this purpose.

Figure 121   Such truing should provide a wheel with a smoothly concentric rotating periphery and the desired edge contour, either flat, rounded, or sharp. For correction of porcelain/alloy marginal discrepancies, a slightly rounded edge as shown is desired.

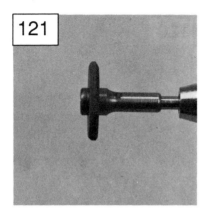

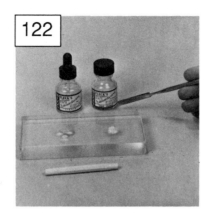

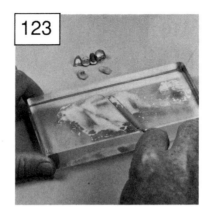

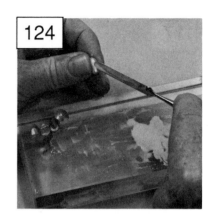

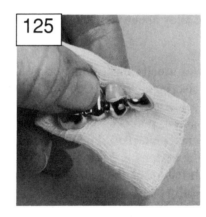

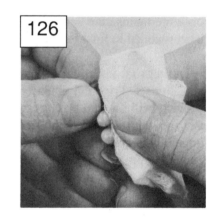

In principle, correction of marginal discrepancies between alloy and porcelain is accomplished by discing or stoning the more prominent surface until it just comes flush with the other material. The disc or stone should always be rotated in a direction from alloy to porcelain, so that the alloy will be drawn against the porcelain. In other words, if the marginal discrepancy was excess porcelain contour, the prominent porcelain surface would be ground until the disc just contacted the adjacent alloy and in one final slow, dragging rotation pulled the alloy against the porcelain. By contrast, any marginal discrepancy due to an excess of alloy may be easily corrected by grinding on the alloy until it just comes flush with the porcelain surface. If this is done slowly, with moderate pressure and a reasonably coarse disc, the alloy will have been dragged tightly against the porcelain margin at the moment these two surfaces become even. How much alloy will drag or, in the case of a slight open-gap discrepancy, how far the alloy will drag depends upon the particular type of alloy that has been used for the casting.

Figures 122 and 123 When gross marginal discrepancies are completed and the facings and framework are carefully cleaned and dried, and all finishing procedures and instruments are identified, the cement mix can be made. The powder and liquid must be mixed properly on a heavy glass slab with a flexible metal spatula. No substitution for these implements can be made. The mixing procedure should follow the manufacturer's directions.

Figures 124 and 125 With a suitable instrument (beaver-tail burnisher or small spatula) the backing window and facing are coated with cement. When pins are involved, the pin holes should be filled with

cement using an explorer tine or small wire. It is very difficult to fill blind pin holes without trapping air. When all surfaces are coated with cement, the facing is pressed slowly and firmly into position. Once almost completely seated, very firm pressure may be applied to the facing to effect its fully seated position.

Figure 126 When the facing is fully seated, excess cement is quickly wiped away.

Figure 127 Any marginal discrepancies must be corrected immediately before the cement hardens. Areas of discrepancy should first be firmly burnished.

Figure 128 Any error remaining after burnishing can be corrected by slow-speed discing with moderate pressure. Again, this is done by

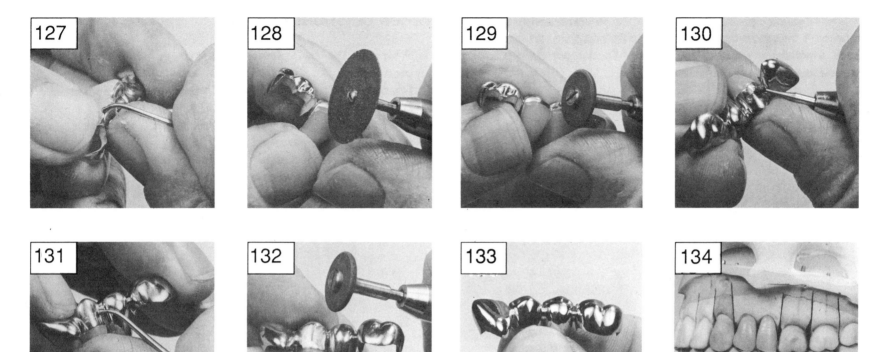

discing the more prominent surface until the two surfaces are just flush. *Always rotate the disc from alloy toward porcelain.*

As soon as the alloy and porcelain surfaces become flush, discing should be stopped and the alloy margin lightly burnished and smoothed by rubbing with a ball or beaver-tail burnisher.

Figure 129   After significant discrepancies have been corrected by discing and burnishing, these areas and any areas of very minor discrepancy may be smoothed using an abrasive rubber wheel. Again rotation should be from alloy to porcelain. Contour (rolling) of the alloy margin may also be done with the rubber wheel. Light burnishing may be repeated at this point if desired.

Figures 130 through 132   If ends of the pins were left exposed, they

too must be finished before the cement completely hardens. This is best done using a small ball-shaped stone. With the stone rotating from pin to alloy and grinding about the entire circumference of the pin, the soft pin metal can be bradded against the alloy casting so that the two are almost welded together. Burnishing and smoothing with a Burlew wheel produces a smooth surface on which the location of the pins is almost imperceptible. This must all be accomplished before the cement hardens; otherwise the cement will serve as a barrier between the two materials.

Figure 133   When all margins are corrected, the cement is allowed to set completely, and final polishing of the bridge is completed. If grinding has been done on the porcelain facings, they should be resmoothed and polished. To avoid disturbing the alloy margin, this is best done by using a small, true-running Burlew wheel that is dipped frequently into a flour-of-pumice paste, or with one of the porcelain-polishing rubber wheels. A high gloss may be imparted to the porcelain surface by using such a polishing wheel at high speed. Special porcelain polishing wheels and pastes are available.

Figure 134   Fabrication is now completed, and the bridge is ready for final delivery to the dentist.

REVIEW QUESTIONS

1. What are the two categories of facings available for pontic construction?
2. Discuss the factors to be considered when contouring a porcelain pin facing.
3. Give the faciolingual dimension of the area of contact for a convex pontic tip on the residual ridge.
4. Discuss the basic techniques available for maintaining the pin holes in the pontic casting when a pin facing is used in a metal bridge.
5. What is the direction of rotation of the discs when finishing the alloy pontic with a porcelain facing present?

SECTION 22

Porcelain-faced Bridges: Interchangeable Facings

MANDIBULAR ANTERIOR PORCELAIN-FACED BRIDGE

In the bridge illustrated in Section 21 the conventional or original technique for the use of porcelain pontic facings was shown using a pin facing and a denture tooth. These facings were completely protected from occlusal forces by the cast backing; thus there was no anticipation that they might have to be replaced due to breakage. However, to accomplish this a significant amount of metal was displayed along the occlusofacial margin of the facing. Patient acceptance of such metal display, especially in the anterior regions of the mouth, is low and steadily decreasing.

The use and design of porcelain facings was modified years ago to eliminate having any alloy on the incisal surface of anterior facings. As one might expect, the result was improved esthetics and increased breakage. To combat the problem of breakage, the idea arose to make facings interchangeable, so that they could be more easily replaced. If the size and shape of facings could be standardized and grooves or slots used for retention (rather than pins), a broken facing could be rather easily replaced by sliding a new facing onto the existing framework. This was the design concept of Steele's interchangeable facings.

Because of their esthetic advantage (little or no display of metal) backed by ease of replacement in the event of breakage (due to the absence of alloy protection of the incisal) these facings became popular and are still used. However, the facility with which these facings can be replaced is significantly jeopardized if they are handled such that a biologically acceptable pontic form is developed.

Figure 1   Pictured in order of their frequency of usage, the Steele's

interchangeable facings are: (1) Flatback, (2) Posterior Trupontic, (3) PBE (Porcelain Biting Edge), (4) Anterior Trupontic, and (5) Side Groove Posterior.

The bridge example shown in this section shows variations in the use and design of the Flatback and Trupontic facings. Further information regarding their use as well as the other interchangeable facing forms is available from the manufacturer.

Possibly the most popular current use of the interchangeable porcelain pontic facing is in the lower anterior bridge. The esthetic potential of the facing-ridge relationship in this area is normally not critical, and the incisal display of metal can be effectively limited depending upon the type of facing used. Some question arises as to the validity of this design in relation to the occlusal forces that are imposed directly on the facing. However, the direction of force is usually such as to take advantage of the support offered by the framework. By comparison, in a maxillary bridge of similar design occlusal forces tend to divorce the facing from the supporting framework. Concern over the direction of occlusal forces is valid because breakage does occur, particularly when the incisal edge is unprotected. However, this same occlusal contact that might break the lower anterior facing would certainly wear resin veneers if they were used, since it occurs on the facial aspect of the facing.

Figure 2   This example involves a six-unit bridge with standard three-quarter crown retainers on canine abutments. Residual ridge contour is

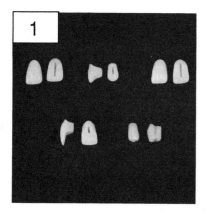 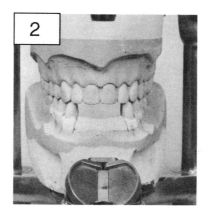 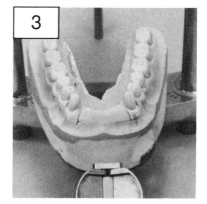 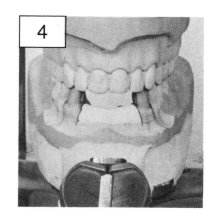

essentially ideal. Working and opposing casts have been mounted on the Hanau articulator via face-bow transfer and centric occlusion record. Adjustment of the instrument for incisal guidance was indicated by the preoperative casts. Horizontal condylar guidance was established by means of a protrusive record (checkbite).

Retainer Development

Figure 3   The working cast has been developed by the double pour section technique to establish removable canine dies. Patterns for the retainers are waxed with special consideration for accuracy of internal adaptation, as these are partial crown retainers.

Figure 4   The retainers are cast and fitted to their appropriate dies, and adjustments are made for proper occlusion. We are dealing with a segmented-group-function occlusion; therefore, the remaining uninvolved teeth provide an index to the occlusal contact of the retainers. However, because these are canines it is imperative that they establish a positive lateral guidance. In addition, because this is an anterior bridge, it is also desirable that the canines function to share protrusive guidance. The retainers must be carefully adjusted at this time to provide accurate guidance during development of the pontics.

Figure 5   Note the mesial and lingual convergence of the abutments. This is quite common for the mandubular canines, and frequently makes it difficult for the dentist to make partial crown preparations that draw and yet are conservatively extended.

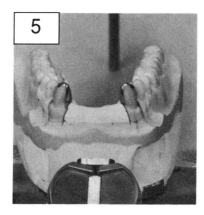 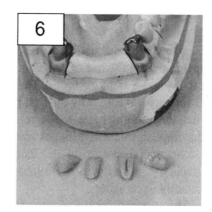

Preparation of Facings

Figure 6   Facings are selected for the pontics. To provide variety in this bridge example, each facing will be developed somewhat differently. (In a practical case, all pontics for a given bridge would probably be of the same design.) The two central incisor pontics will be made using Steele's Flatback facings. The gingival tips developed for these two pontics will be different. The lateral incisor pontics will be made using Trupontic facings with different tip forms.

Figure 7   Trupontic facings are manufactured with two different tip forms, the saddle tip as seen on the left, and the conical tip seen on the right. Both types will be used in this bridge, although the difference matters little, as their tips will be recontoured. In addition to the variety of types of facings and types of pontic tips developed, a different

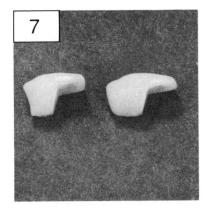

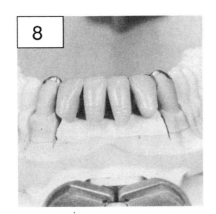

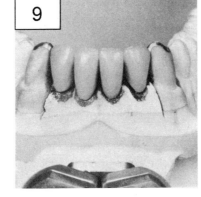

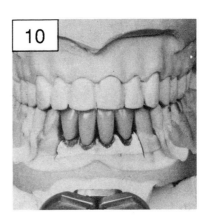

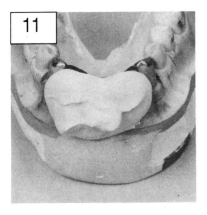

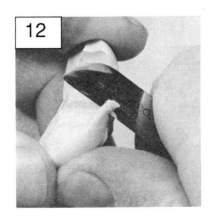

tips are too large and must be adapted. Compressive adaptation of the lower anterior pontic tip against the residual ridge is seldom desired. In fact, *mandibular anterior pontic tips are often made with no tissue contact*. Because it provides a greater learning experience, and because the residual ridge in this situation is quite high (little resorption of bone has occurred), the facing tips will be adapted to the ridge.

Figure 9 The residual ridge is marked with a soft lead pencil to facilitate locating the points of contact of the facing tips. The tips are arbitrarily ground to contour to permit approximate positioning of the facings.

Figure 10 Final adjustments are made to bring the facings into proper position with appropriate inclination and occlusal contact. Note that the midline relationship has been perfectly established. This is desirable, but not critical. Position of the facings is easily maintained by seating them against a strip of utility wax that has been placed on the crest of the edentulous ridge.

Figure 11 When final positioning is established, a quick-set plaster facial index is made.

Figure 12 The index is trimmed to expose the incisal edge of the facings, and to remove any septa that might dislodge the facings upon removal of the index.

Figure 13 Depending upon the amount of vertical overbite, the index is trimmed, if possible, such that the articulator can be fully closed with

technique will be used in developing each of the pontic backings, again for illustrative purposes.

Figure 8 Facings of proper shade and most appropriate size are selected. If a full range of facings is not in stock, proper mold size can be determined by careful measuring of the space or by trial-positioning denture teeth until the correct size is found and then measuring them. In either case, the closest available size can be determined from the manufacturer's mold guide book. If some discrepancy must occur, it is best to order facings slightly too large rather than too small.

The selected facings are grossly positioned to gain some perspective as to their size, mesiodistal width, incisal length, and gingival contour. As shown in this photograph, the mesiodistal width and the incisal configuration of the facings is quite acceptable; however, the gingival

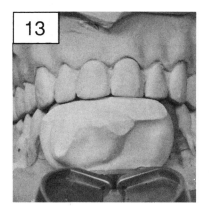
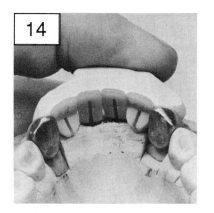
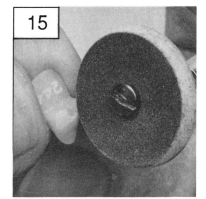
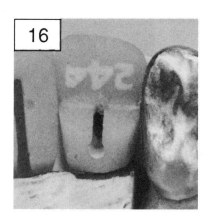

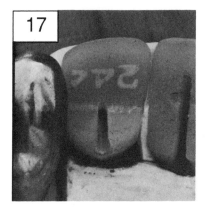
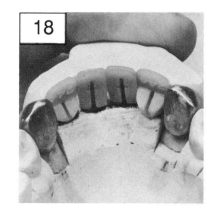

it in position. This may be impractical for some mandibular anterior situations.

Figure 14   This lingual view shows the facings in position in the plaster index. Though not particularly evident in this photograph, the left lateral conical tip Trupontic facing has been modified to provide a convex pontic tip. The right lateral Trupontic facing has been converted from a saddle-type tip to a ridge-lap tip configuration. Both Trupontics are too large in cingulum contour, and will be reduced.

The Flatback facings have no specific tip form other than the facial outline that was established during the initial contouring. Space for developing these tips as part of the cast backing is evident between the facing and ridge.

Figure 15   A fine-grit stone is used to complete the modification of the saddle-tip Trupontic facing to a ridge-lap tip form—slightly concave faciolingually but purposely convex mesiodistally.

Figure 16   The modified ridge-lap-tipped right lateral Trupontic facing is in position on the working cast.

Figure 17   The left lateral convex-tip Trupontic facing is in position on the working cast. This tip is convex both faciolingually and mesiodistally.

Figure 18   With all facings in position, the extension of the proximal bevels on the Trupontics is estimated. Proximal bevels on these facings

should be extended just beyond contact. In ideal alignment, this would mean that adjacent bevels were exactly even with one another. However, if the retainers are overextended (as frequently occurs in the preparation of the mandibular canine for a partial crown), or if the facings are rotated and lapped for esthetics, the bevels are simply extended just beyond the proximal contact point of the retainer so as to permit development of an adequate joint.

Figure 19   Beveling of the linguoproximal angle of the Trupontic facings is accomplished with suitable stones.

Figure 20   The proximal bevels are extended to include the cavosurface angle of the tip shelf. This lingual bevel should encompass the periphery of the post hole.

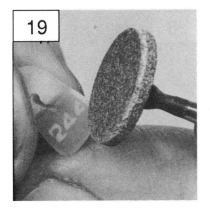

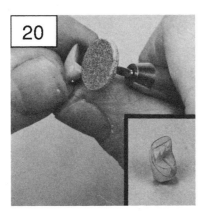

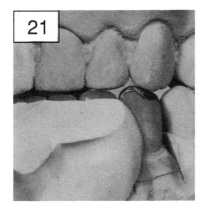

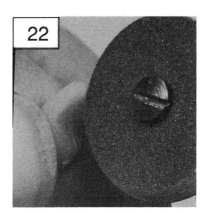

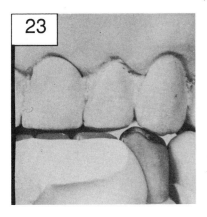

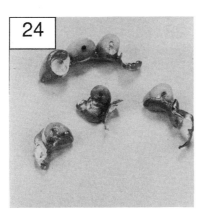

Figure 21　With their tip forms established, the Trupontic facings must be adjusted to provide for occlusal clearance if the incisal of these facings is to be protected with alloy. Because Trupontic facings seat from facial to lingual, the incisal edges can be completely covered by alloy if desired. Depending on the occlusion, it may not be practical to extend the alloy incisal coverage to include the full range of occlusal contact on a lower anterior facing. Therefore, to minimize esthetic loss the facings are usually reduced to provide only about 0.75 millimeter clearance in centric and are aligned to permit harmonious contact on their facial surface during the protrusive excursion.

Figure 22　The incisal must be beveled toward the lingual to permit the Trupontic to draw in line with the post. The angle of the bevel is usually kept minimal (15° to 20°) so as to maintain maximum thickness of the porcelain, because the occlusal load will occur partially on the facing.

Figure 23　Incisal edge clearance must be established in all centric and eccentric relations, though the facial surface of the facing may contact in centric or during excursions. Shown here is the clearance available with the mandible in left lateral functional position. Note the outline form of the alloy coverage on the incisal of the canine abutment. The distal arm of the retainer, which carries the heavy functional load, is much thicker, to resist wear and stress of this functional contact. The esthetically critical mesial arm was prepared to show less metal. Because Flatback facings seat from incisal to gingival, the incisal edges cannot be covered with alloy.

Two different tip forms have been established using the Trupontic facing; a convex tip, and a ridge-lap form. The gingival end of the Flatback facing does not have sufficient dimension to develop a desirable tip form in porcelain. Such form must be established as part of the alloy backing. Unfortunately, the Flatback facing as commonly used is simply shortened to the desired length, a manufactured post inserted into the slot, and the backing waxed and cast.

Figure 24　This approach provides little opportunity to establish a desirable tip contour and results in a poor junction between the facing and post. It is the exposed cement line and irregular contour associated with this poor junction that irritates adjacent soft tissue. Such irregularity in contour is undesirable on any surface of a restoration but is particularly objectionable on surfaces that contact soft tissue.

The result of irregular and rough tip contour is chronic inflammation of the gingival tissue and resorption of bone. This deficiency is effec-

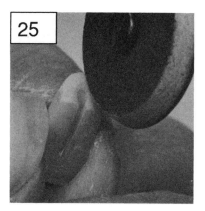

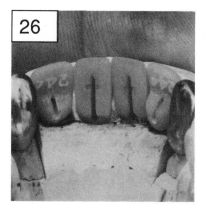

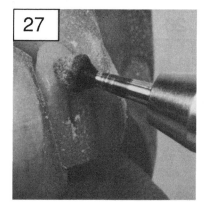

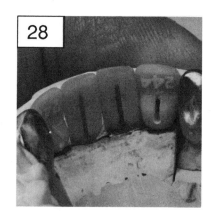

tively overcome by extending the alloy backing to cover the entire gingival end of the facing. In this fashion a smooth, uninterrupted tip contour is established in a convex or ridge-lap form. The disadvantage of this approach is that it limits the interchangeability of these facings. However, it does not totally preclude replacement of a Flatback facing that might be broken, and because of the much more favorable tissue response, this is the only technique for use of the Flatback facing that can be recommended.

An intermediate approach is available, however. The gingival end of the facing can be beveled about the orifice of the slot so as to permit development of an accurate and smooth marginal junction between the facing and backing. Although this approach may provide a rather acceptable result in the initial development of the pontic, it produces an even greater restriction on adequate replacement of the facing in the event of breakage. The gingival tip area of a facing is not visible in the mouth; thus it is essentially impossible to bevel a replacement facing such that there would be accuracy of fit at the hidden junction. However, assuming that the facing would never have to be replaced, this approach represents an improvement over the simple posting procedure, and will therefore, for variety of example, be presented here.

In summary, the tip formed by a Flatback facing with manufactured post is generally unacceptable to soft tissue. This deficiency is effectively overcome by beveling the orifice of the slot, but this makes it extremely difficult for a dentist to replace the facing accurately should that become necessary. A desirable tip surface can be created by completely covering the gingival end of the Flatback facing with alloy. Although this makes replacement of a facing more difficult, it may still be accomplished.

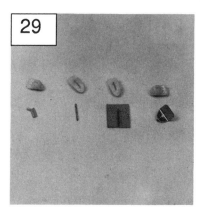

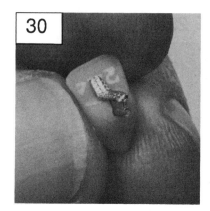

Figure 25   A medium-grit stone is used to surface the entire gingival end of the left central Flatback facing. This will provide a positive cavosurface angle about the edge of the tip and adequate clearance for alloy coverage.

Figure 26   The tip of the left central incisor Flatback facing has been beveled, and clearance is available for full alloy coverage of this surface.

Figure 27   Using a small round stone, the orifice of the slot is beveled to provide a definite finish line for the partial coverage pattern and casting for the right central Flatback facing.

Figure 28   The orifice of the slot on the right central incisor Flatback facing has been beveled, and clearance is available to permit waxing to this finish line.

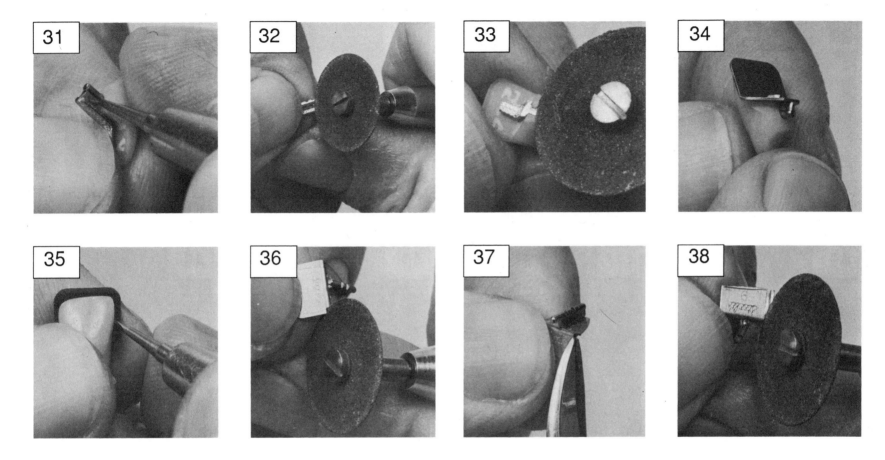

Development of Pontic Backings

Figure 29   A number of options exist for development of backings for these facings. The four different examples shown here represent the major possibilities. A *stock post* will be used in the left lateral Trupontic facing. A *plastic pin* will be used in development of the backing pattern for the left central Flatback facing. A *stock plastic backing plate* will be used in developing the pattern for the right central Flatback facing. A *stock gold post and backing plate* will be used in developing the backing for the right lateral Trupontic.

Figure 30   The stock Trupontic post in position in the facing is illustrated.

Figures 31 and 32   Excess post length is marked with a sharp instrument and cut away with a separating disc.

Figure 33   The post is reseated in the facing and is trimmed flush with the surface of the facing.

Figure 34   The manufactured gold post and backing plate are in position on the right lateral Trupontic facing.

Figure 35   Excess post and plate contour is marked using a sharp instrument.

Figures 36 and 37   A notch is cut with a separating disc to proper depth on either side at the angle of the backing. Excess plate can then be trimmed with shears. If preferred, this excess may be ground away.

Figures 38 and 39   The margins of the grossly trimmed plate are surfaced until they are just short of facing contour.

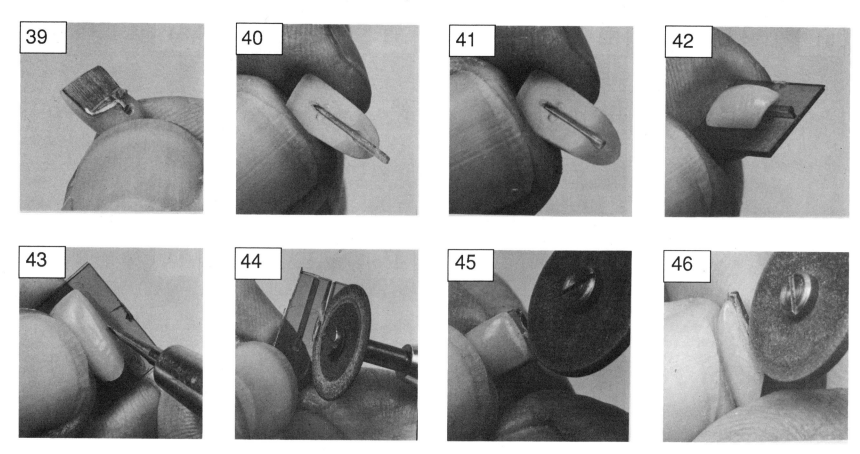

Figure 40 A plastic sprue pin has been reduced such that it can be fully and snugly seated in the left Flatback facing slot.

Figure 41 Excess pin length is marked and removed.

Figure 42 A stock plastic backing has been seated in the right Flatback facing.

Figure 43 Excess is again marked with a sharp instrument.

Figure 44 Excess plate may be removed with a disc or cut with a warm, sharp instrument.

Figures 45 and 46 With the backing plate reseated on the facing, excess is trimmed flush with the lateral surfaces of the facing. If the

marginal adaptaion of the trimmed plastic backing plate is not ideal, the plate may be trimmed short of facing outline so that the margins may be developed in wax.

Figure 47 Some excess backing is left at the incisal edge.

Figure 48 Using the plaster facial index, the facings are reseated in the working cast and are ready for the development of the backing patterns. In review, note that there is a metal post, a plastic post, a plastic backing plate, and a metal backing plate.

Figure 49 All posts and backing plates are removed to permit application of die lubricant preparatory to waxing.

Figures 50 and 51 The metal post for the left lateral Trupontic backing

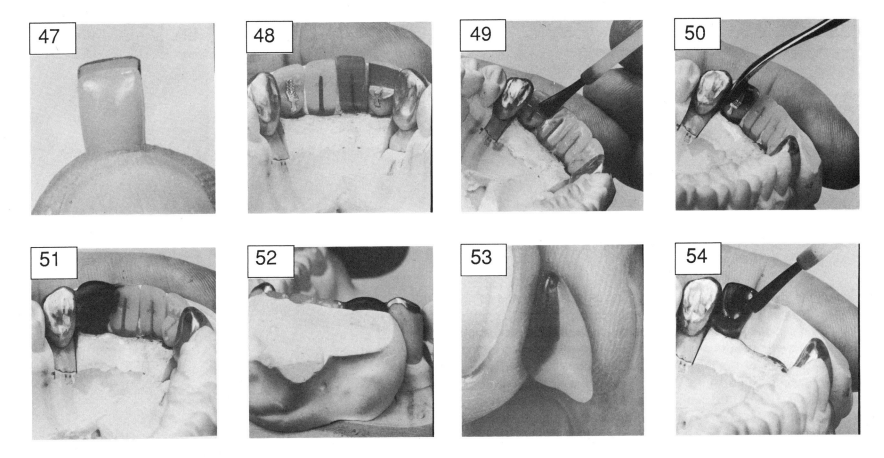

has been repositioned and waxing of the pattern initiated. Wax addition may be accomplished with the facing either in or out of the working cast. However, it is easier to establish relationships with the facing in the working cast.

Figure 52 Wax is extended to cover the incisal edge, and occlusal relationships may be established at this time.

Figure 53 With gross wax-up completed, the pontic is removed from the working cast to complete the backing pattern.

Figure 54 The left lateral incisor Trupontic with backing pattern in position is replaced on the working cast, and die lubricant is applied before developing the backing pattern for the left central incisor pontic.

Figure 55 The left central incisor Flatback facing is lubricated, the post is reinserted, and the assembly is repositioned in the working cast ready for development of the backing pattern. Wax is applied and the pattern developed as before.

Figure 56 The waxing sequence is repeated until all backing patterns are completed. The pontics are then repositioned in the working cast for final evaluation of marginal extension. If corrections are necessary, the pontics may be repositioned or the margins may be reprepared and backing patterns altered accordingly. If facing position is changed, a new plaster facial index is made.

Figure 57 The incisal edges are covered with a slight excess of wax. Note that the facioincisal aspect of the Trupontic wax patterns has not

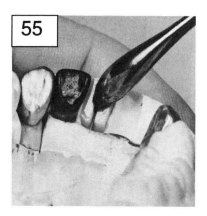
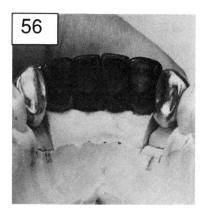
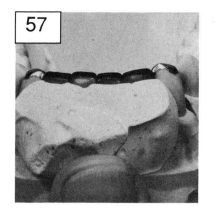
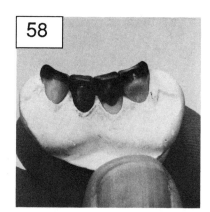

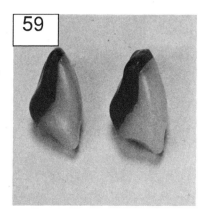
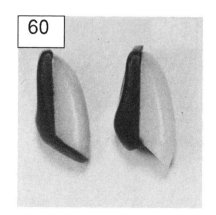

been rolled but has been carved in line with the facial surface of the facings.

Figure 58   The variety of tip designs that have been developed are shown. To review, the left lateral Trupontic facing has been developed with a contoured porcelain convex tip; the left central Flatback facing has been developed with a pattern for full-alloy-coverage convex tip; the right central incisor Flatback facing has been developed with a beveled margin about the orifice of the slot and a ridge-lap tip form, and the right lateral Trupontic facing has been developed with a contoured porcelain ridge-lap tip. Clinically speaking, the form of each of these tips is acceptable, but the design as it relates to the material used is ideal in only one example. Only the full-alloy-coverage convex tip of the left central Flatback facing provides a potential for ideal tissue compatibility. The junction line between facing and backing on the right central Flatback pontic, though a distinct improvement over the straight posting technique, is still undesirable because this union will be in contact with soft tissues. The two Trupontic facings provide excellent potential form but cannot be considered desirable in that the porcelain is not glazed. If highly polished, these tip surfaces may prove acceptable, but plaque retention is inevitable. A low-fusing glazing medium could be applied to these surfaces, but it is soluble in many mouths.

Figure 59   This proximal view shows an excellent example of the contrast between convex and ridge-lap pontic tip forms. Note also that the occlusal wax margins have been carved in line with the facial surface of the facings and left flat. Rolling will be accomplished after the casting is completed.

Figure 60   Proximal outline form of the two Flatback facing pontics is shown. Note the contrast between the full and partial tip coverage. The incisal portion of the backing pattern for the Flatback facings has been left slightly overextended, to protect the facings. The premise is that, after casting, occlusal adjustment will leave the incisal edge of the facing inclined facially. If the backing alloy is reduced in keeping with this incline, it will extend to a higher level than the facings. Theoretically, this causes the alloy backing to receive the greater portion of the incisal load. Practically speaking, there is some question as to how effective this might prove to be in any given situation; however, at least maximum support of the facing is established.

Figure 61   This illustration emphasizes the difference in path of draw of the two types of facings. The faciolingual path of draw of the Trupontic facing permits alloy coverage of the incisal edge. In fact, it

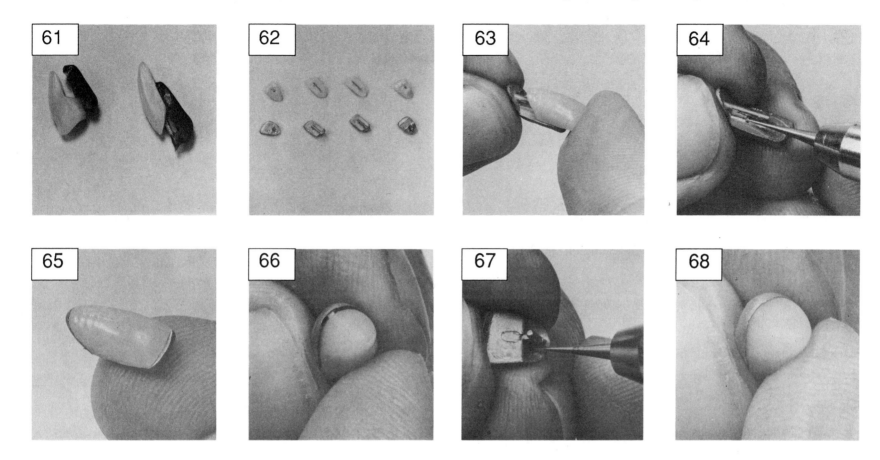

would also permit coverage of the gingival tip surface, if desired. Such design would make this usage very similar to the procelain-faced crown or denture-tooth facing. The incisogingival path of draw of the Flatback facing does not permit coverage of the incisal edge of the facing. However, as demonstrated, the gingival end may be covered to whatever extent desired.

The backings are now ready to be cast. Sprues are attached just above the cingulum bulge on such backing patterns; 10- or 12-gauge sprues are appropriate, and they should be directed slightly toward the incisal edge. Maximum compensation in casting is indicated. The backings should be cast with the same type of alloy used for the retainers.

Figure 62   The backings have each been cast and sprues removed.

Figure 63   Each casting is carefully inspected for any defects, and the facing is gently trial-seated. Force can easily result in fracture of these facings, particularly the Flatback facing. Some interference is frequently encountered in seating such facings on their backings.

Figure 64   There is a natural tendency for some slight rounding of sharp internal angles in a casting. Because porcelain is absolutely nonyielding and does not abrade, relief of these angles in the casting may be necessary to overcome restrictions in seating. Relief may be easily accomplished with small round or flame-shaped burs.

Figure 65   If the castings have been adequately compensated, the facing should seat completely and quite accurately once isolated conflicts have been relieved. This photograph shows one of the Flatback facings seated in its backing.

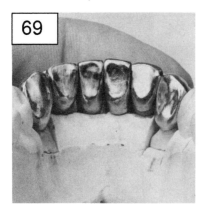

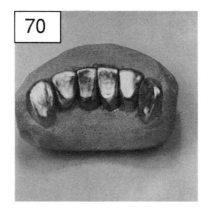

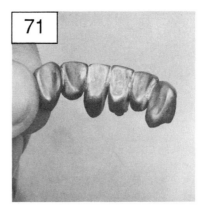

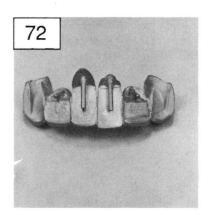

Figure 66 Similar conflicts may arise in seating the Trupontic facing and its backing.

Figure 67 Again these conflicts usually occur in the area of the internal angles about the post.

Figure 68 Slight relief should permit complete and accurate seating of these facings in their backings.

Soldering

Figure 69 When all facings have been completely seated in their respective backings and margins verified, the units are reassembled in the working cast by means of the plaster facial index. Position of the units should be carefully examined, and any desired changes made at this time. It will prove helpful to stabilize the pontics in this position by applying utility wax against their lingual surfaces so that the plaster index may be removed for examination of facial contour and marginal extension.

Figure 70 When all units are in final accurate position, a lingual plaster index is made for soldering investment transfer. Practically speaking, it is impossible to maintain open airways through the joint areas of such units. Hence special care should be taken in cleaning the joint areas and sealing the interproximal areas with sticky wax prior to investing. For the inexperienced technician, it is wise carefully to contour the wax placed in the gingival embrasures so that investment can extend into the embrasures and prevent solder from flowing too far

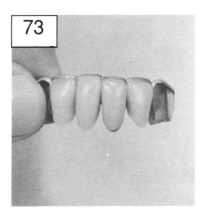

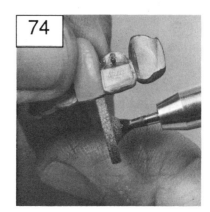

gingivalward. The experienced technician will leave these embrasures open and control the extension of solder by the amount that is applied. This latter approach is shown here.

It is also wise, especially for the inexperienced technician, to accomplish the union of such a bridge in two stages. In this case, all joints will be soldered during one operation. This illustration shows the units invested, ready to be soldered.

Figure 71 The bridge is shown after soldering and pickling, but before any contouring has been done. The neat, well-formed joints are evidence that this soldering operation was done by an experienced technician.

Figure 72 This facial view of the assembled bridge clearly shows the very close approximation of adjacent backing margins.

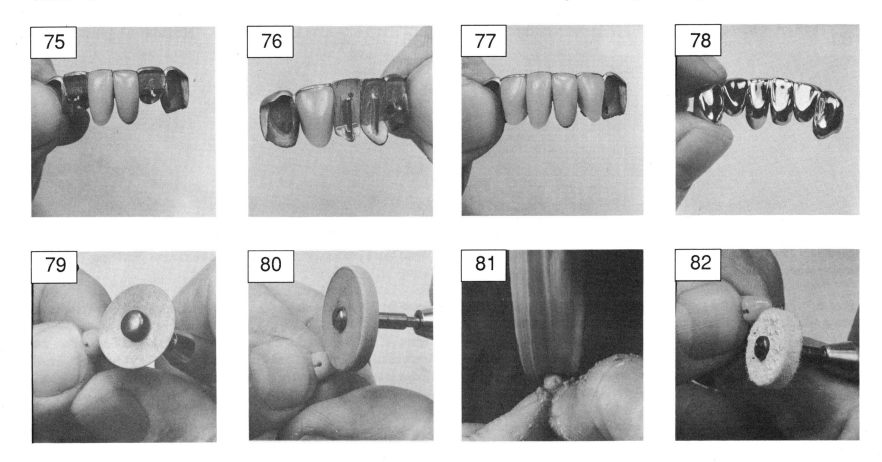

Figure 73 The facings are seated in the framework to ensure accuracy of their position. Note that the gingival embrasures are completely open. No solder has been allowed to extend into the gingival embrasures; as a result, no metal is visible between the pontics.

Finishing

Figures 74 and 75 The excess alloy at the incisal of the two central Flatback facings is reduced and smoothed to reasonable contour. Final finishing of these incisal margins is *not* done at this time.

Figures 76 and 77 The lateral Trupontic facings are fitted in position, and any necessary gross marginal corrections are made. Final finishing of the margins of the facing, especially at the incisal, should *not* be completed at this time.

Figure 78 The bridge is ready to be delivered to the dentist for trial insertion. Porcelain facings are never cemented prior to checking the framework in the mouth. The dentist will verify the adequacy of proximal contacts, make necessary occlusal adjustments and, if indicated, alter gingival tip contours. If the bridge does not seat or if one of the retainers is inadequate, the dentist will desolder a joint or section the bridge. Hence cementation of facings prior to trial insertion may result in their loss.

Figure 79 When the bridge is returned to the laboratory for finishing, final polishing of the porcelain Trupontic tips must be accomplished. This polishing should not involve the area of the backing margin. If corrections of tip contour have been made, roughened areas are surfaced and shaped with appropriate Carborundum or sandpaper discs.

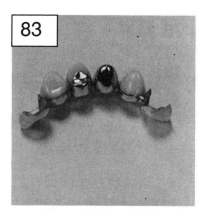

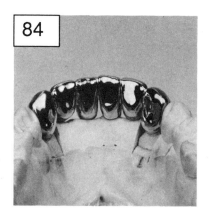

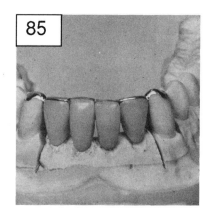

Figure 80   The surface is then smoothed with Cratex or other rubber abrasive wheels.

Figure 81   Final smoothing may be done with flour of pumice and a wet rag wheel, or one of the special porcelain-smoothing wheels.

Figure 82   Polishing to a high gloss may be accomplished with a minim felt wheel and a porcelain polishing agent or with one of the manufactured polishing wheels especially designed for this purpose.

The facings are now ready for cementation and final finishing of margins.

Figure 83   This photograph of the gingival surface of the finished bridge shows the variety of tip forms that have been developed. In review, the left lateral pontic has a convex porcelain tip developed from a conical-tip Trupontic facing. The left central pontic has a convex alloy tip. The right central incisor pontic demonstrates a ridge-lap tip formed both by alloy and porcelain. Note that the junction line between these two materials will be in contact with soft tissue. The right lateral pontic has a porcelain ridge-lap tip formed from a saddle-tip Trupontic facing.

Figure 84   A lingual view of the completed bridge on the working cast.

Figure 85   This facial view contrasts the display of alloy on the Trupontic lateral facings and the Flatback central facings. The finished bridge is ready for delivery to the dentist.

REVIEW QUESTIONS

1. List the types of interchangeable facings that are available.
2. The tip formed by a Flatback facing with a manufactured post is generally unacceptable to soft tissue. How is this deficiency effectively overcome? What is the disadvantage of this procedure?
3. List four possibilities for the development of backings for the slot-type interchangeable facings.
4. Describe the variety of tip designs that may be developed with the slot interchangeable facings.

SECTION 23

Resin-faced Bridges

For many years the only veneering materials for fixed partial dentures were manufactured porcelain facings and denture teeth. Once acrylic resin was developed for this purpose, its use became very popular. It proved to be a versatile material, easy to manipulate, and only modestly demanding in terms of framework design. Resin veneers are easily repaired both in and out of the mouth, and shade potential has become quite acceptable. Two significant disadvantages persist, wear and color instability. Acrylic resin wears rapidly when in occlusal contact. Abrasion by foodstuffs and toothbrushing is also significant. Over time resin also absorbs oral fluids, which cause it to become foul and to change in color. In recent years the techniques and materials for bonding porcelain to metal have become available, and because porcelain is stable this combination of materials has become very popular. Nevertheless acrylic resin is still used and preferred by some as a veneering material.

MAXILLARY ANTERIOR RESIN-FACED BRIDGE

The example of basic technique presented here is a maxillary anterior six-unit bridge (canine to canine) that shows a variety of pontic framework design. As in most exercises presented in this manual, the variety is used for illustrative purposes. Under normal circumstances, all pontics in a given bridge would of course be of a similar design.

Figure 1 The canine preparations have been recorded by a full arch rubber impression made in a custom tray.

Figure 2 The detail of the standard three-quarter crown preparations and the edentulous ridge has been faithfully reproduced.

Figure 3 The maxillary working cast has been mounted on a semiadjustable articulator by means of a face-bow record. The opposing cast has been related in centric occlusion, and a protrusive record has been made to permit adjustment of horizontal condylar guidance in the instrument. Anterior guidance has been set via preoperative casts and checked to ensure clearance of posterior tooth contact during these excursions. Because this dentoform presented a segmented-group-function occlusion, lateral guidance was set in accordance with the functional guidance of the remaining uninvolved posterior teeth.

To facilitate establishing form and size of the pontics, plastic (resin) denture teeth have been selected for trial positioning on the working cast.

Retainer Development

Figure 4 The denture teeth have been grossly positioned on the working cast. With some understanding of the size and position of the pontics, patterns for the retainers can be knowledgeably developed. The patterns are carefully developed to ensure maximum internal adaptation and to provide proper contact in functional excursions.

Figure 5 The patterns have been invested and cast in standard fashion for three-quarter crown retainers, and are pictured here seated on their respective dies in the working cast.

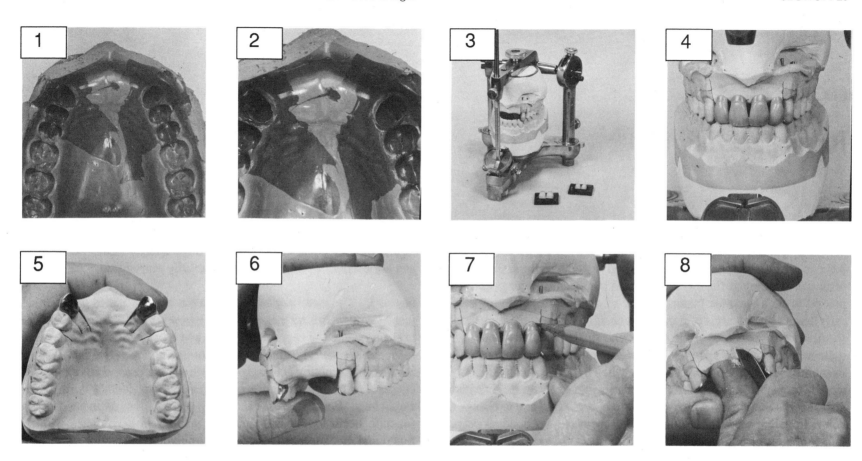

Figure 6 This photograph shows the proximal and incisal configuration of the retainers.

Development of Pontic Framework

Figure 7 The denture teeth are repositioned on the working cast, and their gingival tip outline is traced with a sharp pencil to permit evaluation of contour.

Figure 8 Presuming that the work authorization so dictates, the residual ridge of the working cast is lightly relieved to develop a slight concavity as outlined in the area of each pontic tip. This will permit placement of a convex tip firmly against the ridge. The objective is to have positive contact of the pontic tip along its faciogingival edge with minimal (0.5 millimeter) compression of tissue.

The work authorization may instead call for a modified ridge-lap tip design, with or without ridge relief.

Figure 9 In addition to serving as a visual aid in determining pontic size and position, the plastic denture teeth can be used in a number of ways to develop the pontic patterns. They may also be used as a facing for the pontic, as will be demonstrated in one pontic for this bridge. The first objective in the use of denture teeth for development of pontic patterns is to establish correct position and size.

Figure 10 The denture teeth are shown here after gingival surfaces have been contoured to permit adaptation to the edentulous ridge. Position of the teeth is good, but they are too long gingivally. The surface of the cast is blackened with a soft lead pencil. The areas on the

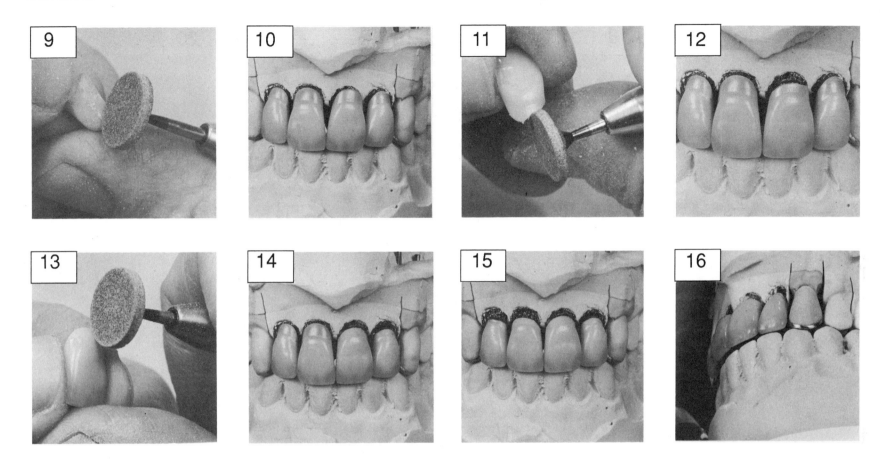

plastic teeth requiring reduction are marked by pressing and slightly rotating the teeth against the blackened ridge.

Figure 11   The gingival collar, or neck of the tooth, is reduced to establish appropriate length.

Figure 12   The left central incisor tooth has been reduced to a better level.

Figure 13   The facial surface of the tooth is contoured to eliminate the cervical line.

Figure 14   This photo shows the recontoured left central and lateral incisors contrasted with the uncorrected right central and lateral incisors.

Figure 15   The replaced teeth are esthetically compatible with the adjacent teeth.

Figure 16   The teeth have been arranged to provide the desired occlusal relationship. Note the contact of the left lateral incisor when the articulator is moved into the left functional excursion.

Figure 17   Continuity of arch form has also been established by this position. If desired, such teeth could easily be lapped or rotated for esthetic reasons.

Figure 18   Baseplate or inlay wax is neatly added between the necks of the teeth and the cast.

Figure 19   The wax is carved to create ideal tooth contour.

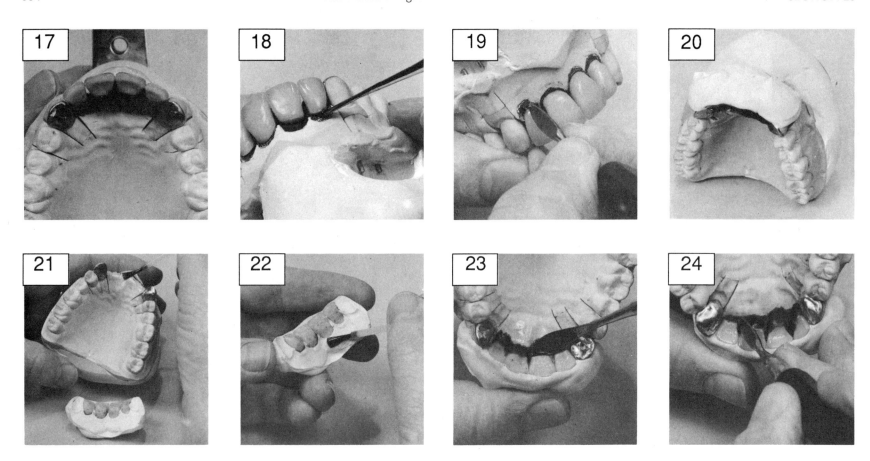

Figure 20 When facial contour is correct, gypsum separator is applied to adjacent teeth and land area, and a quick-set plaster index is made over the denture teeth and adjacent cast.

Figure 21 The plaster index and teeth are removed, and all wax debris is cleared from the working cast and plaster index. Die lubricant is applied to the ridge area of the working cast.

Figure 22 Die lubricant is also applied to the plaster index, but *not* to the denture teeth.

Figure 23 The index and teeth are repositioned on the working cast, and inlay wax is added to complete the lingual contour of the pontics.

Figure 24 This wax addition is carved to create ideal contour of the pontic tips.

Figure 25 The completed lingual contours of the pontics are illustrated. If necessary, wax could be added to the linguoincisal surface of the teeth to create proper occlusal contacts. When contour is complete, gypsum separator is applied to the working cast.

Figure 26 Quick-set plaster is mixed and placed to form a lingual index.

Figure 27 This illustration shows a facial view of the lingual index in position on the working cast.

 Several possibilities exist at this point for development of the pontic patterns. First, the plastic denture teeth may be used as patterns for the cast pontic backings. This is done by grinding away the facial surface to establish the desired window outline and retention form. The plastic

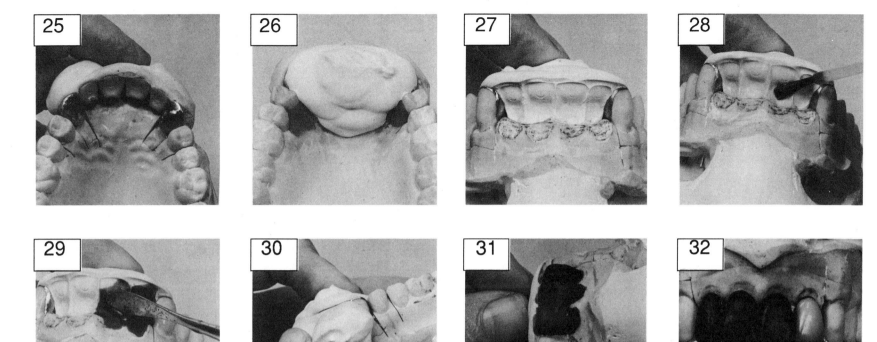

tooth is then sprued, invested, burned out, and cast just as a wax pattern. This is a simple method of making pontic and other noncritical patterns. However, the use of resin patterns is not generally recommended as they tend to expand and distort the mold during burnout.

A second possibility is to grind away the lingual half of each denture tooth and use the facial portion as a facing. The basic procedure is the same as for porcelain-faced pontics. However, proper retention must be developed in the backing pattern, because the resin facing must be bonded to the backing by addition of self-curing or heat-cure acrylic, rather than cement. This technique offers the advantage of having a manufactured shade and form for the veneer. With the broad range of molds and shades of plastic denture teeth now available, the potential for establishing pontic veneers by this technique is virtually unlimited. However, when molds or shades are inadequate, or when space is critical, the processed resin veneer is best used.

The third possibility is to use the denture teeth to make a mold from which the pontic patterns can be formed.

Techniques for use of a denture tooth as a facing and for developing a mold to form the pontic patterns are illustrated in developing this bridge.

Figure 28   Die lubricant is applied to the lingual index in preparation for addition of wax to form the pontic patterns.

Figure 29   Wax is flowed into the index and against the edentulous ridge area.

Figure 30   As wax is built to excess in each given pontic area, the facial index is positioned to mold the pontic form. Thus, the lingual index, facial index, and cast function as a mold to form the pontic patterns.

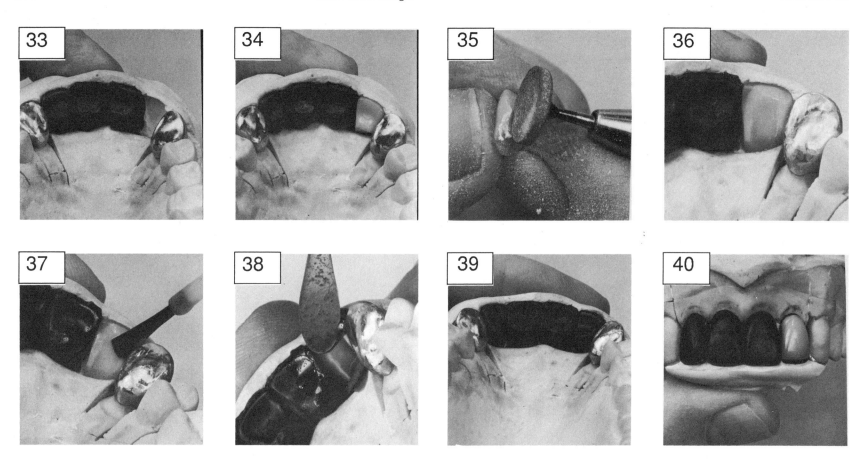

Figure 31   One unit at a time, wax is added and molded with the facial index to develop the complete tooth form.

Figure 32   The right lateral and both central incisor patterns have been molded. The left lateral incisor has been left uninvolved to serve as a facing.

Figure 33   Lingual contour has been formed by the lingual plaster index.

Figure 34   The left lateral incisor denture tooth is positioned in the plaster index.

Figure 35   The lingual surface of this tooth is reduced to create the desired thickness and peripheral outline of the facing.

Figure 36   The facing must be thick enough to maintain shade and permit retention form to be developed. Proximal bevels must be established to permit formation of adequate joints without display of alloy. Gingival and incisal finish lines are established to permit the desired alloy coverage of these surfaces. In this example both incisal and gingival surfaces will be covered with alloy. The gingival surface of the facing has been relieved to permit full alloy coverage with the finish line at the faciogingival angle. The incisal edge has been relieved to provide 1 millimeter clearance for alloy at the facioincisal angle. Proper inclination of the bevel provides even greater clearance lingually.

Figures 37 through 39   When preparation of the facing is complete, die lubricant is applied and the pattern for the backing formed.

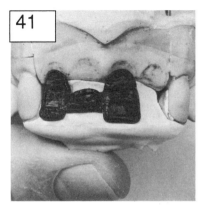

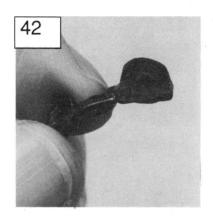

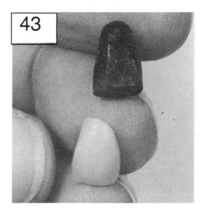

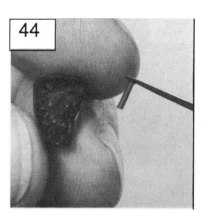

Figure 40 Because of their poor resistance to wear, resin veneers must be protected with alloy to provide a durable occlusal or incisal surface. The esthetic disadvantage of this design is obvious. As a result, several designs are employed in the development of occlusal or incisal surfaces for resin veneer crowns and pontics. For instructional purposes, three basic designs are presented in this bridge. (1) The first is full alloy coverage, used for the two lateral incisor pontics. (2) The second is full resin coverage, employed for the right central incisor pontic. (3) The third is a compromise between the first two, and consists of forming the lingual half of the incisal edge in alloy, and the facial half in resin. This design is used on the left central incisor and is the commonly used design for processed resin veneers.

The gingival surface presents essentially the same possibilities. The gingival tips may be formed entirely of alloy or entirely of plastic, or a junction between the two may occur in the region of the tip surface. There is little justification for locating a junction line between two materials in the area of tissue contact. These junctions invariably produce irregularities and roughness that invite the collection of foreign material and irritate the soft tissue. Of the other two possibilities, the all-resin tip is most commonly used. Even so, there is still some question regarding the effect of long-term contact of resin pontic tips with soft tissue. In addition to the problem of tissue response, another significant disadvantage presented by the all resin pontic tip is that in the event of breakage or other failure of the pontic it is extremely difficult to repair the bridge in the mouth and redevelop proper contour and smoothness of the resin tip. Repairs are simple, however, if the

pontic tip is formed with alloy. Examples of both alloy and resin tip construction are presented here.

Figure 41 The facial of the pontic patterns that were molded by the facial and lingual plaster indexes are carved to establish the desired extension of the veneer. The veneer "cut-backs" are extended proximally to avoid display of any metal, but adequate bulk for strength of the joint areas is maintained.

Retention for the resin pontic veneer is easily made by creating undercut grooves and pits. As with a veneered crown, wire loops, beads, or pickups may be employed if desired. A peripheral or bezel lock is common to both the pontic and resin-veneer crown. Such an undercut groove about the periphery of the backing creates a mechanical lock that prevents separation of the plastic from the alloy at the external junction line.

Note that the right lateral incisor backing is developed with alloy coverage of the incisal and gingival surfaces. The right central incisor pontic backing is designed for an all-resin incisal and gingival surface. The left central incisor pontic backing is designed with an alloy gingival tip and an incisal edge that will be half alloy and half resin.

Figure 42 This enlarged view of the left central backing shows the undercuts placed for retention.

Figure 43 The denture tooth facing is separated from its backing pattern. Provisions must be made for mechanical retention of the facing

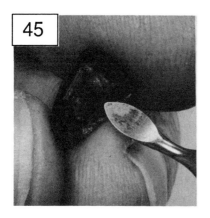

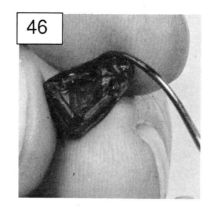

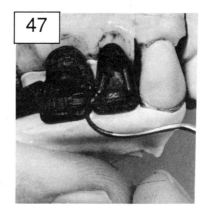

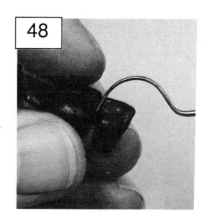

in the backing. This may be done in conventional manner by placing undercut grooves, pits, beads, or loops in conjunction with the peripheral groove. For demonstration purposes, still another form of retention is used here for this backing: a ridge-lock.

Figure 44 A short length of 18-gauge round or half-round wax is cut to appropriate length. If half-round wax is used, its convex surface is adapted to the backing.

Figure 45 The wax ribs are positioned on the backing close to but not touching the peripheral undercut. They may be held in place by tacky liquid, by lightly flaming them before they are placed, or by carefully luting them to the backing.

Figure 46 Luting is done with an explorer tine to avoid eliminating the undercut groove on either side of the wax rib.

Figure 47 The backing is in position, with round wax ribs on the proximal and incisal borders of the window. This backing pattern is luted to the rest of the framework pattern so that the pontic frame may be cast in one piece.

Figure 48 By careful use of the warm explorer tine, the lingual surface of the junction between the facing backing and the rest of the framework pattern is carefully filleted.

Figure 49 The pontic framework may be invested at a convenient water/powder ratio, as dimensional accuracy is not critical. Note that

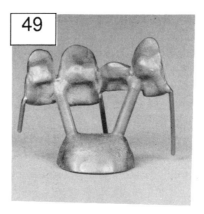

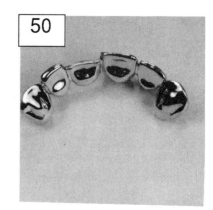

only two supply sprues have been used. This is because the bulky patterns provide an open mold cavity. At least one additional supply sprue would be indicated if there were thin sections in the pontic pattern. Attachment of the sprues to the joint areas between patterns is justified when using two sprues only if they are filleted adequately to provide direct supply to the thicker units of the pattern and if the casting can be made with assurance that there will be no shrink spot porosity. In this example large-diameter (8-gauge) sprues were used and open vents were placed at adjudged terminal flow points. Sound spruing, venting, investing, and casting techniques assure sound, accurate, porosity-free castings.

After casting, the sprues were removed and the pontics grossly finished. The framework was carefully repositioned on the working cast using the lingual plaster index. The bridge was invested and

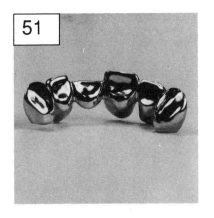
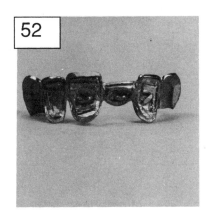
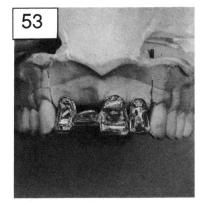
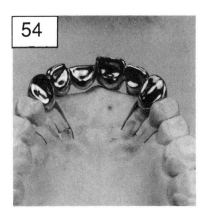

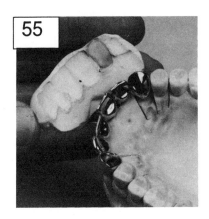
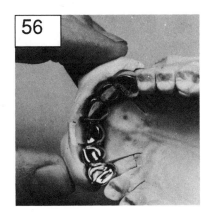
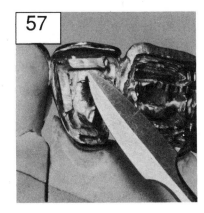
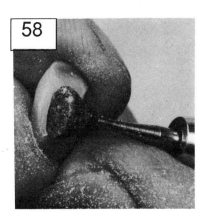

soldered in conventional manner. The completed framework was occluded, surfaced, and polished.

Figure 50 Note the normal configuration of the lingual embrasures.

Figure 51 Note the correct gingival embrasure forms and the smoothly filleted contour of the joint areas.

Figure 52 The framework has been carefully cleaned and the retentive features within the backings have been refined by machining with appropriate burs. Note the peripheral undercut on each backing. Also evident are the metal loops in the central region of the right lateral and central and left central backings.

Figure 53 The framework is repositioned on the working cast before

developing the veneers. The various incisal edge designs are evident in this photograph (compare **Figure 40**).

Figure 54 Note the ridge relationship of the smoothly convex alloy tip surfaces. The right central tip will be formed with resin.

Developing Resin Veneers

Figures 55 and 56 The facial index with the left lateral facing in place is repositioned on the working cast. Note that it does not seat completely. This is to be expected, because the retentive ribs were placed after the facing was removed from the backing pattern.

Figure 57 The round metal ribs have been ground flat on their exposed surfaces, leaving an undercut groove on either side. This pro-

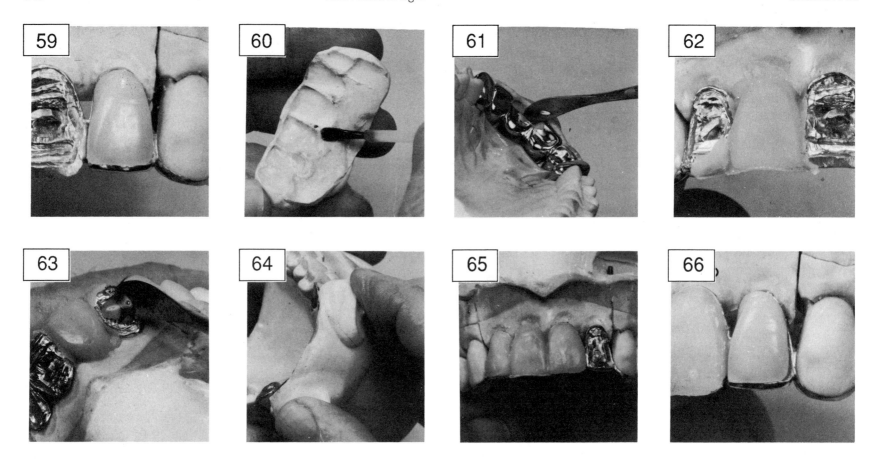

vides opposed undercuts on either side of the ribs; more importantly, it also provides directly opposed undercuts between the rib and the peripheral undercut.

Figure 58 The lingual surface of the facing is freely relieved in the area of the ribs to permit its repositioning. The peripheral margin of the facing is relieved as little as possible.

Figure 59 Overrelief of the lingual surface of the facing is not critical and may be desirable, as it provides more room for packing resin that will lock the facing to the cast framework. Relief should not, however, be so excessive as to influence shade.

Figure 60 Die lubricant is applied to the plaster index and to the working cast adjacent to the pontic frame.

Figure 61 Ivory wax is added to the pontic framework to establish the veneer patterns.

Figure 62 By adding wax to one unit at a time, the veneers may be molded to contour with the plaster facial index.

Figures 63 through 65 This procedure is repeated until gross patterns have been developed for each pontic.

Figure 66 The facing for the left lateral is repositioned in the framework. Note that alloy is exposed in the embrasure between the lateral facing and the canine retainer. This unesthetic display of alloy can be eliminated by altering the contour of the lateral facing.

Figures 67 through 69 Die lubricant is applied to the adjacent canine

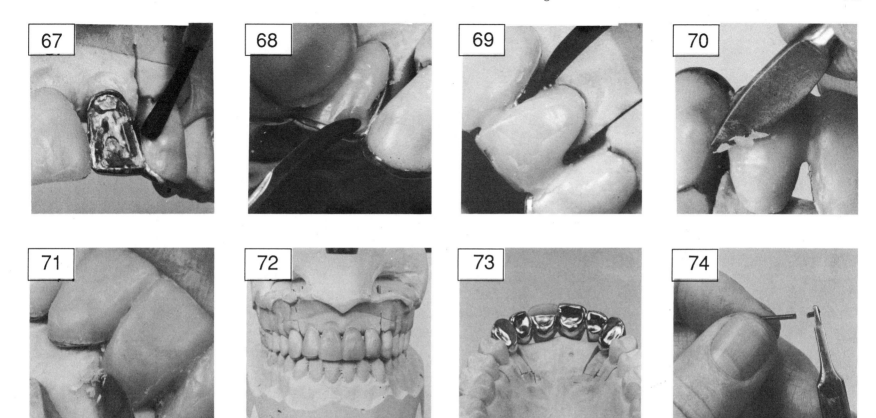

die, and ivory wax is added about the periphery of the facing to close the facial embrasure.

Figure 70   The wax addition is carved to redefine the embrasure and establish the correct outline form.

Figure 71   The gross patterns for the other veneers are refined. Any desired facial markings are made in the wax patterns at this time.

Figure 72   Patterns for the veneers and refinement of the facial contours have been completed.

Figure 73   This lingual view shows the incisal and gingival configuration for the right central veneer.

When facings are used for veneers, provision must be made to retain these in the upper half of the processing flask. Their exposed contour is not usually sufficient to permit this (as it does when processing a denture).

Figures 74 through 77   A simple means of retaining the facing in the upper portion of the flask is to attach a short segment of a plastic sprue pin to the surface of the facing. A small mix of autopolymerizing resin is made, and a small drop is placed in the center of the facing surface. A 3- to 4-millimeter segment of plastic sprue pin is placed in the drop of resin, which cures quickly.

Figure 78   Because of their curvature, acrylic veneer bridges involving the anterior segment are difficult to process in a denture flask. Special sectional flasks are available for this purpose.

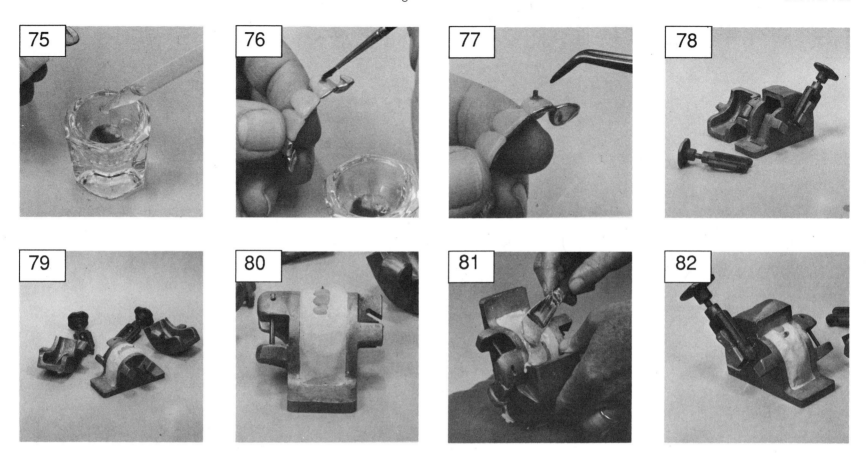

Figure 79 With wings of the flask removed, plaster is placed in the central curved portion of the flask and the bridge frame positioned to permit proper access to its curvature. Ideally the bridge will be embedded to a level even with the junction between framework and veneer. Any unit not being veneered will be completely invested. Some skill and finesse is required to accomplish this step of the investing procedure. Either quick-set plaster, regular plaster, or a combination of the two may be used for this pour, depending upon the skill and experience of the technician. The consistency of the plaster is the key to success in accomplishing the investing procedure.

   If difficulty is encountered, one alternative is to fill the central portion of the flask with plaster and wait for initial set. At this point, a trench somewhat larger than the bridge frame is carved in the plaster. The set plaster is then saturated with water, a small mix of plaster added in the ditch, and the bridge carefully positioned.

Figure 80 The surface of the investing plaster must be reasonably smooth and devoid of undercuts and must be contoured to avoid interference with the flask wings. A gypsum separator is painted on the exposed plaster surfaces.

Figure 81 A flask wing is positioned and securely attached to the flask. Dental stone (Hydrocal) is used for the upper flask halves. A firm, creamy mix of stone is carefully vibrated into the wing, first through its port and then through the access at the open end of the wing.

Figure 82 Before final set, the stone in the first wing pour is trimmed flush with the metal boundary of the wing. Do not mar the veneer pattern.

Figure 83 Gypsum separator is again applied in preparation for the second wing pour.

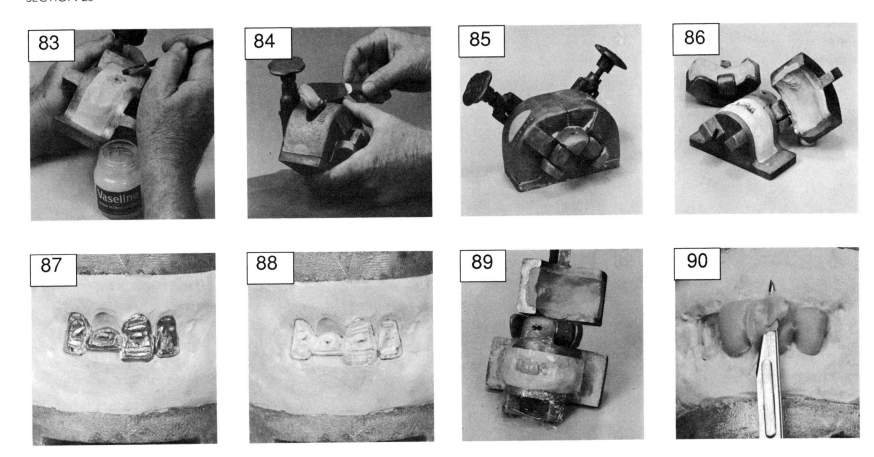

Figure 84   The second wing is securely attached to the flask. This pour of stone must be accomplished entirely through the wing port.

Figure 85   Excess stone at the port area is wiped smooth, and the wing pours are allowed to set (1 hour minimum).

Figure 86   When the stone has set, the flask is disassembled. Though not evident, the left lateral facing has remained in a wing of the flask.

Figure 87   All wax is removed from the bridge frame by flushing with boiling water. All wax and gypsum debris must be removed.

Figure 88   All alloy to be veneered is completely covered by opaque, following the manufacturer's instructions. Opaque is also added to the backing that will receive the facing. The opaque surface should not be handled or contaminated in any manner prior to the application of the body resin.

Figure 89   Depending upon the brand of resin used, body resin of proper shade is mixed and placed according to the manufacturer's directions. The result of a trial closure with wet cellophane in place is shown here. If necessary, additional body material may be added to ensure complete filling of the mold and uniform compression on the material. Note that the cellophane has kept the fresh resin from contacting the facing.

Figure 90   When the framework design results in thick areas of resin adjacent to thin areas, some adjustment must be made to compensate for the shade discrepancy that will occur due to variation in volume. In this bridge the right central incisor backing has no alloy in either the

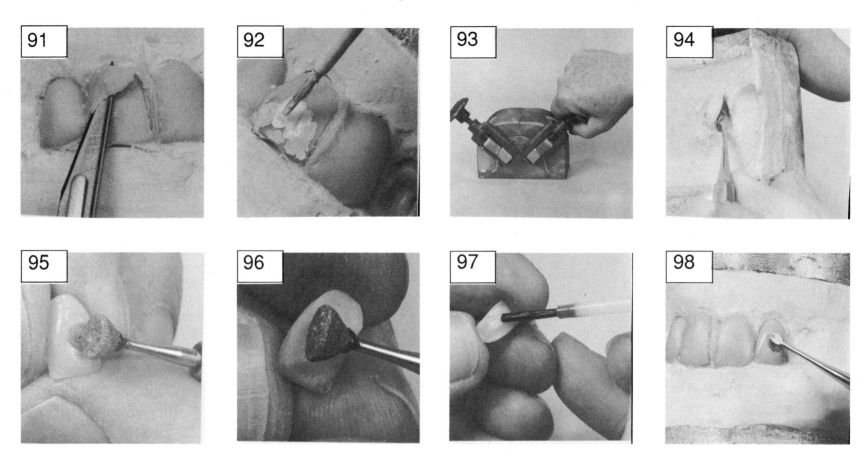

gingival tip or incisal edge area; the shade in these areas will be quite different from that of the adjacent central pontic, which has alloy backing the entire facial surface. This discrepancy in shade may be overcome by cutting back the body resin to a level even with the surface of the adjacent central backing. The incisal half of the material is being cut back with a very sharp number 11 scalpel blade.

Figure 91   The gingival portion is reduced in the same manner.

Figure 92   Opaque is now added to the surface of the "cut-back" body resin. The objective is to establish an opaque layer even with that of the adjacent pontic, so that the veneer-opaque relationship will be the same for all units. Only resinous opaquing material may be used in this manner.

Figure 93   When the opaque layer has gelled to the extent that it will not flow, body material is reapplied and trial-packed.

When the flask is reopened, cut-backs are made for the addition of the incisal color blend, which is added and trial-packed as desired.

Figure 94   Before final closure, the left lateral facing must be removed from the upper wing of the flask.

Figure 95   The segment of plastic sprue pin that was used to hold the facing in the flask wing is removed, (1) to prevent conflict in closing the wing of the flask over the facing, (2) to avoid locking the facing in the upper wing when it is to be removed after curing, and (3) to permit covering the facing with cellophane during curing. A small nub of the

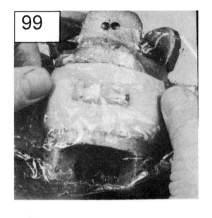

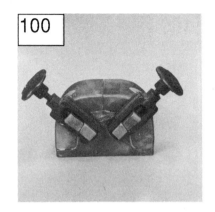

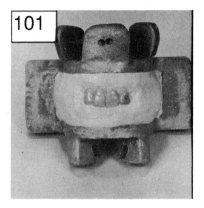

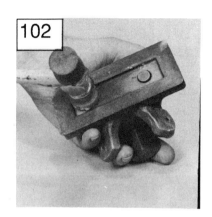

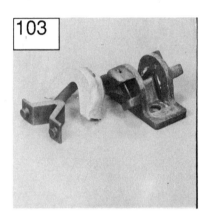

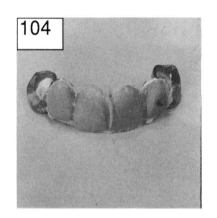

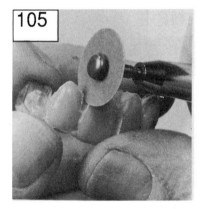

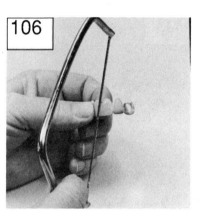

sprue pin and the adjacent resin material serves as an index for facing position.

Figure 96　The lingual surface of the facing is ground to ensure a clean surface for bonding with the processed resin.

Figure 97　Monomer is applied to the clean, ground surface.

Figure 98　The facing is positioned in the framework preparatory to final closure.

Figure 99　Wet cellophane is stretched over the uncured resin veneers to avoid wrinkles.

Figure 100　The flask is closed with the cellophane in place, and the bridge is cured following the instructions of the manufacturer.

Figure 101　The veneers have been processed, and the flask wings are removed. Correction of discrepancies in form or shade, or placement of stains can be easily accomplished at this point by appropriate cut-back, placement of new material, and reprocessing.

Figures 102 and 103　When processing is complete, the bridge is deflasked by first tapping the knockout lugs on the back of the flask.

Figure 104　Care must be taken in deflasking the bridge to avoid damaging the critical margins of the partial crown retainers. Note the limited amount of adherent flasking material, and the remnant of the sprue pin on the lateral facing.

Finishing the Bridge

Figure 105　The flash of resin is removed using appropriate discs,

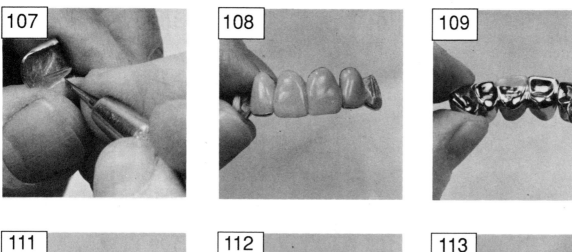
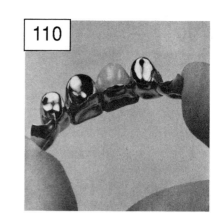
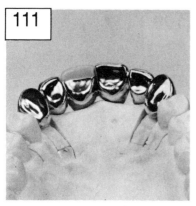
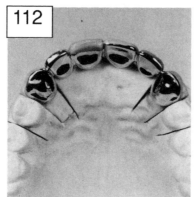
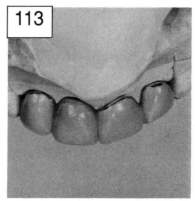
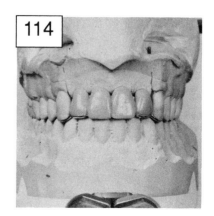

stones, burs, and hand instruments. The sprue pin remnant on the left lateral incisor facing is also removed.

Figure 106 A very thin die saw blade or disc may be used to redefine interproximal embrasures.

Figure 107 Appropriate hand instruments are used carefully to remove excess resin adjacent to the margin of the retainers.

Figure 108 Rough edges and junctions between resin and alloy are carefully smoothed with fine rubber wheels and then with minim felt wheels and pumice. The veneers are then lightly buffed with whiting or a similar final polishing compound, to provide a high gloss.

Figure 109 The alloy framework, which was smoothed before processing the veneers, is easily polished to a lustrous finish.

Figure 110 Special care should be taken to ensure smooth, highly polished convex tip surfaces.

Figure 111 This lingual view of the bridge shows the minimization of soft tissue contact that can be achieved by using convex pontic tips with adequate linguogingival embrasure form. The juncture line between alloy and resin on the right central pontic will not be in contact with the soft tissue of the edentulous ridge.

Figure 112 Adequate lingual contour is provided to deflect foodstuffs. Cingulum contour of central incisor pontics must sometimes be exaggerated to protect the incisal papilla.

In review, note the variety of incisal design: full alloy coverage on the lateral incisor pontics; full acrylic coverage on the right central pontic; and the split incisal edge design on the left central incisor pontic.

Figure 113   The alloy pontic tips extend just facial to the point of tissue contact.

Figure 114   The junction line between alloy and acrylic at the gingival tip is not evident when viewed from the facial. Note the uniform distribution of alloy displayed on the incisal of the canine retainers and lateral incisor pontics. After final occlusal equilibration, the alloy on the incisal of the lateral pontics may be rolled so as to become less evident. The finished bridge is now ready for delivery to the dentist.

REVIEW QUESTIONS

1. Describe the three basic designs of the incisal or occlusal surface for resin veneer pontics.
2. Discuss the design of the resin veneer gingival pontic tip surface with regard to the type of materials that can be used.
3. What procedure is necessary for alloy extension on the incisal of resin veneer pontics so that the alloy is less evident in the mouth?

Interconnectors and Telescopic Construction in Fixed Bridges

The original concept for the use of nonrigid connectors in fixed bridges was to permit the use of intracoronal restorations that might not have sufficient retention to serve as retainers for a rigid bridge. The common example was a bridge from premolar to molar with a full crown retainer on the molar and, for esthetic reasons, an inlay as the premolar retainer. Such inlays frequently came loose. It was surmised that the use of a nonrigid connector in the anterior joint would relieve stresses applied to the inlay and thus reduce the incidence of failure of these retainers. This was the basis for the original term "broken-stress bridge," which is still broadly used. Other advantages were asserted, but as it is not appropriate to debate the philosophy of this concept here, suffice it to say that there are many fallacies in this premise. As a result, such a construction is seldom indicated for the purpose of "breaking stress."

Nonrigid connectors are now used instead to facilitate placement of a bridge on abutments that cannot be prepared to draw together. They are also used to join segments of very large bridges, thus facilitating their fabrication and/or repair. Should a problem occur in one of the segments that can be removed, this segment can be remade without jeopardizing the entire bridge. In such situations, the bridge should be termed "nonrigid," rather than "broken-stress," even though the latter name is commonly employed.

Where draw cannot be established between abutments, two basic approaches are available for development of a fixed bridge: the use of a nonrigid connector, or the use of a telescopic crown. Many modifications of these designs have been developed. A basic technique for developing the most common form of nonrigid connector and a basic example of a telescopic retainer are presented here.

NONRIGID BRIDGE

To identify the fundamental rationale and technique for use of interconnectors, a basic "do-it-yourself" example is shown. Examples of variations using prefabricated interconnectors are also shown.

Hand Formed Interconnector

Figure 1 The most common example of the nonparallel abutment problem is the tipped mandibular molar.

Figure 2 It is clearly evident that the two abutment preparations do not draw together in that their long axes are not parallel to one another. Because the axial walls of the molar crown preparation are short, grooves have been placed on the facial and lingual surfaces to enhance retention. These grooves are exactly in line wih the path of draw of this abutment preparation.

Figure 3 This occlusal view, taken exactly in line with the direction of the grooves in the molar preparation, demonstrates their parallelism and clearly shows the lack of parallelism between the two abutment preparations. To permit placement of a fixed bridge in this area, the anterior retainer will be developed with a semiprecision tapered-keyway interconnector. A male lug will be developed as part of a hygienic pontic. Together with a female keyway in the anterior retainer, this will constitute a nonrigid connector for the bridge. Note the box prepared in the distal of the premolar abutment to provide room for development of the keyway.

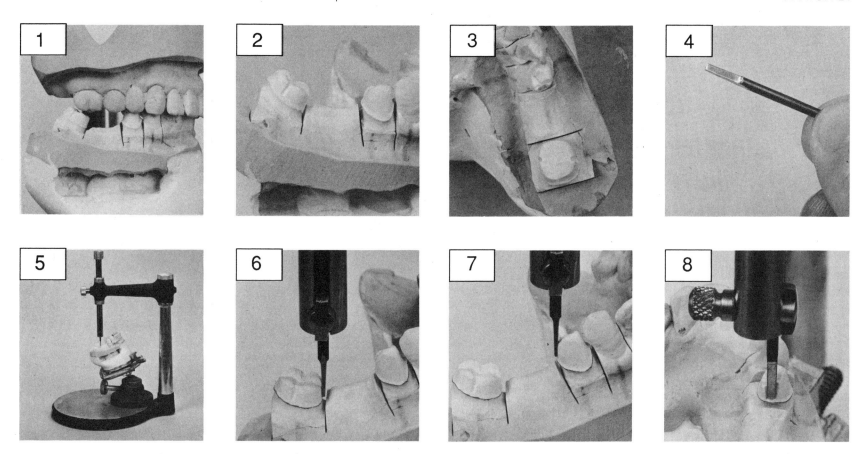

Figure 4   A mandrel to form a keyway in the wax pattern has been fashioned from the shank of a straight handpiece steel bur. It is approximately 2 millimeters wide and essentially parallel along its edges, and tapers from 1.5 to 1 millimeters in thickness over a length of 6 to 8 millimeters.

Figures 5 and 6   The mandrel is mounted in a surveyor, and the working cast is positioned on the surveyor table such that the path of draw of the molar abutment is parallel to the mandrel. The mesial surface of the molar preparation is the most critical in terms of establishing parallelism and a path of insertion for the bridge.

Figure 7   Once the correct orientation of the working cast has been established, the table is moved to bring the mandrel into position on the distal of the premolar abutment.

Figure 8   The mandrel is positioned in close approximation to the recess that has been developed in the premolar abutment to accommodate the keyway. A minimum clearance of 0.3 to 0.5 millimeters should be maintained.

Figures 9 and 10   When the final position has been determined, the mandrel and die are lubricated in preparation for development of the pattern.

Figures 11 and 12   The mandrel is again positioned to establish the correct relationship with the premolar die. Wax is carefully flowed between the die surface and mandrel, and the crown pattern is built up to gross form.

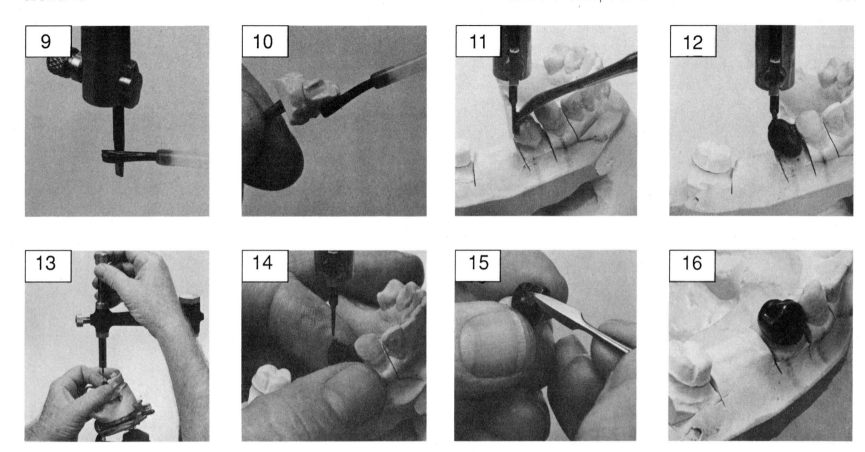

Figures 13 and 14 With the wax pattern and die held in position, the mandrel is carefully withdrawn from the pattern.

Figures 15 and 16 Occlusion is established, and the pattern is carved to final contour in conventional manner.

Figure 17 Carving or addition of wax about the orifice of the keyway can be safely accomplished with the mandrel repositioned by hand.

Figures 18 through 20 With a spade mandrel in the surveyor, the working cast is brought into position to permit carving of a guiding plane on the distal surface of the retainer pattern.

Figure 21 The flat surface thus created will be parallel to the path of

insertion of the keyway and will permit close apposition of the pontic surface when the bridge is completely assembled. A wall thickness of 0.75 to 1.0 millimeter must be maintained.

Figure 22 With the mandrel again hand-positioned, a notch is carved through the occlusal marginal ridge aspect of the keyway to provide sufficient room for connection of the lug with the body of the pontic. This notch can be as much as one-half to two-thirds the faciolingual width of the keyway and extended to within 1.5 millimeters of its length.

Figures 23 and 24 The walls of this notch may be slightly flared and beveled to facilitate positioning of the lug.

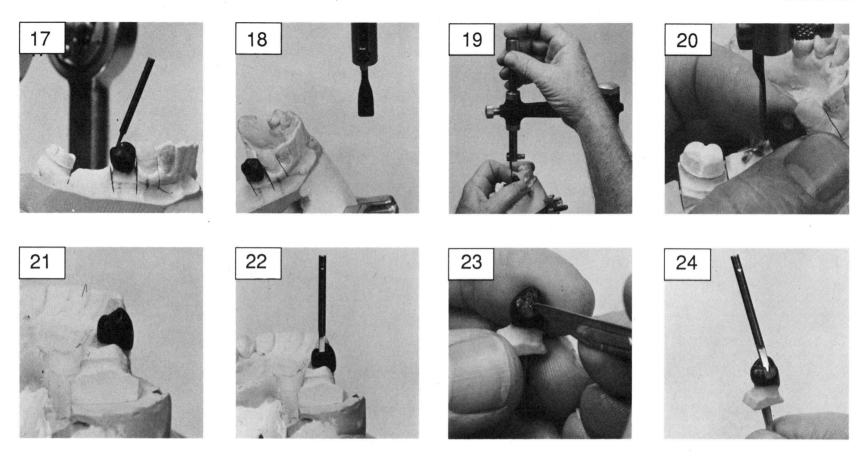

Figure 25   After verification of internal and marginal adaptation, the premolar retainer is ready to be cast.

Figure 26   After the retainer is cast, it is carefully cleaned and inspected for any defects and then seated on the die for verification of marginal accuracy. Ideally no correction of the keyway rest should be necessary. However, if blebs are present they can be removed with fissure burs and the internal surfaces of the keyway machined smooth with finishing burs.

Figure 27   The casting is positioned in the working cast for evaluation and correction of proximal and occlusal relationships.

Figure 28   The pattern for the molar retainer is developed in a conventional manner.

Figure 29   The pattern for the pontic is developed in a conventional manner. It is grossly adapted to the distal of the premolar, then positioned and joined to the molar pattern.

Figure 30   Die lubricant is applied to the keyway in the premolar retainer.

Figures 31 through 33   Wax is added and firmly molded into the keyway rest. If desired, this lug pattern may be removed and inspected for adaptation and final evaluation of keyway form. Many technicians prefer to form the lug with Duralay resin, leaving sufficient extension to be embedded in the pontic pattern.

Figures 34 and 35   With all units (dies, patterns, and casting) accu-

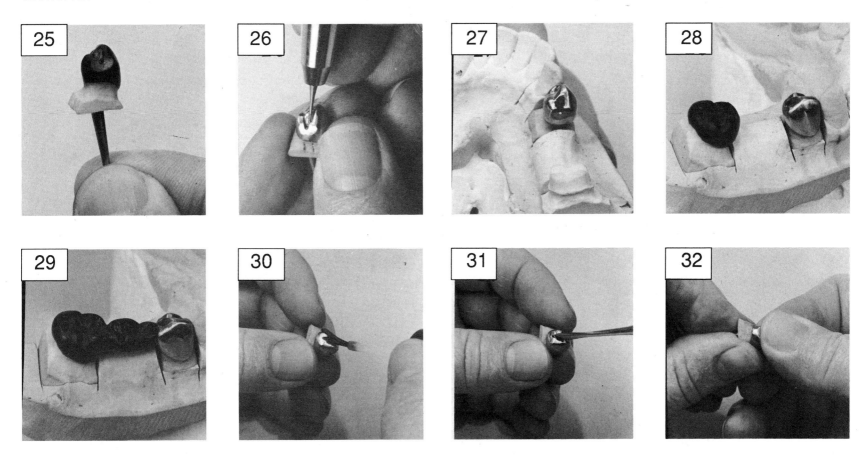

rately seated in the working cast, the pontic and lug patterns are united with due care to maintain or develop adaptation of the pontic pattern to the flat distal surface of the premolar retainer.

Figures 36 and 37   The pattern assembly is removed for inspection. Note the relatively parallel surfaces of the lug and pontic.

When the pattern is totally accurate, it is invested and cast in keeping with full crown technique.

Figures 38 through 41   The castings are occluded, contoured, surfaced, and polished in conventional manner. Special care should be given to finishing the margins about the keyway, providing as smooth a junction as possible to minimize the collection of debris.

After trial insertion and completion of any necessary corrections, the dentist will usually have the patient wear the bridge "temporarily seated" for a number of days. The bridge is then permanently cemented by first placing the premolar retainer, then placing the molar and pontic.

Prefabricated Interconnector

Most interconnectors today are made from preformed plastic patterns that can be incorporated into the wax-up and cast as part of the bridge. The most popular of these is the Ney Mini-Rest (J. M. Ney Co., Hartford, CT).

Figure 42 shows the interlocking pyramidal form of the Mini-Rest.

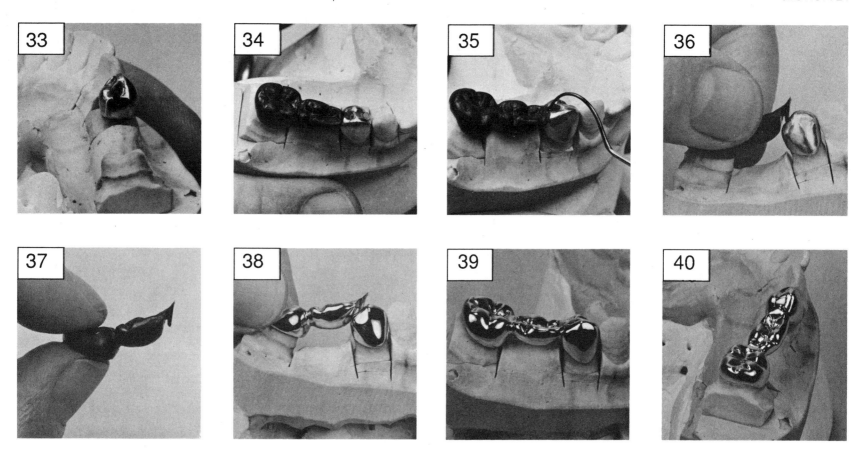

Figure 43 Conventional use of such patterns involves incorporating the female portion in the distal aspect of the anterior component of the bridge, and the male portion in the distal component. This works quite well when the anterior abutment is a large tooth that permits preparation sufficient to allow incorporation of the female within a reasonably normal crown contour. However, anterior abutments are normally premolars or canines, and these teeth frequently are not large enough to permit such dimension of preparation. In addition, if the interconnector is being used to accommodate a marked discrepancy in path of draw between anterior and posterior abutments, the necessary inclination of the connector will cause the anterior retainer to be grossly overcontoured gingivally.

Figure 44 One means of overcoming the problem is to incorporate the interconnector within the body of the pontic. By moving the connector away from the retainer, normal contour of the distogingival margin of the retainer can be maintained. The disadvantage of this approach is that it places the interconnector out in the span of the bridge, where it is subject to greater "bending" or "buckling" load rather than the shear loading that occurs when it is immediately adjacent to the abutment. This is also very tedious to accomplish in veneered pontic situations.

Figure 45 An alternate possibility for improving contour is to invert the male portion of the connector and attach it to the distal surface of the anterior retainer. Especially when the connector must be inclined to accommodate a more mesially oriented path of draw of the posterior abutment, such design permits maintenance of the gingival embrasure space. This illustration contrasts a conventionally placed interconnec-

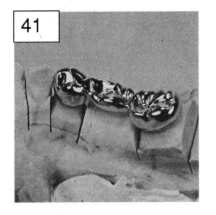

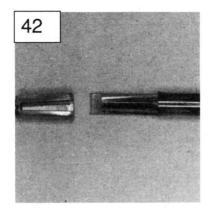

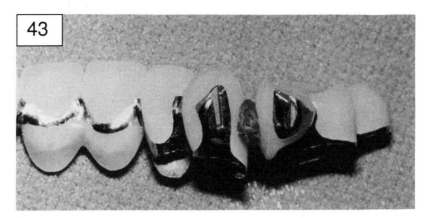

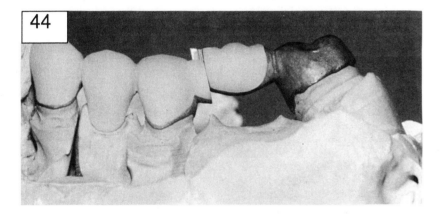

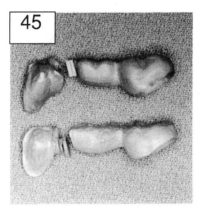

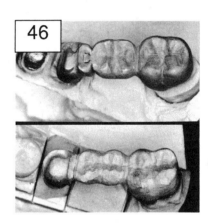

tor (top) with distally extended inverted male connector (bottom). Note the difference in contour at the area of the distogingival margin of the anterior retainer.

Figure 46 An additional advantage of this design is that the junction line of the male/female connection is not exposed on the occlusal.

Figure 47 However, this means that this juncture is exposed gingivally, which is not desirable if the pontic is in contact with tissue in this area.

Figures 48 through 50 These photographs illustrate the need for an interconnector to accommodate discrepancy in draw between anterior and posterior abutments. The male connector has been inverted and attached to the distal of the anterior retainer with no encroachment on

gingival embrasure space. With both anterior and posterior components in place, the junction line forms an almost normal facial embrasure.

THE TELESCOPIC BRIDGE

The second method of developing a bridge for nonparallel abutments is to use a telescopic crown. A *telescopic bridge* is so termed when one or more of its retainers is developed in two telescoping sections. The first section, which covers and seals the prepared tooth surface, is called a *thimble* or *coping*. It establishes marginal seal and contour and provides a retentive surface form over which a conventional crown—the *overcasting*—can be fitted. The coping can be contoured to provide a path of draw quite different from that of the preparation on which it is

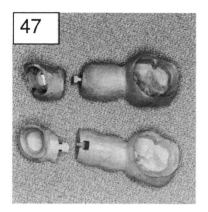

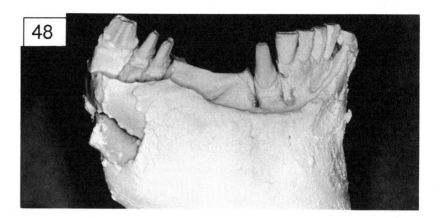

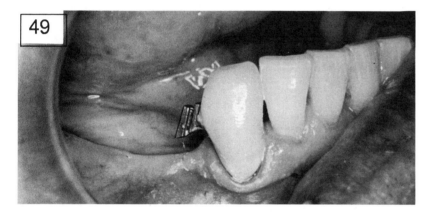

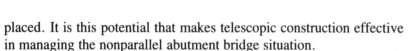

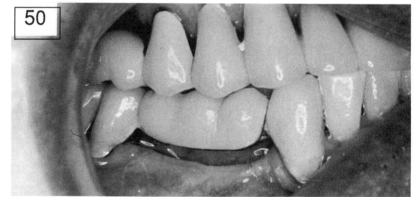

placed. It is this potential that makes telescopic construction effective in managing the nonparallel abutment bridge situation.

Telescopic construction is also extensively used for the so-called *periodontal prosthesis*. These are usually extensive bridges or splints (often full arch) made for patients who have suffered extensive loss of bone around their remaining teeth due to periodontal disease. Each tooth is restored with a primary coping that is permanently cemented. The bridge (or splint) is then placed with temporary cement such that it can be removed if necessary. Should the periodontal involvement of a tooth progress to the extent that it must be forfeited, the bridge or splint is removed; the tooth is extracted; and with the involved retainer converted to a pontic, the bridge is replaced. The facility and economic advantage of such design in case of abutment failure is obvious. Coverage of this use of telescopic construction is beyond the scope of this manual.

The disadvantages of telescopic construction are the bulk required to have two castings fitted over a tooth, the difficulty of fitting one casting to another, and the increased initial expense of such construction.

Figures 51 through 53 The technique for development of a single telescopic retainer bridge to accommodate draw is demonstrated here using the same cast that was employed for the nonrigid bridge.

Figure 54 A thimble pattern is developed on the tipped molar abutment, providing full contour only in the marginal area. A minimum thickness of 0.5 millimeter must be maintained in thinner areas.

Figure 55 The working cast is positioned on a surveyor such that the path of draw of the anterior abutment is parallel to a spade or dowel mandrel.

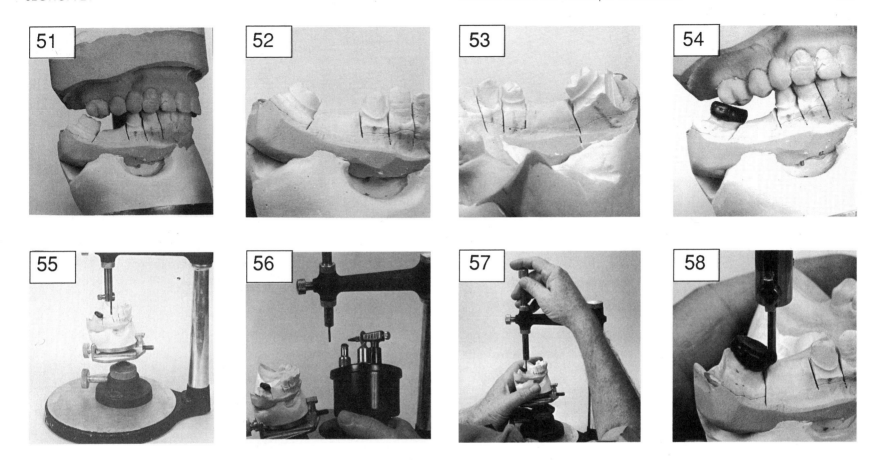

Figures 56 through 58 The mandrel is warmed and positioned against the mesial surface of the thimble pattern such that this surface is carved parallel to the path of draw.

Figure 59 The result should be a surface that curves faciolingually in keeping with tooth contour but is flat occlusogingivally in a plane parallel to the path of draw of the anterior abutment. Ideally, sufficient length should be available without having to carry the plane thus created beneath the crest of the gingival tissue.

Figures 60 and 61 The surveyor mandrel may also be used to parallel portions of the facial, distal, and lingual surfaces of the thimble.

Figures 62 and 63 If possible, it is desirable to prepare the distal surface of the thimble such that it is parallel with the mesial surface to

provide maximum retention for the crown. However, gaining such parallelism often requires marked overextension of the distal contour of the final crown. If such is the case, retention in lieu of, or in addition to, a parallel distal contour may be gained by grooves or ridges placed in the facial and lingual surfaces of the thimble. To ensure their parallelism, such grooves are best placed with a dowel mandrel in the surveyor.

Figure 64 Note that as the axial surfaces have been carved, a rather heavy chamfer margin has been developed about the circumference of the thimble approximately 1 millimeter above the preparation margin. If adequate length of the axial walls permits, this margin should be maintained at a supragingival level. The final result should be a wax pattern for a thimble that provides accurate internal and marginal adaptation with the preparation, adequate length of parallel axial surfaces to retain the overcasting crown that will serve as the distal retainer for the

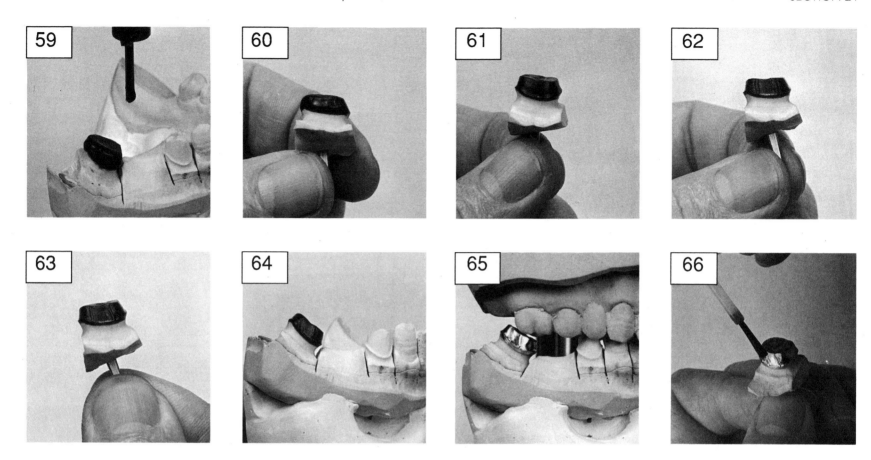

bridge, and a minimum of 1.5 millimeters occlusal clearance for development of normal occlusal contour in the crown.

Figure 65　The thimble is cast as per full crown technique. After thorough cleaning and inspection, the casting is seated on its die and positioned in the working cast. Adequacy of path of draw of the various axial surfaces may be verified on the surveyor if desired. In particular, the facial and lingual grooves should be machined to provide definition and slight taper for draw. Occlusal clearance is verified, and the casting is refined through the rubber-wheel stage.

Figures 66 and 67　Die lubricant is applied to the thimble, and wax is added for development of the crown pattern. It will quickly be noted that waxing against alloy is quite different from waxing against a stone

die. Because the alloy does not absorb the wax lubricant, some time should be allowed for the vehicle to evaporate and excess should be blown away. Because of the surface texture and temperature of the alloy, wax tends to warp away from the alloy surface. To overcome this tendency, some technicians prefer to warm the casting before wax is applied by the flow-on technique. Others prefer to dip the thimble into molten wax, on the premise that total circumferential coverage will cause the wax to shrink toward the alloy surface. Whatever technique is adopted, accuracy of internal adaptation must be verified before the pattern is completed.

Figure 68　Occlusal and axial contours are established in a conventional manner. Marginal accuracy is as important as for the conventional crown.

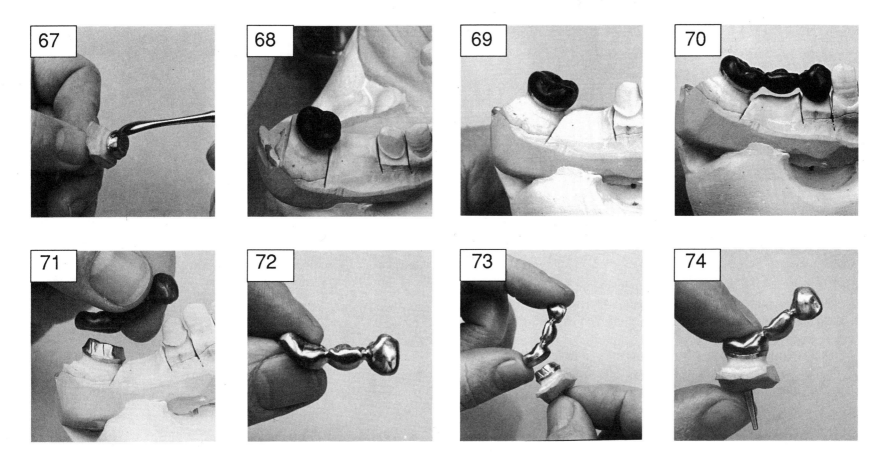

Figure 69   When the pattern for the telescopic overcasting is developed, the bridge may be completed in segments or as a one-piece casting.

Figure 70   Because construction of bridges shown previously has been segmented, the pattern for this bridge has been developed in one piece, as a contrasting example.

Figure 71   When withdrawal of the pattern is assured, it is sprued, invested, and cast as per full crown technique.

Figures 72 through 74   After thorough cleaning and inspection, accuracy of fit of the telescopic crown is verified.

Figure 75   The bridge is then placed on the working cast to verify the accuracy of relationship.

Figures 76 and 77   Discrepancies in the alloy-to-alloy margin between thimble and crown can be eliminated by burnishing and surfacing with appropriate discs and stones.

Figure 78   The bridge is smoothed and finished in conventional manner. The surface of the thimble should *not* be polished, as the dentist will probably prefer to lightly stone this surface to ensure maximum mechanical bonding of the cement.

The dentist will place the bridge in the mouth by first cementing the thimble, and then cementing the bridge over the thimble and the anterior abutment.

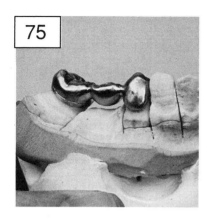
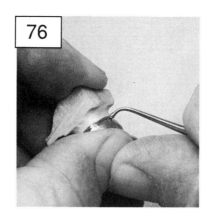
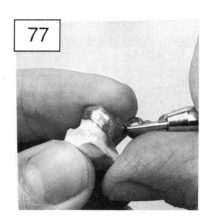
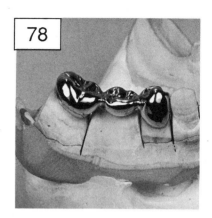

REVIEW QUESTIONS

1. What are two basic methods for the development of a fixed bridge where the abutments cannot be prepared to draw together?
2. What is the minimum thickness of a thimble or coping for a telescopic bridge?
3. What additional measures of retention are available in preparing the thimble portion of a telescopic crown if the distal surface cannot be made parallel to the mesial surface?

INDEX